Gynecologic Cancer

A Clinicopathologic Approach

Denis Cavanagh, M.B., Ch.B.(Glas.), F.A.C.O.G., F.A.C.S., F.R.C.O.G.
Professor of Obstetrics and Gynecology
Director of Division of Gynecologic Oncology
American Cancer Society Professor of Clinical Oncology
University of South Florida College of Medicine
Tampa, Florida

Eugene H. Ruffolo, M.D., F.A.C.O.G., F.C.A.P.
Clinical Professor of Pathology and Obstetrics and Gynecology
University of South Florida College of Medicine
Director of Pathology, Tampa General Hospital
Director of Pathology, Humana Women's Hospital
Tampa, Florida

Donald E. Marsden, M.R.C.O.G., F.R.A.C.O.G.
Senior Lecturer in Obstetrics and Gynaecology
Director of Gynaecologic Oncology
University of Tasmania
Hobart, Tasmania, Australia

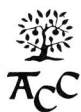

APPLETON-CENTURY-CROFTS/Norwalk, Connecticut

0-8385-3530-5

Notice: Our knowledge in clinical sciences is constantly changing. As new information becomes available, changes in treatment and in the use of drugs become necessary. The author(s) and the publisher of this volume have taken care to make certain that the doses of drugs and schedules of treatment are correct and compatible with the standards generally accepted at the time of publication. The reader is advised to consult carefully the instruction and information material included in the package insert of each drug or therapeutic agent before administration. This advice is especially important when using new or infrequently used drugs.

Copyright © 1985 by Appleton-Century-Crofts
A Publishing Division of Prentice-Hall, Inc.

All rights reserved. This book, or any parts thereof, may not be used or reproduced in any manner without written permission. For information, address Appleton-Century-Crofts, 25 Van Zant Street, East Norwalk, Connecticut 06855.

85 86 87 88 89 / 10 9 8 7 6 5 4 3 2 1

Prentice-Hall of Australia, Pty. Ltd., Sydney
Prentice-Hall Canada, Inc.
Prentice-Hall Hispanoamericana, S.A., Mexico
Prentice-Hall of India Private Limited, New Delhi
Prentice-Hall International, Inc., London
Prentice-Hall of Japan, Inc., Tokyo
Prentice-Hall of Southeast Asia (Pte.) Ltd., Singapore
Whitehall Books Ltd., Wellington, New Zealand
Editora Prentice-Hall do Brasil Ltda., Rio de Janeiro

Library of Congress Cataloging in Publication Data

Cavanagh, Denis, 1923–
  Gynecologic cancer.

  Includes index.
  1. Generative organs, Female—Cancer. I. Ruffolo, Eugene H. II. Marsden, Donald E. III. Title
[DNLM: 1. Genital Neoplasms, Female. WP 145 C377g]
RC280.G5C38 1985   616.99'465   85-1328
ISBN 0-8385-3530-5

Design: M. Chandler Martylewski

PRINTED IN THE UNITED STATES OF AMERICA

*For their patience during its preparation,
we dedicate this book to Margaret, Marina and Katherine.*

Contents

Preface ix
1. Cancer of the Vulva 1
2. Cancer of the Vagina 41
3. Cancer of the Cervix 59
4. Carcinoma of the Endometrium 129
5. Sarcomas of the Uterus 179
6. Cancer of the Fallopian Tube 205
7. Epithelial Carcinoma of the Ovary 213
8. Primary Nonepithelial Ovarian Cancer 271
9. Gestational Trophoblastic Neoplasia 305

Index 341

Preface

This book has been written to fulfill the need for a short textbook which emphasizes the importance of clinicopathologic correlation in the area of gynecologic oncology. It embraces all aspects of the diagnosis and management of gynecologic malignancies. Special stress has been laid on the importance of an accurate histopathologic diagnosis before treatment is undertaken. Particular attention has been given to the quality of the photomicrographs, illustrating the importance of grading and even histopathologic subtyping with regard to treatment-planning and prognosis. In 1974 the American Board of Obstetrics and Gynecology established the Division of Gynecologic Oncology and began to issue certificates of special competence in this subspecialty. In recent years the ABOG has also laid great emphasis on patient management problems based on clinicopathologic correlation. These events have led to an increased appreciation of the importance of establishing a diagnosis as accurately as possible before proceeding with the treatment of patients with gynecologic cancer. If any further stimulus was needed, the present medicolegal climate has supplied this.

The book had its origin in a series of book chapters written for the *Obstetrics and Gynecology Annual* edited by Dr. Ralph M. Wynn and published by Appleton-Century-Crofts. The chapters have been updated and are written in such a way as to be of practical value to the general gynecologist, as well as the gynecologic oncologist and the pathologist with a special interest in premalignant and malignant lesions of the female genital tract. The book will be particularly helpful to the community hospital pathologist, who is often expected to supply not only an accurate diagnosis but up-to-date references on almost every subject.

All of the chapters have been written by the authors in an effort to keep contradictions to a minimum. A special effort has been made to supply references which are keyed to the text, and which will provide a reader with an opening for a more detailed review of the subject matter covered.

x PREFACE

For numerous helpful suggestions we owe thanks to our colleagues Dr. Hora Praphat, Dr. William Roberts, Dr. Philip Townsend, Dr. John Shepherd, Dr. Thomas McDonald, Dr. Peter Bryson, Barbara J. Wisniewski, RNC, and Dr. Richard Anderson. In addition, we would like to thank Dr. Harvey Greenberg, Dr. Gerry Sokol, Dr. Robert Miller and Dr. Allan Katz, our colleagues in Radiation Oncology at Tampa General Hospital, and Bayfront Medical Center. We also thank our colleagues Drs. Essman, Songster and Davis of the Department of Pathology at Bayfront Medical Center.

For assistance in collecting pertinent professional and public educational materials we are grateful to the Florida Division of the American Cancer Society, most particularly to Bob Wichman, John Carbonneau and John Schoppman.

For their assistance in the typing of the manuscript we thank Anne Housley and Mary Anderson, and for his assistance with proofreading we thank Mr. William McNab.

For their help and patience throughout the preparation of the manuscript we thank the staff of Appleton-Century-Crofts, particularly Kathy Drasky and Nancy McSherry-Collins.

D.C.
E.H.R.
D.E.M.

Gynecologic Cancer

CHAPTER 1
Cancer of the Vulva

Invasive cancer of the vulva is not common. It accounts for 0.3 percent of all female cancers in the United States, with an incidence rate of 1.5 per 100,000 females in the country. There are approximately 500 deaths per year from this malignancy in the United States, which account for 0.3 percent of all female cancer deaths.[1] As this is predominantly a disease of old age, the steady increase in life expectancy has brought vulvar cancer into a more prominent place among vulvar malignancies, and in the last 30 years there has been a concentrated attack on the problem.[2-7] Most epidemiologic studies show no influence of parity, marital status, or race on the incidence of vulvar malignancy.[8,9] Certain skin changes appear to be associated with the development of this disease and chronic vulvitis is often present. Exposure to coal tar derivatives has some influence on the development of vulvar cancer. The use of x-ray therapy for the treatment of benign lesions of the vulva may sometimes be associated with the development of vulvar cancer, although it is possible that the underlying condition was the causative factor. The location of these lesions on the skin surface might be expected to facilitate early diagnosis, but in fact a significant proportion of patients present with advanced stage disease.[10] In our own experience, over one-third of patients had spread of the tumor beyond the vulva at the time of diagnosis, and in 38 percent the diagnosis was not made for more than a year from the onset of symptoms.[7] The delays were due not only to the reluctance of the patient to seek help, but were also often related to failure of the physician consulted to biopsy lesions before prescribing local ointments. Furthermore, the treatment of this malignancy usually calls for extensive surgery and, because the disease usually occurs in elderly women, there is often a tendency to treat them less than adequately. It cannot be overemphasized that the diffuse lymphatic drainage of the vulvar area makes radical surgery mandatory if good results are to be achieved. The majority of vulvar cancers are squamous cell carcinomas. Adenocarcinoma, Paget's disease, basal cell carcinoma, malignant melanoma, and sarcoma together constitute less than 10 percent of vulvar cancers.

VULVAR DYSTROPHIES

The term "vulvar dystrophy" replaces a variety of terms such as leukoplakia and kraurosis vulvae. The classification of vulvar dystrophies recommended by the International Society for the Study of Vulvar Diseases is shown in Table 1.

Although vulvar cancer has been commonly reported in association with these conditions, a causal relationship has rarely been established and when it has, there has always been associated epithelial atypia.[11] Most hyperplastic dystrophies show no evidence of atypia and are what most dermatologists would call neurodermatitis. Microscopically, they are associated with epithelial hyperplasia and hyperkeratosis (Fig. 1). However, the gross appearance of the lesions may change over time, depending on the extent to which the patient scratches the vulva and the amount of moisture in the area. The changes may extend onto the thigh. The lesions are sometimes elevated, with thickened tissues, colored white or red. The lesions should be biopsied before treatment is undertaken. An example of an atrophic dystrophy (lichen sclerosus et atrophicus) is shown in Figure 2. A toluidine blue test is useful, though it is not necessarily accurate in the presence of hyperkeratosis, where false-negatives may occur, or excoriation, which may lead to false-positive results. The test involves applying 1 percent aqueous toluidine blue to the vulva, and after 1 minute, washing it off with 1 percent acetic acid. Sky blue areas should be biopsied.

Pruritus vulvae is the predominant symptom associated with all vulvar dystrophies, and may be due to degeneration and inflammation around the terminal nerve fibers. Hyperplastic lesions are generally associated with intense itching, whereas with lichen sclerosus the pruritis is usually mild. Itching and scratching lead to excoriation and secondary infection, and so the appearance of the vulvar skin may be quite variable.

TABLE 1. VULVAR DYSTROPHIES

Hyperplastic
    Benign epithelial hyperplasia (neurodermatitis or lichen simplex)
    Atypical epithelial hyperplasia (dysplasia)
Atrophic—lichen sclerosus et atrophicus (LSA)
Mixed—LSA with foci of epithelial hyperplasia
    Without atypia
    With atypia

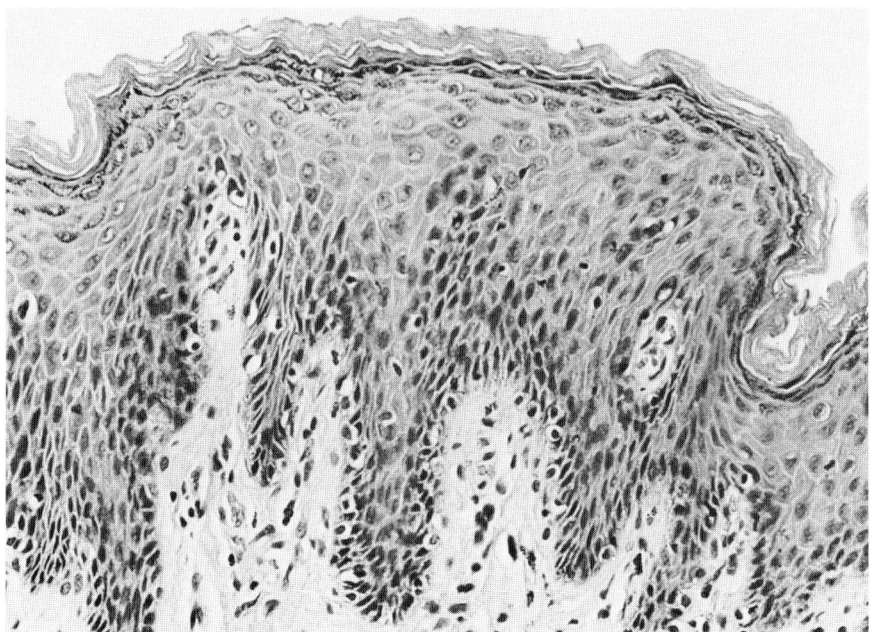

Figure 1. Vulvar dystrophy of the hyperplastic type without atypia. Beneath an orthokeratotic layer, the epithelium is acanthotic, exhibiting orderly maturation to the surface without any atypical or dysplastic changes.

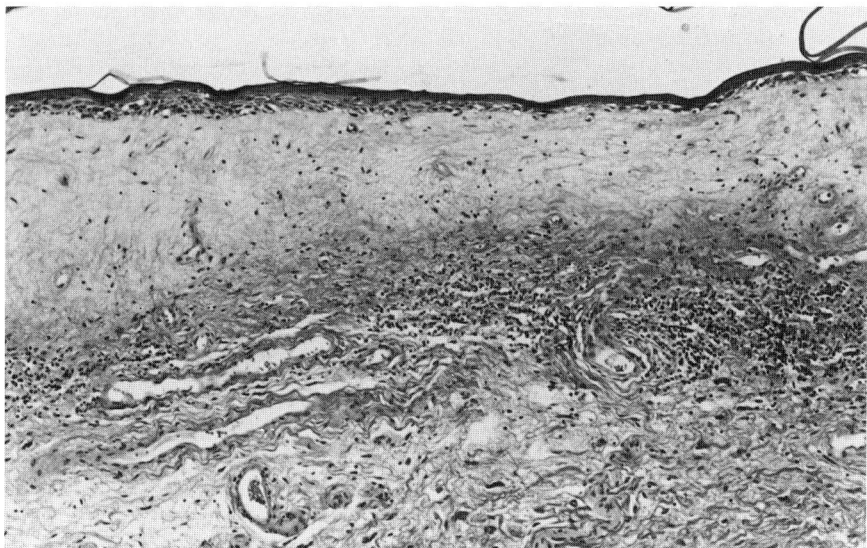

Figure 2. Vulvar dystrophy of the atrophic type (lichen sclerosus). The epithelium is atrophic, demonstrating vacuolar degeneration at the epidermal-dermal interface. The superficial dermis appears edematous, and later sclerotic, over a band of chronic inflammatory reaction.

Management
There are 4 basic principles of treatment in the management of patients with vulvar dystrophies: (1) The patient should avoid the use of deodorants, perfumes, and douches, and even baby powders should be used with care. (2) A nonirritating soap should be used in the area and should be washed off thoroughly after bathing. The area should be dried carefully by dabbing rather than rubbing, and if necessary, a blow dryer should be used. (3) The patient should be encouraged to wear cotton pants, or no pants at all, so that there is adequate evaporation of sweat from the area. (4) A histopathologic diagnosis should be established by biopsy and treatment undertaken on the basis of the biopsy.

Technique of Vulvar Biopsy
There are 4 steps in this technique: (1) The area should be cleansed with an antiseptic solution and 1 percent lidocaine should be infiltrated under the skin using a 26-gauge needle. (2) A 4-mm cutaneous punch biopsy instrument is pressed against the skin over the recently made wheal and rotated so as to give a circular skin incision. (3) Using fine tissue forceps with teeth, traction is applied to the circular area of skin and this is freed using small pointed scissors. (4) Monsel's solution is applied to the area and pressure is maintained for 6 to 12 minutes. A 2-0 chromic catgut suture of mattress type may be inserted to stop bleeding, but it is rarely necessary.

Treatment
Hyperplastic dystrophy without atypia is best treated with a corticosteroid cream such as 2 percent hydrocortisone cream. In atrophic or mixed dystrophy, or lichen sclerosus et atrophicus, a 2 to 5 percent mixture of testosterone propionate in petrolatum jelly gives good results if massaged thoroughly into the vulvar area 2 to 3 times daily. This usually results in a thickening and softening of the vulvar tissues with relief of the pruritus vulvae. Once a patient has obtained relief from pruritus, testosterone cream should be applied locally once or twice a week indefinitely.

If atypia (dysplasia) is noted in a lesion, it should be widely excised. All patients with chronic vulvar dystrophy should be examined every 3 months and biopsies taken of any gross lesions or toluidine blue-positive areas. Colposcopy is of little value in inspection of the vulva because observations of vascular patterns are not so helpful as in the cervix. Thus, a magnifying glass is just as useful as long as the vulva is examined under a bright light. In the past a simple vulvectomy was commonly done for vulvar dystrophy, but it is now thought that this should only be done if the patient has intractable pruritus or if extensive atypia has developed.

VULVAR INTRAEPITHELIAL NEOPLASIA

Vulvar intraepithelial neoplasia (VIN), including VIN 3 and carcinoma in situ (Bowen's disease), is apparently on the increase.[12] Also, it is now being seen more frequently in patients in the 20 to 40-year age group. It is possible that some of these cases are morphologic VIN caused by viral infections and this may explain why many of the changes regress spontaneously. It is these factors together with the increase in the emphasis on sexual fulfillment which have led to the more conservative management of this condition. This trend toward more conservative management is further supported by reports stating that in the young patient, carcinoma in situ of the vulva rarely progresses to invasive disease.[13]

Diagnosis

Pruritus vulvae is the most common presenting symptom but many patients with VIN are asymptomatic. The lesions vary considerably in gross appearance and may present as thickened white patches, brown pigmented papules, or red granular lesions. The toluidine blue test should be used to pick up suspicious areas on the vulva, but unfortunately it is frequently negative in the presence of hyperkeratotic lesions.

Lesions classified as vulvar intraepithelial neoplasia include cases of squamous cell carcinoma in situ (formerly Bowen's disease, erythroplasia of Queyrat, and carcinoma simplex) as well as cases of vulvar Paget's disease. The latter will be considered separately because it presents special problems. Carcinoma in situ of the vulva (Fig. 3) in its simplest form is a disorder characterized by cellular abnormalities that extend through the full thickness of the epithelium (not including the more superficial keratinized layer).[14]

Deoxyribonucleic acid patterns ascertained by microspectrophotometry were aneuploid in 92 percent of the cases studied by Friedrich and coworkers and 10 percent of their patients with aneuploid lesions had spontaneous regression of tumor with replacement of abnormal areas by euploid epithelium.[15] In reviewing a group of 50 patients treated over the period 1967 to 1977, these authors also pointed out several interesting features. Patients' ages ranged from 14 to 81, with a mean age of 39 years and a modal age of 30 years. Seventy-six percent of the patients were premenopausal. They found an association with sexually transmitted disease in 60 percent of the patients and an association with other malignancies (in situ or invasive) in 30 percent.

Management

A variety of types of management have been used, with the choice depending upon the type of lesion, surface area involvement, and the age of the patient. The most commonly used methods of treatment are wide excision, total vulvectomy, local chemotherapy, and laser surgery.

Wide Excision. This is now generally regarded as the treatment of choice, but the entire lesion must be removed or the disease will be likely to recur. Even when multiple foci of disease are present, if the clitoris is not involved, multiple areas of wide excision may be valuable. Indeed, it is sometimes possible to remove the entire vulva but leave a noninvolved clitoris, and this too is worth considering in the young patient.

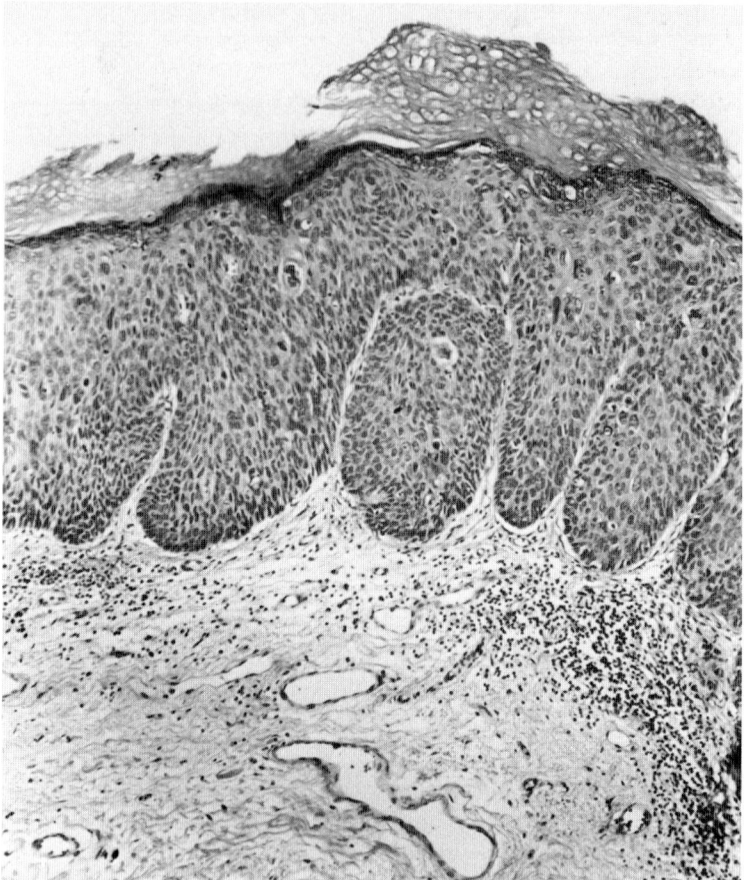

Figure 3. Squamous cell carcinoma in situ of the vulva. Notice the complete lack of maturation and presence of malignant cytologic changes involving the entire thickness of the epithelium but not extending through the basement membrane.

Total Vulvectomy. This is used where the lesions are very extensive or where they are associated with intractable pruritus in the older woman. We believe that the vulvectomy should be carried down to the fascia, especially when an area of invasive carcinoma is suspected in the midst of an extensive in situ lesion. A "simple vulvectomy," which usually consists of removing the skin of the vulva by cutting through the fat, is unanatomic and no less debilitating than a total vulvectomy. Following total vulvectomy, the application of skin grafts is rarely necessary although this has been suggested by some.[16] "Simple vulvectomy" with skin grafting is called a "skinning vulvectomy." We consider it an unsatisfactory procedure. Whether vulvectomy or wide excision is used, a margin of approximately 1 cm should be obtained on the lesion to reduce the possibility of recurrence.

Local Chemotherapy. This is usually in the form of 5 percent 5-fluorouracil. This treatment is used in young women because it is more conservative than excision. It is essential that representative biopsies be obtained prior to treatment. The 5-fluorouracil cream (Efudex) is supplied in 25-g tubes. It is applied to the lesions twice daily for 6 to 8 weeks. It produces a pronounced irritation with erythema and this is followed by local ulceration. The treatment can be repeated in 6 to 8 weeks if necessary. This method of treatment is generally thought to be unsatisfactory and recurrences are common.[14,17]

Laser Therapy. This has recently been introduced for use in the management of vulvar dystrophy and vulvar intraepithelial neoplasia. Ablation of abnormal tissue can be attained using the CO_2 laser without mutilation, and treatments can be used repeatedly if necessary. As pointed out by Lobraico, the amount of cellular ablation of dystrophic tissue by the CO_2 laser determines the outcome of the treatment.[18] Limiting the destruction to the surface epithelium by low power density over a short period of time may fail to remove the underlying causative factor in the dermal layer. To achieve optimal results, a depth of 5 to 7 mm of tissue destruction must be attained. Moving the laser light at multiple angles of cut with high power density over increased periods of time will help achieve uniformity in depth of destruction. Rapid movement of the laser beam reduces the carbonization and keeps the operative field clean.

Following laser therapy of the vulva, the patient will have discomfort for the first 24 hours and later may complain of a burning sensation in the vulva. The patient may have difficulty in emptying her bladder, and a self-retaining urethral catheter or suprapubic catheter may be necessary for several days. The areas treated by the laser are tender to touch and will remain so until all of the treated areas are healed. Thus, the laser site should be treated as a third-degree burn even though thermal coagulation may extend over 600 μ beyond the impact zone. The end result is, however, generally satisfactory, with scarring being minimal. However, more experience with the CO_2 laser will be necessary before its use in vulvar dystrophy and intraepithelial neoplasia can be adequately evaluated. As with local chemotherapy, it is absolutely essential that adequate diagnostic biopsies have been obtained before laser therapy is carried out.

Our own experience, based on the observation of over 100 cases of carcinoma in situ of the vulva, leads us to believe that in general the most satisfactory method of treatment is wide local excision. This procedure is usually not disfiguring in the young woman as there is adequate elasticity in the vulvar tissues to allow satisfactory, cosmetically acceptable closure of all but the largest defects. In our experience, there is no difference in recurrence rates between patients treated with wide excision and those treated by total vulvectomy. Whatever mode of therapy is chosen, careful follow-up is mandatory, with biopsies being employed freely whenever an abnormal area is detected.

Further Investigation

Finally, it should be noted that in up to 40 percent of women with carcinoma in situ of the vulva, in situ or invasive carcinoma of the cervix or vagina will precede, coexist with, or be found after the diagnosis of the vulvar lesion. Accordingly, it is extremely important that all patients with vulvar carcinoma be investigated cytologically and colposcopically for these conditions.

PAGET'S DISEASE OF THE VULVA

This is a special type of vulvar intraepithelial neoplasia and is similar to the lesions found in the breast. The patient's chief complaint is usually pruritus vulvae, but occasionally pain and bleeding may be present. The disease affects the labia majora and may appear as a bright red scaling and slightly elevated lesions with some white patches present. The skin is usually indurated.

A diagnosis is made by biopsy and the microscopic picture is typical. There are multicentric foci of large clear Paget cells in the epidermis (Fig. 4). In up to 10 percent of the cases an adenocarcinoma is present in underlying apocrine glands. Paget's disease may also be accompanied by invasive adeno-

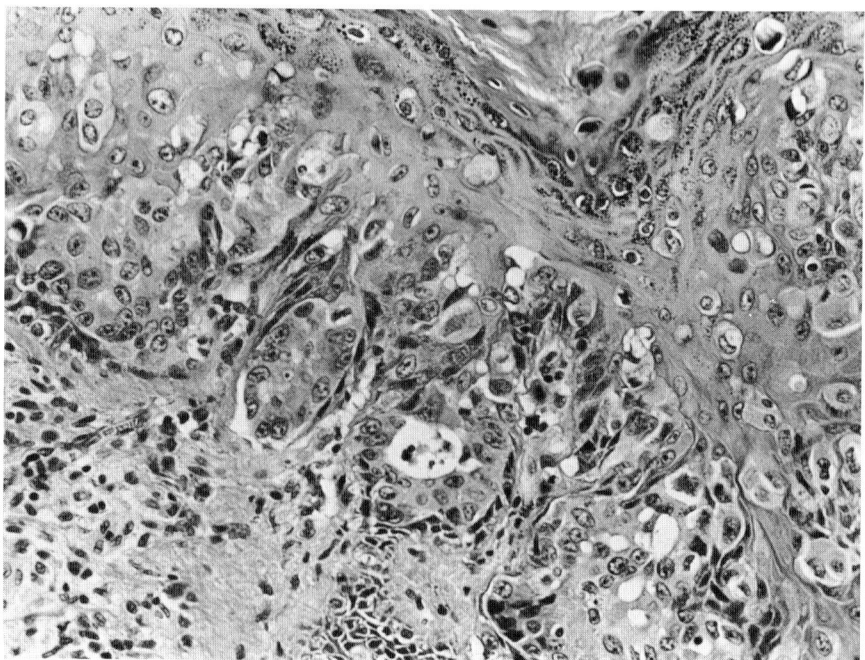

Figure 4. Paget's disease of the vulva. Malignant glandular cells are found within the benign squamous epidermis. They are seen as large, pale, single cells in the upper strata, as well as in groups forming glands with lumina in the lower portion of the epidermis.

carcinoma. A definite diagnosis can be made using special stains (Alcian blue) to identify mucopolysaccharides in the Paget cells. It must be kept in mind that although most patients with Paget's disease of the vulva have the same prognosis as other patients with vulvar intraepithelial neoplasia, those with concomitant adenocarcinoma have a poor prognosis. Boehm and Morris[19] have reported that approximately 50 percent of those patients with involvement of apocrine glands with carcinoma have lymph node metastases, and there are almost no 5-year survivors. Creasman and associates[20] have also emphasized that in the presence of the adenocarcinoma the minimal treatment for Paget's disease of the vulva is radical vulvectomy with bilateral inguinal lymphadenectomy.

Management
The treatment of Paget's disease of the vulva should be a total vulvectomy, and multiple sections should be cut of the specimen in search of an apocrine gland carcinoma. If this is found, then a bilateral regional node dissection can be carried out as a second stage of the procedure.

"MICROINVASIVE CARCINOMA OF THE VULVA"

"Microinvasive carcinoma of the vulva" has never been well defined, so there is considerable disagreement with regard to the criteria for diagnosis and the mode of treatment. A variety of terms have been used for this condition, such as "superficial carcinoma,"[21] "early invasive carcinoma,"[22] and "microinvasive carcinoma". The latter term was originally used to describe invasion of 5 mm or less into the stroma[23] (Fig. 5). As already stated, there is no general agreement regarding the type of surgical treatment required for patients with these lesions,[22-26] as some authors have reported a 10 percent incidence of inguinal lymph node metastasis in patients with 5 mm or less of stromal invasion.[24] Friedrich and Wilkinson[27] reviewed the reports of 14 authors and found that, of a total of 306 cases reported where the depth of invasion was 5 mm or less, the incidence of positive inguinal nodes was 11 percent. It was essentially unchanged when lesions invading 3 mm or less were considered, but for lesions invading 2 mm or less the incidence was of the order of 0.5 percent.

Conservative Treatment
Radical vulvectomy with bilateral groin lymphadenectomy has been the treatment of choice for invasive vulvar carcinoma, but the morbidity produced by this procedure with regard to both body image and sexual function has led to attempts to find an alternative approach for the "microinvasive" lesions. This has included attempts to preserve the vulvar tissue without sacrificing curability even when possible metastatic disease exists.[26] To ensure that the price of conservatism is not too great, however, the depth of the lesion alone should

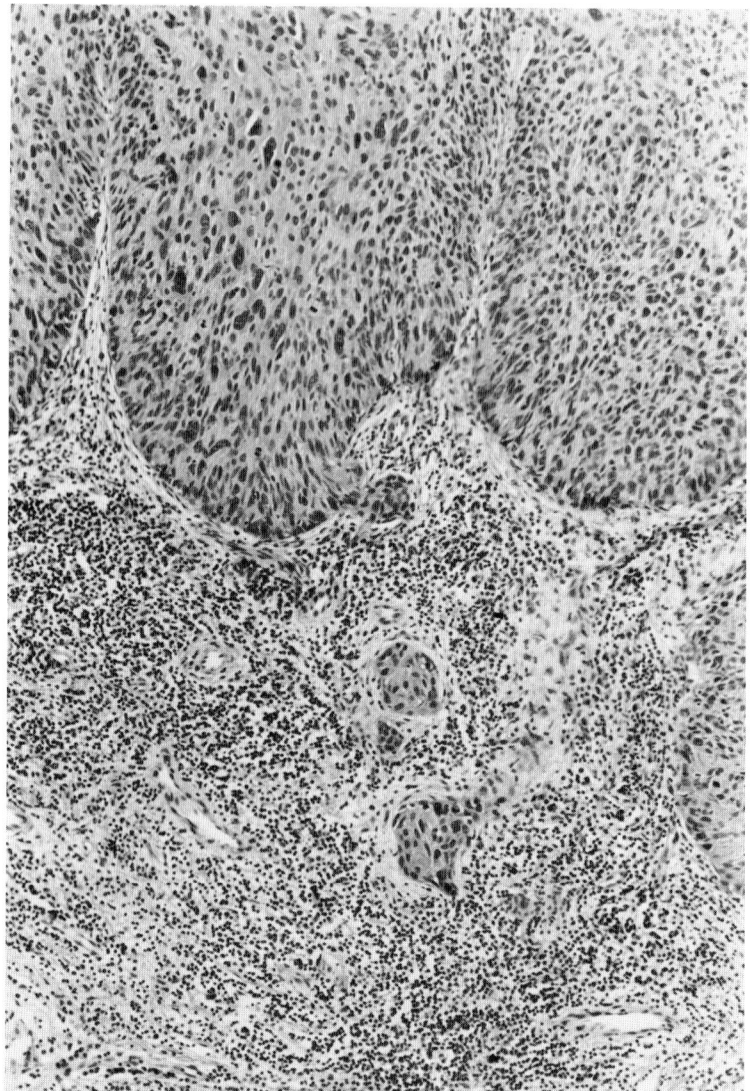

Figure 5. Microinvasive carcinoma of the vulva. There is a tongue of carcinoma extruding through the basement membrane into the underlying stroma. Also noted in the stroma are discrete foci of invasive carcinoma surrounded by chronic inflammatory cells.

no longer dictate the mode of treatment for "microinvasive" vulvar carcinoma. Many other factors must be included when a conservative approach is being considered. These factors are the depth of stromal invasion, the size of the lesion, the presence of lymphatic or vascular permeation, the degree of tumor differentiation, and the presence or absence of nodal involvement.

Depth of Stromal Invasion. In a series of 117 patients with Stage I squamous cell carcinoma, Iversen et al. reported that when invasion was less than 1 mm, there was no case of vessel invasion or death from cancer.[26] In their patients, Magrina and coworkers[6] reported that tumors that invaded the stroma for less than 2 mm showed no microscopic confluence and no lymphatic permeation; none had positive nodes and none died of the disease. In these patients, the incidence of positive nodes with tumors invading the stroma for 3 mm or less was 3 percent as compared with 10 percent when the invasion was 5 mm or less. The depth of invasion was also studied by Kabulski and Frankman.[28] Of six patients with the depth of invasion 1 mm or less, none died from the carcinoma or had metastasis to the groin lymph nodes. Of 17 patients with the depth of invasion more than 5 mm, 9 who had lymph node metastasis died from their carcinomas. Five of 17 patients with a depth of invasion of 1.1 to 5.0 mm had lymph node metastases and 3 of the women in this group died of the carcinoma. Thus, it appears that microinvasion may be considered to have low metastatic potential only up to a depth of 2 mm of stromal invasion.

Size of Lesion. Magrina and coworkers[6] found 20 patients with lesions smaller than 1 cm. All of these showed less than 5 mm of stromal invasion and all were grade 1 or 2. Although four showed confluence and one showed lymphatic permeation, none of the patients had positive nodes and none died of their disease. It is noteworthy, however, that three developed vulvar recurrences. Even more significantly, of their patients with lesions measuring 1 to 2 cm, 10.4 percent had nodal metastases. This suggests that the crucial factor is tumor cell burden, this being related to both the depth of invasion and surface area of the lesion. Tumor cell bulk is difficult to assess, whereas depth of invasion and size of lesion are easy to measure. From the data available it is evident that when a microinvasive lesion is over 1 cm in size, it should not be considered to be early disease.

Lymphatic and Vascular Permeation. There was no clear relation between depth of invasion and occurrence of vessel permeation in the study reported by Iversen and coworkers.[26] However, when vascular involvement was present, it seemed to increase the extent of lymph node metastasis. Of 15 women with vessel invasion with the primary lesion, 6 (40 percent) had lymph node metastases, whereas only 2 of 61 women (3 percent) without demonstrable vessel invasion had lymph node metastases. Parker and associates[22] also found a positive correlation between vascular involvement and lymph node metastasis. They recommended the exclusion of those patients with vascular invasion from the group of patients with early invasive carcinoma of the vulva, and stated that these cases should not be managed conservatively. In contrast, Magrina et al. found no statistically significant difference when they related lymphatic permeation to nodal involvement, recurrence, and survival in their patients.[6] These workers did not observe vascular permeation and thus could not relate this to outcome. Iverson and coworkers also demonstrated a positive correlation between vascular permeation, lymph node metastases, and an increased mortality rate.[26] Thus, from the data available, it appears that the presence of lymphatic or vascular permeation removes a microinvasive lesion from the realm of low metastatic potential.

Tumor Differentiation. Most pathologists use the Broders' grading system for estimating the degree of differentiation in patients with squamous cell carcinoma. Grades 1, 2, 3, and 4 have been described, with a spectrum from well to poorly differentiated tumors. In the uterine cervix, large cell keratinizing, large cell nonkeratinizing, and small cell carcinomas are described. In 1973, Jakobsson and colleagues described a multiple criteria grading system for squamous cell carcinoma.[29] This takes into account the degree of keratinization, nuclear differentiation, mode of invasion, and the host cellular response. Barnes et al. stated that patients with extensive overlying intraepithelial neoplasia invading the stroma as isolated foci or groups of cells, and cases of well-differentiated verrucous carcinomas that infiltrate the stroma with pushing borders and a prominent host inflammatory response may be managed conservatively.[30] However, they emphasize the importance of confluency and point out that tumors with the confluent or spray pattern of infiltration are usually more aggressive cancers, which require a more radical approach. Kabulski and Frankman[28] divided their patients into groups by using a scoring system based on the pattern, differentiation, appearance of the nuclei, and mitotic activity. They found that the tumors with a low score had a much better prognosis than those with a high score. Parker and associates[22] considered cellular anaplasia as indicating an unfavorable prognosis. In Way's[3] series, 35 percent of the patients with well-differentiated tumors had positive lymph node metastases, in contrast to 62 percent of the patients with anaplastic carcinomas. Magrina and coworkers[6] found that 20 of 106 patients who had 1 cm lesions all had well-differentiated (grade 1 and 2) lesions; none of them had positive nodes and none died of their disease. Thus, well-differentiated microinvasive lesions have low metastatic potential.

Nodal Involvement. It has been universally accepted that lymph node metastasis has an unfavorable prognosis, so that the findings of positive superficial inguinal nodes call for a more extensive removal of nodes from groins and pelvis, or perhaps radiotherapy.

Treatment

Surgery is the treatment of choice for "microinvasive carcinoma" of the vulva. The extent of the surgery depends on the careful study of the biopsy specimen and the clinical findings. Parker and associates[22] suggested the following approach: (1) excisional biopsy of the vulvar lesion and careful inspection and cytologic evaluation of the cervix and vagina for a possible second primary tumor; (2) histopathologic evaluation of the biopsy with reference to depth of invasion, vascular channel involvement, and cellular anaplasia; (3) radical vulvectomy without lymphadenectomy if invasion is present to 5 mm or less without vascular channel involvement or cellular anaplasia; (4) radical vulvectomy and lymphadenectomy if greater than 5 mm of invasion or if any vascular involvement or cellular anaplasia is seen; and (5) staged lymphadenectomy if a patient is selected for radical vulvectomy only but the surgical specimen reveals residual disease with vascular involvement or cellular anaplasia. Iversen and coworkers proposed hemivulvectomy as the primary treatment for women with tumors infiltrating less than 1 mm and without vessel invasion.[26] If the infiltration is deeper than 1 mm, they believe that hemivulvectomy should be combined with ipsilateral inguinofemoral lymphadenectomy, because groin metastasis seems to occur predominantly ipsilaterally. However, when the tumor is located in the midline, they believe it is necessary to perform radical vulvectomy with bilateral groin lymphadenectomy.

DiSaia and colleagues considered radical vulvectomy for the young patient to be an overly aggressive approach.[25] They reviewed 79 cases of invasive squamous carcinoma of the vulva treated with radical vulvectomy and bilateral inguinal lymphadenectomy. It was noted that the deep femoral group of lymph nodes was never positive in the absence of ipsilateral positive superficial inguinal lymph nodes. Thus, they suggest that a conservative approach should be used if the primary lesion is 1 cm or less in diameter, confined to the vulva or perineum, with focal invasion limited to 5 mm in depth, without vascular channel invasion, and without cellular anaplasia. After the biopsy, the next step would be to remove the superficial inguinal nodes. This would allow an assessment of these nodes for metastatic disease. If the nodes are negative for metastasis, a wide local excision of the vulvar skin could then be performed with a margin of 2 cm of normal skin on all sides of the primary lesion. Adequate subcutaneous tissue should be taken, especially beneath the primary lesion. A split thickness skin graft may be utilized but it is rarely necessary. Although the approach is a logical one, whether it will preserve a satisfactory curability rate calls for the study of many more cases and it will require a long follow-up period.

In 1984, the debate over the use of the term "microinvasive" carcinoma continues, but the recommendations of the 7th International Congress, International Society for the Study of Vulvar Disease are as follows:

> The Subcommittee believes that the term "Microinvasive cancer of the vulva" is misleading and dangerous when taken with its current definition. These lesions are known to be associated with lymph node metastases, recurrence, and death. Such behavior is similar to that of Stage I cancer of the vulva. Consequently, we recommend that the term "Microinvasive cancer of the vulva" be discontinued. We also recommend that the designation Stage I A cancer of the vulva be used for a small group of lesions of the vulva and that for the purposes of study these lesions be solitary and confined to a maximum of 2 cm diameter and 1 mm depth of stromal invasion.[31]

INVASIVE SQUAMOUS CELL CARCINOMA OF THE VULVA

Invasive squamous cell carcinoma of the vulva is sometimes referred to as epidermoid carcinoma but this is an undesirable term. The overall incidence is 3 to 5 percent of gynecologic cancers in women.[32] However, there are marked regional differences in incidence largely depending upon the median age of the population served and the referral pattern. At the University of South Florida, invasive squamous cell carcinoma of the vulva accounts for approximately 10 percent of gynecologic malignancies treated.

Epidemiologic Factors

It is generally believed that parity, marital status, and racial differences have no etiologic relation to this cancer.[8,9] There is agreement that invasive squamous cell carcinoma is typically a disease of the postmenopausal woman. In the authors' experience, age has ranged from 24 to 92 years with a median age of 67 years. In reviewing the epidemiologic profile, race, parity, and weight appear to play a significant part. Our "high-risk" patient is typically white and weighs approximately 150 pounds. Other coexistent problems noted have been diabetes (12 percent), syphilis (6 percent), invasive cervical carcinoma (4 percent), other cancers (3 percent) and venereal granulomatous disease (3 percent). Two of our patients were pregnant at the time the diagnosis of carcinoma of the vulva was made, and so it is important to inspect the vulva for suspicious lesions even during pregnancy. It is particularly important to investigate these patients for other types of malignancies because some authors have reported associated malignancies in 16 to 40 percent of cases of squamous cell carcinoma of the vulva.[33]

Carcinoma of the cervix is the type of malignancy most frequently associated with carcinoma of the vulva; thus it is important to obtain a Papanicolaou smear of the cervix and a biopsy of any lesions of the cervix in patients with vulvar malignancy. Also, it is equally important to inspect the vulva carefully on follow-up visits in patients who have been treated for carcinoma of the cervix. It has been suggested that this represents a field phenomenon in which the carcinogenic influence may be expressed in any area from the cervix to the perianal skin.[34]

As already mentioned, vulvar dystrophy is commonly found in association with squamous cell carcinoma of the vulva and this has been reported by many authors.[35,36] However, this does not establish a cause and effect relationship between vulvar dystrophy and invasive carcinoma of the vulva. As already mentioned, the vast majority of dystrophic vulvar lesions regress, and so should not be treated as premalignant lesions. The association that we mentioned with venereal disease in our patients has been reported by other authors.[36]

Diagnosis

The most common symptom is pruritus vulvae; pain, discharge, and bleeding are less commonly reported. The patient becomes aware of a lesion on her vulva, but despite the superficial nature of the lesion, patient delay in seeking medical help is common. In our series, there was patient delay of over 12 months in 99 of 296 patients (33 percent), and 4 patients did not consult the first physician until the lesion had been present on the vulva for over 10 years. Rutledge and coworkers[32] reported that 60 percent of their patients were aware of a vulvar mass or "sore" for an average period of 10 months prior to treatment. In 30 percent of their cases there was a physician delay of 3 months or more, and 25 percent had been under medical treatment without having a biopsy. Boutselis reported a patient delay of 26.6 percent and a physician delay of 25.5 percent with an average delay of 3 to 9 months.[37] Garcia and Boronow reported that in their series, patient delay ranged from 1 month to 8 years and physician delay from 2 to 12 months.[38] Parker and coworkers[22] reported that the duration of symptoms was 3 months or more in 70 percent of their patients, 6 months or more in 50 percent, and 12 months or more in 30 percent. These findings underscore the need for patient and physician education with regard to the early diagnosis of carcinoma of the vulva. Physicians must be made more aware of the importance of having a biopsy diagnosis before treating vulvar lesions, and should be aware of the value of a toluidine blue test for selecting biopsy sites. Biopsy of the vulva is a simple procedure that can be performed in any physician's office or clinic.

Site of the Primary Lesion

The lesions involve the labia majora in approximately two-thirds of the cases. In one-third of the cases the lesions involve the clitoris, labia minora, or posterior fourchette and perineum. Most lesions are located in the anterior part of the vulva; the lesions may be exophytic or ulcerated. The lesions vary from small to very large, depending mainly upon the length of delay in diagnosis. Advanced lesions may have a fungating appearance (Fig. 6). The presence of edema is a bad prognostic sign because it indicates the probability of lymphatic obstruction with tumor.

Histopathology

The histopathologic types seen in 296 patients are given in Table 2. The most common invasive lesion is a well-differentiated squamous cell carcinoma showing epithelial pearls (Fig. 7). We believe that any lesion over 1 cm in diameter with stromal invasion over 3 mm, or any lesion showing lymphatic

TABLE 2. HISTOPATHOLOGY OF CARCINOMA OF THE VULVA

Type	Patients
Squamous carcinoma	272 (92%)
Adenocarcinoma	12 (4%)
Melanoma	12 (4%)
Total	296

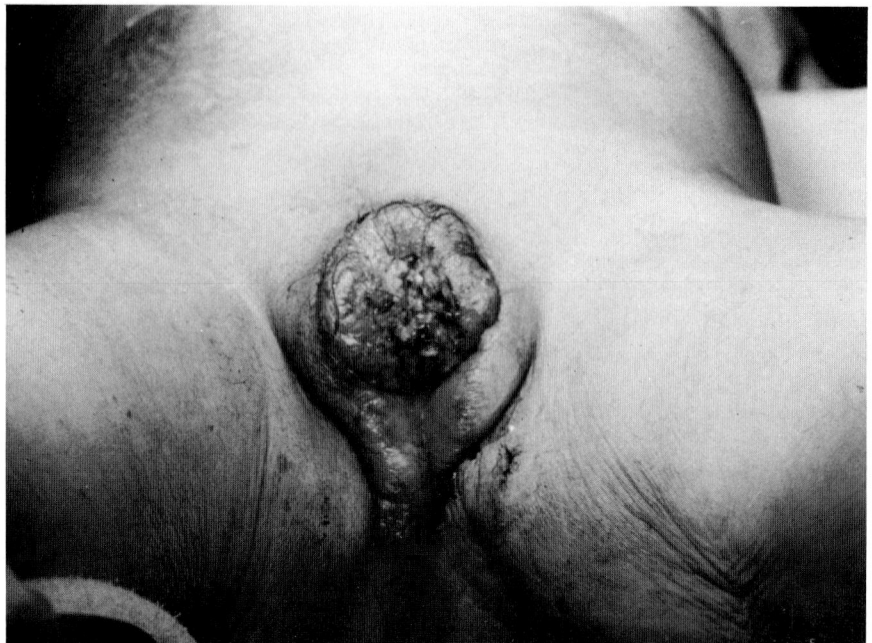

Figure 6. Squamous cell carcinoma of the vulva presenting as a fungating lesion of the clitoris.

or vascular permeation, should be classified as Stage I B (TIB) and should be treated by radical surgery. Less well-differentiated tumors occur and may be more common in the vestibule or clitoral areas. In squamous cell carcinoma of the vulva, perineural involvement with tumor is commonly seen. Multicentric lesions are common and have been seen in 30 percent of our patients with invasive carcinoma. It is important to recognize that microscopic foci of carcinoma may exist in areas of the skin that are grossly normal, and that some false-negatives occur with the toluidine blue test.

Routes of Spread

Squamous cell carcinoma of the vulva may spread by the lymphatics, the vascular system, or the interstitial spaces. By far the most common route of spread is by the lymphatics. The lymphatics of the labia drain upward to the inguinal lymph nodes. The lymphatics that drain the posterior fourchette and perineum drain in a similar manner, but their proximity to the anus allows for posterior drainage to the anal region and pelvic lymph nodes. Also, there are channels that drain the clitoris to the deep pelvic nodes, but it is emphasized that direct spread to the deep nodes without involvement of the superficial nodes is rare from any area of the vulva. The lymphatics of the vulva are numerous and tend to cross the midline. The regional lymph nodes include: (1) the superficial inguinal nodes, (2) deep inguinal nodes, (3) superficial femo-

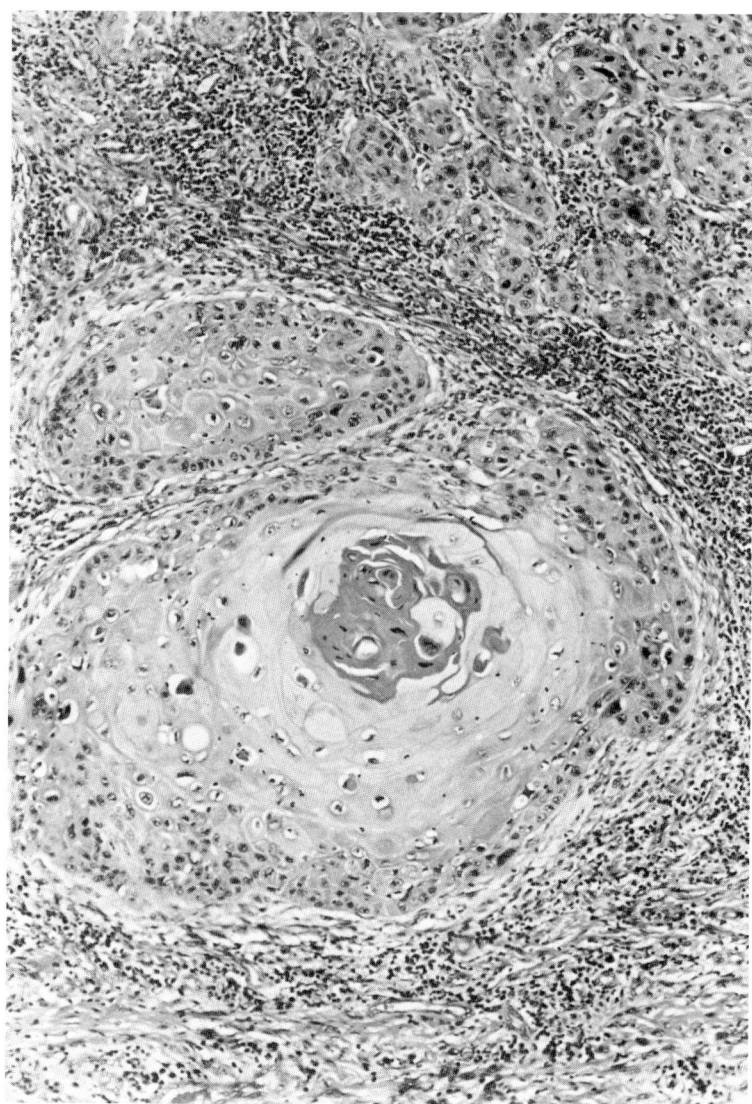

Figure 7. Invasive squamous cell carcinoma of the vulva. This is a well-differentiated keratinizing carcinoma lying deep in the underlying stroma, well beyond the 3 mm limit.

ral nodes, (4) deep femoral nodes (include Cloquet's node), and (5) deep pelvic nodes (external iliac, obturator, and internal iliac nodes). The superficial inguinal nodes are the primary nodal group for the vulva and can serve as "sentinel" nodes. This is of great practical importance, and its recognition has led to a change in surgical management, with the trend away from routine pelvic lymphadenectomy in the absence of positive nodes in the groins. Ultimately, the lymphatic drainage is to the para-aortic nodes, but these are rarely involved except in advanced disease.

The incidence of positive lymph nodes in reported series varies from 21 to 58.8 percent. In most of the reported series both inguinal and pelvic lymphadenectomies were performed (Table 3). There is generally a positive correlation between tumor size and the incidence of lymph node metastases, but this is by no means invariable. Collins and associates[39] found positive nodes in 20 percent of patients with vulvar lesions that were less than 3 cm in diameter and 71 percent when the lesions were over 3 cm in diameter. The presence of palpable groin nodes is worth noting on the physical examination.

Rutledge and coworkers[32] reported that 88 percent of patients with palpable groin nodes had nodal metastasis. On the other hand, Morley reported a 25 percent error in preoperative evaluation of groin nodes.[4] In our own experience when the groin nodes are palpable, about 50 percent will have nodal metastasis, whereas when the nodes are not palpable after careful examination, only 8 percent will have positive nodes.[40] We think that careful palpation of the groin nodes is an important part of the physical examination.

Clinical Staging

The approved classification is that of the International Federation of Gynecology and Obstetrics (FIGO). This is based on an analysis of tumor (T) by size and location, node (N) status by palpation, and distant metastases (M) as ascertained by palpation of the pelvis and by radiologic investigation. This classification is given in Table 4. There are two problems with this classification as we see it. First, it is complex and thus will not be used universally. Second, it is evident that a lesion of the perineum is probably not so significant as a lesion of the clitoris, and yet, the former lesion will be classified as Stage III (T3). In general, the facts are that the patient's prognosis is good if a

TABLE 3. INCIDENCE OF POSITIVE NODES

Author	Number of Cases	Percent Positive Groin and Pelvic Nodes	Percent Positive Pelvic Nodes
Taussig (1938)	65	46.2	7.7
Cherry and Glucksman (1955)	95	44.2	—
Green et al. (1958)	238	58.8	6.7
Stening and Elliot (1959)	50	40.0	12.0
Way (1960)	143	42.0	16.1
Macafee (1962)	82	40.2	—
Collins et al. (1963)	71	31.0	8.5
Rutledge et al. (1970)	101	47.6	11.1
Boutselis (1972)	60	40.0	12.0
Morley (1976)	374	37.0	—
Green (1978)	142	38.0	1.4
Krupp and Bohm (1978)	195	21.0	4.6
Curry et al. (1980)	191	30.0	4.7
Cavanagh et al. (1981)	133	40.0	12.0

TABLE 4. CLINICAL STAGING[a]

Stage	T	N	M	
Stage I	T1	N0	M0	All lesions confined to the vulva,
	T1	N1	M0	with a maximal diameter of 2 cm or less and no suspicious groin nodes
Stage II	T2	N0	M0	All lesions confined to the vulva,
	T2	N1	M0	with a diameter greater than 2 cm and no suspicious groin nodes
Stage III	T3	N0	M0	Lesions extending beyond the vulva
	T3	N1	M0	but without grossly positive groin nodes
	T3	N2	M0	Lesions of any size confined to the vulva
	T1	N3	M0	and having suspicious grossly positive
	T2	N3	M0	nodes
Stage IV	T3	N3	M0	Lesions extending beyond the vulva with
	T4	N3	M0	grossly positive nodes
	T4	N0	M0	Lesions involving mucosa of rectum,
	T4	N1	M0	bladder, or urethra, or involving
	T4	N2	M0	bone
	M1A			All cases with distant or palpable deep
	M1B			pelvic metastases

[a] Approved by FIGO, 1979.

lesion is less than 2 cm in diameter, if the nodes are negative for metastatic tumor, and if there is no spread beyond the pelvis. Thus, one of the most important factors influencing prognosis is the clinical stage of the disease, and we believe that, as with carcinoma of the ovary, accurate staging can be accomplished only postoperatively. Some consideration should be given by the FIGO cancer staging committee to this idea.

In our series of 296 patients treated surgically, and retrospectively placed in the FIGO classification, 124 (41 percent) were in Stage I, 76 (26 percent) were in Stage II, 69 (24 percent) were in Stage III, and 27 (9 percent) were in Stage IV. Thus one-third of our patients had Stage III or IV disease at the time of initial diagnosis, and this again emphasizes the need for improved education of both physicians and patients with regard to the importance of early diagnosis.

Clinical Course of the Disease

Squamous cell carcinoma of the vulva is generally a slow-growing lesion that ultimately spreads to the groin and pelvic lymph nodes and remains localized in these areas for a considerable period of time. Ultimately, the pelvic lymph nodes become involved and metastasis to the common iliac and para-aortic lymph nodes may lead to ureteral obstruction; furthermore, ultimately para-aortic nodal involvement with distant metastases is present. Recurrences are usually associated with disease in the vulva or the groin and are often the result of inadequate resection. The most common causes of death are uremia from bilateral ureteral obstruction, hemorrhage from rupture of vessels involved with tumor, and sepsis. Any patient with a vulvar lesion that is resectable should be treated; otherwise the patients not only die, but they die in abject misery (Fig. 8).

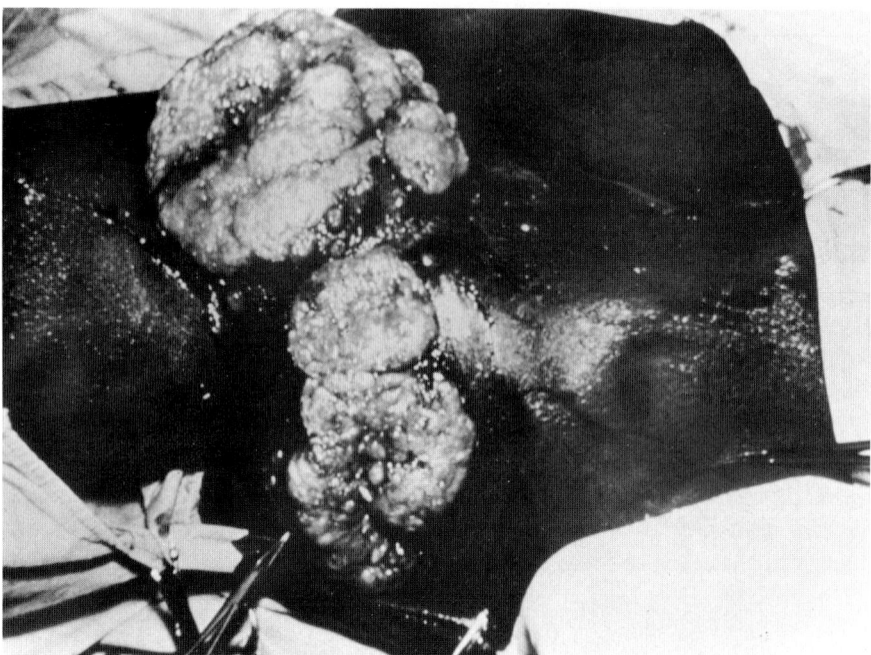

Figure 8. Carcinoma of the vulva with massive involvement of the right groin nodes presenting as fungating tumor.

Pretreatment Investigation

When a patient with vulvar carcinoma is seen, a thorough investigation should be undertaken. On the basis of our experience to date, we recommend the following studies:

1. Routine studies to include a complete blood count, urinalysis, biochemical profile, serum electrolytes, serology, blood urea nitrogen, and 2-hour postprandial blood sugar.
2. Papanicolaou smear of cervix, colposcopy of cervix and vulva, toluidine blue test, and biopsy of vulvar lesions or toluidine blue positive areas.
3. Screen for granulomatous diseases of the vulva if there is any significant possibility that these are present.
4. X-ray of chest, intravenous urogram, and barium enema.
5. Examination under anesthesia, cystoscopy, and sigmoidoscopy. Colonoscopy should be performed if indicated, and this should usually be done without anesthesia to minimize the chance of perforation.
6. A liver scan should be performed and if suggestive of metastatic disease, a laparotomy should be performed prior to radical vulvectomy.
7. X-rays of skull and long bones, or bone scan, should be performed if indicated.

8. Lymphography, sonography, and computerized axial tomography should only be done in selected cases. It is especially important to avoid lymphography unless a good indication is present because it may increase the risk of cellulitis in a lymphedematous limb at a later date.

Management

Provided the disease is resectable, it is generally agreed that the best treatment for invasive squamous cell carcinoma of the vulva should be nothing less than extensive excision of the vulva with bilateral groin lymphadenectomy. The primary lesion and groin nodes should be removed in continuity. The operation may be carried out under local anesthesia, or epidural anesthesia, if the patient is not fit for general anesthesia. In our opinion, the following are the most important points to be achieved at the operation of radical vulvectomy with bilateral regional lymphadenectomy:

1. A "horned" incision should be used so as to remove the skin over the inguinal lymph nodes. The tips of the horns will rest on the anterior superior iliac spines, with the upper part of the incision being interspinous in location, and the lower part extending along the inguinal skin creases and into the labiocrural folds so as to clear all lesions by 1 to 2 cm (Fig. 9). Recently we have been performing the groin node dissections in selected patients with early lesions through separate incisions in each groin, rather than using the "horned incision," with good results.
2. The lymph nodes should be removed with the vulvar specimen, with continuity of the labiocrural lymphatics being maintained within the specimen.

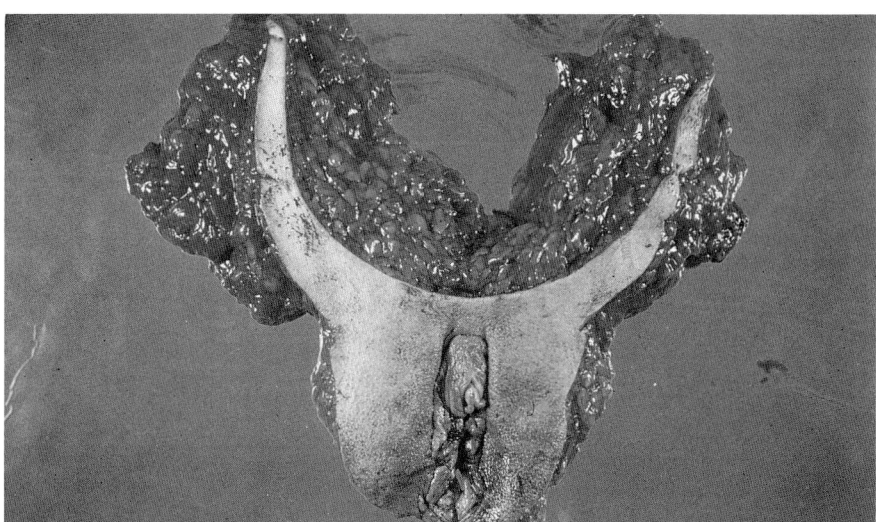

Figure 9. Vulvectomy specimen obtained using the "horned" incision.

3. The mons pubis should be removed with special attention being paid to this excision if the clitoris is involved.
4. The dissection should be carried down to the fascia so that all tissues are removed superficial to the urogenital diaphragm.
5. Resection of the vagina, urethra, anus, or even bone is required if the tumor has involved these sites.
6. Bilateral transplantation of the sartorius muscles is carried out to protect the femoral vessels. Fixation to the inguinal ligaments is obtained with 2-0 polyglactin sutures.

Using two teams, and starting with a bilateral groin dissection, the operation can be completed in 2 to 4 hours depending upon the experience of the team and the lesion being dealt with. The treatment of our patients is individualized depending on their general condition and the extent of the disease, and the type of treatment is categorized as curative or palliative. Details are given in Table 5.

Curative Treatment. When the patients receiving potentially curative treatment are considered, certain trends have become apparent as our experience with the disease has increased. Although radical vulvectomy with bilateral groin and pelvic lymphadenectomy was performed in 120 of 285 patients, there is now a trend away from this operation. Radical vulvectomy with bilateral groin lymphadenectomy was performed in 132 patients, and there is an increasing tendency to use this operation with liberal frozen sections being obtained of the groin lymph nodes. If a positive lymph node is found in the groin, then both extraperitoneal areas are explored unless a contraindication is evident. With adequate sampling of the groin nodes, we believe that the

TABLE 5. TREATMENT FOR CARCINOMA OF THE VULVA

	Patients
A. For Cure:	
Radical vulvectomy, bilateral groin and pelvic node dissection	120
Radical vulvectomy and bilateral groin node dissection	132
Total vulvectomy	20
Radical vulvectomy, bilateral groin and pelvic node dissection and exenteration	13
Total	285
B. Palliative:	
Radical vulvectomy and bilateral groin node dissection	1
Partial vulvectomy	10
Total	11

chance of having a positive pelvic node in the presence of negative groin nodes is remote, and we have not found a single case among 120 patients. Total vulvectomy was performed in 20 patients because it was believed that the patients were unfit for a more extensive procedure and the groin nodes were not palpable. Radical vulvectomy with bilateral groin and pelvic lymphadenectomies and exenteration was carried out in 13 patients, because it was thought that the disease was too extensive to be treated by radical vulvectomy with regional lymphadenectomy (Fig. 10). Unlike the situation with cervical carcinoma, it is usually possible to preserve either the bladder or the rectum, and total exenteration was necessary in only 1 of our 13 patients. Positive nodes were found in 83 of 210 patients (40 percent). The pelvic nodes were

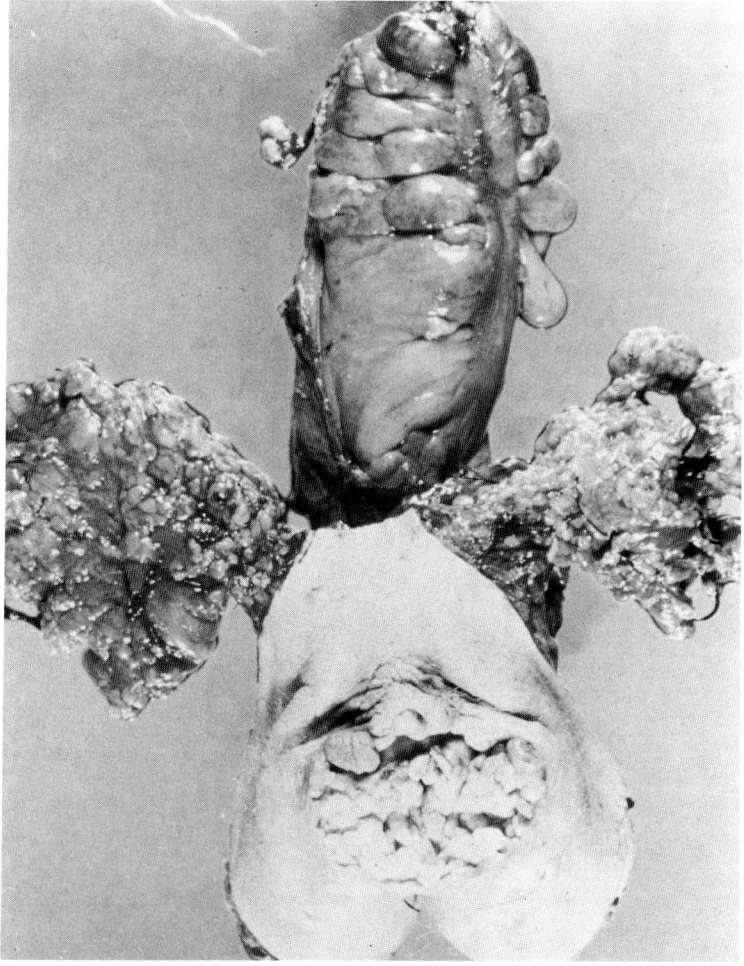

Figure 10. Extensive vulvar carcinoma involving the rectovaginal septum necessitating radical vulvectomy with posterior exenteration.

positive for metastatic disease in 16 of 133 patients (12 percent). A review of the literature reveals positive nodes in 21 to 59 percent of patients with 1.4 to 16 percent having positive pelvic nodes (Table 3).

Palliative Treatment. This was in the form of radical vulvectomy and bilateral groin dissection in one patient who was having recurrent hemorrhage from fungating nodes in the right groin. (Fig. 8). The patient's quality of life was much improved following the operation, but she died 18 months later of pulmonary metastasis. Partial vulvectomy was carried out in 10 patients because they were thought to be unsuitable for radical surgery.

Postoperative Mortality and Morbidity

There were no intraoperative deaths, but 16 of 296 patients (5.4 percent) died within 28 days of operation. Ten of these deaths were caused by pulmonary embolism, one by myocardial infarction, and one by postoperative osteomyelitis of the pubis with fulminating septicemia in a patient treated 15 months previously with radiotherapy (Table 6).

The main cause of morbidity in the 252 patients who received a radical vulvectomy and groin dissection was groin wound breakdown. This occurred in 179 of 210 patients (85 percent). Recently this has been reduced to approximately 20 percent with the use of the "horned" incision, and by undermining the abdominal wall and bringing it down toward the groins and symphysis pubis. If the wound does break down, it is cleansed with hydrogen peroxide and honey dressings are applied three times daily.[41] This leads to a clean granulating wound within a short period of time (Fig. 11), and only one patient has required skin grafting in the past 12 years. Femoral vessel rupture occurred on four occasions early in the series, but the routine use of bilateral sartorius muscle transplantation has eliminated this complication. Persistent lymphedema was a serious problem. This occurred in 22 of 210 patients (10 percent). If cellulitis is present, it should be treated with penicillin. Otherwise, elevation of the legs appears to be the most effective method of dealing with this troublesome complication. The operative treatment of lymphedema is unsatisfactory at this time. Within about 2 years, collateral lymphatic pathways become established and the situation improves, provided the legs have not been allowed to become chronically edematous.

TABLE 6. POSTOPERATIVE MORBIDITY AND MORTALITY IN CARCINOMA OF THE VULVA

A. Mortality	16 of 296 (5.4%)
B. Morbidity	
1. Groin wound breakdown	184 of 266 (69%)
2. Femoral vessel rupture	
Arterial	3 of 266 (1.2%)
Venous	1 of 266 (0.4%)
3. Chronic lymphedema	23 of 266 (8%)

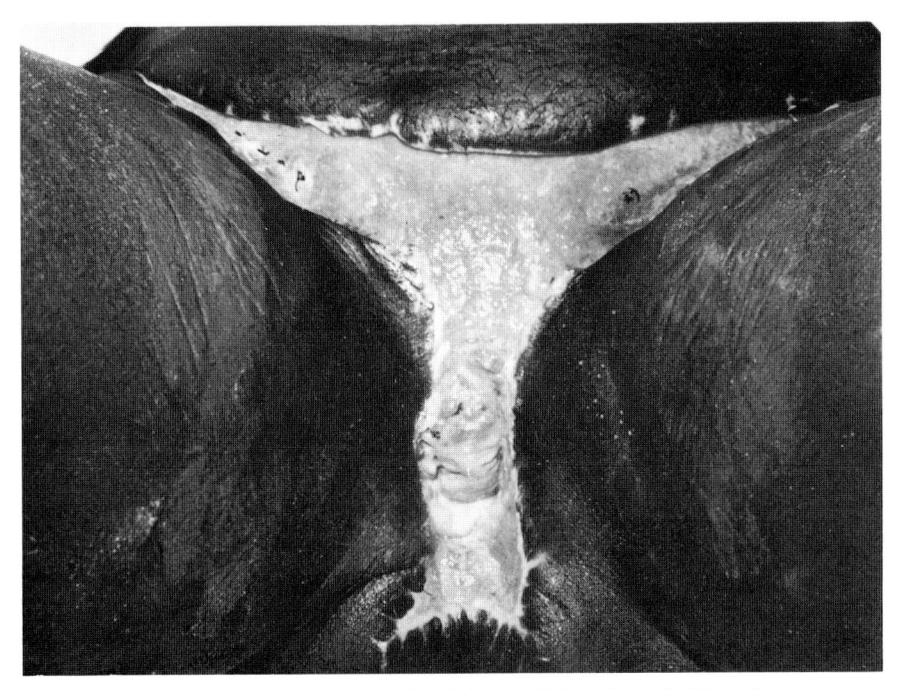

Figure 11. Patient with extensive breakdown of interspinous incision, 3 weeks after radical vulvectomy. The patient was treated with honey dressings three times daily and shows a clean granulating wound.

Results

In our series of 296 patients treated surgically, the absolute 5-year survival was 84 percent for Stage I, 61 percent for Stage II, 28 percent for Stage III, and 50 percent for Stage IV. It is of considerable interest that although only 9 of 30 patients (30 percent) with Stage III or Stage IV disease survived for 5 years, 5 of 10 patients with Stage IV disease treated with exenterative procedures survived 5 years. Thus, it is believed that there is a definitive place for this procedure in selected cases. With positive lymph nodes, the absolute 5-year survival rate was 33 percent and with negative nodes 69 percent. The overall absolute 5-year survival rate was 61 percent. As pointed out by Shingleton and associates[42] when assessing 5-year survival rates, it is important to differentiate between absolute survival rates and reports based on the modified life table method. The absolute 5-year survival rate for all cases treated by radical vulvectomy with lymphadenectomy ranges from 50 to 70 percent. In the series from M.D. Anderson Hospital reported by Rutledge and colleagues,[32] the 5-year survival rate for 139 patients treated for cure was 83 percent using the modified life table method. Patients often have intercurrent disease, which plays a large role in the survival rate. In this series 53 patients with negative inguinal nodes were followed for 5 years or more and none of them developed a recurrence. Thirty-three patients had positive nodes and

TABLE 7. FIVE-YEAR SURVIVAL RATES FOR CARCINOMA OF THE VULVA

Series	Status of Nodes	Number of Patients	Percent Surviving 5 Years Positive	Percent Surviving 5 Years Negative
Way (1960)	Positive	45	42	—
	Negative	36	—	77
Macafee (1962)	Positive	33	33	—
	Negative	49	—	70
Collins et al. (1963)	Positive	19	21	—
	Negative	32	—	69
Franklin and Rutledge (1971)	Positive	33	39	—
	Negative	53	—	100
Morley (1976)	Positive	64	39	—
	Negative	130	—	92
Krupp and Bohm (1978)	Positive	40	36	—
	Negative	154	—	91
Green (1978)	Positive	46	33	—
	Negative	61	—	87
Benedet et al. (1979)	Positive	34	53	—
	Negative	86	—	81
Cavanagh et al. (1981)	Positive	83	33	—
	Negative	127	—	69

13, or 39 percent, survived for 5 years free of disease. Of 16 patients with positive pelvic nodes, 4 survived 5 years.

A review of the literature from 1960 reveals that the 5-year survival rate in patients with positive nodes ranges from 21 to 53 percent (Table 7). With pelvic nodes positive, it ranges from 12.5 to 37.5 percent (Table 8). Most authors agree that radical vulvectomy should be accompanied by bilateral inguinal lymphadenectomy, but Morris disagrees with this.[5] The rationale for

TABLE 8. FIVE-YEAR SURVIVAL RATES FOR PATIENTS WITH POSITIVE PELVIC NODES

Series	5-Year Survival Rate (%)
Way (1957)	2/9 (22.2)
Green et al. (1958)	2/16 (12.5)
Way (1960)	3/8 (37.5)
Merrill and Ross (1961)	1/3 (33.3)
Collins et al. (1963)	1/6 (16.7)
Franklin and Rutledge (1971)	3/12 (25.0)
Morley (1976)	1/6 (16.7)
Currey et al. (1980)	2/9 (22.2)
Cavanagh et al. (1981)	4/16 (25.0)
Total	19/85 (22.4)

this therapeutic approach is based on his observation that the contralateral inguinal nodes are rarely positive when the ipsilateral inguinal nodes are negative. Morris advocates analysis of the ipsilateral inguinal nodes and avoidance of a contralateral inguinal lymphadenectomy when the ipsilateral inguinal nodes are negative for tumor. This view is not generally held, but in 1981 it received support from Iversen and coworkers[26] in Norway. Certainly this conservative approach is worth keeping in mind in the management of poor-risk patients.

Most authors have abandoned pelvic lymphadenectomy and the consensus at this time is that the pelvic nodes should be removed only if (1) the inguinal lymph nodes are positive; (2) the clitoris is involved in the lesion; (3) the urethra, vagina, or anus is involved; (4) the patient has a melanoma of the vulva; or (5) a carcinoma of the Bartholin's gland is present.

Recurrence

Recurrences may be local or involve distant metastases. The distant metastases usually appear within the first 2 years after treatment. Local recurrences usually involve the vulva or the groin nodes. Pulmonary metastases are not uncommon in late disease. The treatment of recurrence is difficult. Multiple local excisions should be attempted and interstitial radiation may be useful as a palliative procedure for local control. To date chemotherapy has proven to be of little value whether used regionally[43] or systemically.

The Place of Radiotherapy

In our series of 236 patients one-third of them had Stage III or IV disease; thus, the best way of improving overall results will be by earlier diagnosis and the judicious use of surgical treatment tailored to meet the needs of the individual patient. It has been suggested that local surgery, or radiotherapy, or both, will give results as good as radical vulvectomy and regional lymphadenectomy but the data do not appear to bear this out (Table 9). Frischbier and Thomsen[44] reported on 118 patients treated with 16 MeV Betatron from 1955 to 1964 with a 5-year survival rate of 43 percent. However, most authorities believe that radiation has a place only as ancillary therapy even with the newest techniques and equipment. We believe that primary radiotherapy should be reserved for patients who have medical contraindications to radical surgery or tumor that has extended beyond the scope of surgical extirpation even by pelvic exenteration.

Daly and Million[45] have suggested that patients with squamous cell carcinomas of the vulva and negative nodes be treated with radical excision of the vulva followed by elective radiation therapy to the groins and pelvic nodes up to and including the hypogastric nodes. They employ a 60 cobalt source, 80 cm source-skin distance (SSD), and split field treatment. They report minimal subcutaneous induration, minimal diarrhea, and no evidence of lymphedema of the lower extremities. These authors suggest that this concept of therapy is practical and believe that it is probably an improvement on vulvectomy with

TABLE 9. FIVE-YEAR SURVIVAL RATES FOR VULVAR CARCINOMA BY TREATMENT REGIMENS

Series	Radiotherapy Alone	Vulvectomy Alone	Radical Vulvectomy and Lymphadenectomy	Radical Vulvectomy and Exenteration
Smith and Pollack (1947)	16.7[a]	47.6	52.6	—
Huber (1953)	19.2	39.4	36.4	—
Taussig (1940)	4.8	8.3	58.5	—
Lunin (1949)	20.0	25.0	100.0	—
Brandstetter and Krataeluvill (1961)	10.3	17.6	58.3	—
Frischbier and Thomsen (1971)	43.0	—	—	—
Boutselis (1972)	33.0	0	66.6	—
Green (1978)	—	—	64.0	—
Cavanagh et al. (1981)	0	—	61.0	47.0

[a] All figures expressed in percent.

bilateral node dissection. However, there is considerable disagreement about this.

Morley[4] has suggested that patients with positive superficial nodes might be treated with pelvic irradiation giving a dosage of 5000 to 7000 rads to the whole pelvis rather than performing a pelvic lymphadenectomy. This seems to be a reasonable approach and we are using this approach in some of our more debilitated patients. After all, it is evident that in management we must have a broad general plan but with enough room for variation to suit an individual patient.

The Place of Immunotherapy

There is as yet no place for immunotherapy, but it seems reasonable that agents such as *C. parvum* might be useful in conjunction with radical surgery, and a controlled study is required for evaluation.

VERRUCOUS CARCINOMA OF THE VULVA

Verrucous carcinoma is a slow-growing, locally invasive neoplasm described by Buschke[46] in Germany in 1896 and subsequently by Buschke and Löwenstein[47] in 1925. They believed it had a predilection for the prepuce of the penis and it was designated giant condylomata acuminata of Buschke–Löwenstein. In 1948, Ackerman described such lesions as verrucous carcinoma, a variant of squamous cell carcinoma.[48] Goethals and colleagues[49] in 1963 and Kraus and Perez-Mesa[50] in 1966 reported on two large series of patients with verrucous carcinoma involving 55 and 105 patients, respectively. All lesions involved the oral cavity and larynx except 2 patients in Kraus's series who had vaginal and vulvar lesions. Judge[51] in 1969 reported another giant condyloma acuminatum involving the vulva and rectum. Since then 13 more cases of verrucous carcinoma of the vulva have been reported.[52–56]

Verrucous carcinoma of the vulva is an uncommon disease with less than 20 cases having been reported. However, as it is looked for, its frequency will undoubtedly increase. The ages of the patients range from 21 to 85 with a mean age of 53 years. There is no obvious predisposing factor. Two patients seen by us had findings compatible with prior lymphogranuloma venereum of the vulva and they were in the younger age group. In 1958 Green[2] also reported that 13 vulvar carcinoma patients who had granulomatous disease had developed their cancers 15 to 20 years earlier than did patients in the nongranulomatous group. The significance of this correlation is unknown.

In most instances the lesion begins as a warty, fungating, slow-growing tumor. It is commonly misdiagnosed as condyloma acuminatum and often local treatment with podophyllin is applied. The treatment is further delayed by the patient because of the unimpressive, slow growth of the lesion. The patient usually seeks medical attention only when the tumor extends over a large area, causing local destruction and deep penetration. Associated infection is common. The benign microscopic appearance sometimes creates a diagnostic problem. Judge concluded that the clinical appearance and behavior of the lesion was the best diagnostic guide.[51] Both pulmonary metastasis and death from recurrent tumor have been reported. When biopsy is performed, multiple samples with adequate tissue should be obtained.

Kraus and Perez-Mesa[50] distinguished the lesions in the genital area from benign condylomata acuminata by the absence of the central connective tissue core in the papillary processes of a verrucous carcinoma. They also noted that the clinician tends to overdiagnose the lesions on gross inspection and the pathologist to underdiagnose the lesions on histologic examination.

Surgery is the treatment of choice for verrucous carcinoma. Adequate excision is the key to the successful treatment, since most of the recurrences occur because of inadequate primary surgery. The application of podophyllin to these tumors is of no value;[57] nor are applications of topical 5-fluorouracil,[55] cryosurgery, and fulguration.[54,55] Radiation therapy is ineffective. Ackerman reported that 8 of 14 tumors recurred following irradiation,[48] as did 7 of 10 that were irradiated in the series reported by Goethals and associates.[49] Kraus and Perez-Mesa[50] reported 17 patients with verrucous carcinoma who received irradiation therapy; 11 patients had recurrences and 4 lesions underwent anaplastic transformations; 2 patients were unresponsive to radiation therapy. Gallousis[54] noted the histologic transformations of verrucous carcinoma of the vulva into a sarcomatoid pattern following irradiation therapy.

Surgery is currently superior to other treatments. Wide excision is effective only when the lesion is small and single. Radical vulvectomy with bilateral groin dissection is the treatment of choice for verrucous carcinoma of the vulva although the place of lymphadenectomy is debatable. Lymph node metastasis is uncommon with verrucous carcinoma, but when Gallousis reviewed the literature, he was able to find 11 of the 119 patients with nodal metastasis.[54] Sonck reported a case of proven distant pulmonary metastasis.[53] Radical vulvectomy, or even an exenterative procedure, is indicated when the tumor involves the bladder, anus, or rectum. Attention should be paid to the increased postoperative infection associated with the tumor. Preoperative antibiotic treatment, local cleansing procedures, and aggressive postoperative antibiotic therapy should be considered to avoid the serious infections to which these patients appear to be predisposed.

BASAL CELL CARCINOMA OF THE VULVA

This condition is rare. The lesion usually occurs on the labia majora and may have an area of central ulceration. A basal cell carcinoma is well circumscribed and rarely involves lymphatics. The typical microscopic picture is shown in Figure 12. The treatment of choice is wide excision. The results are excellent.

ADENOCARCINOMA OF THE VULVA

Adenocarcinoma of the vulva is one of the rarest types of gynecologic malignancy. It usually arises from Bartholin's gland (Fig. 13). The patients tend to be younger than women with squamous carcinoma of the vulva. The symptoms are similar but the disease is often present for a long time before the lesion on the vulva is evident. The diagnosis can be made only if a biopsy is obtained in the area.

Bartholin's gland adenocarcinoma has often spread via the lymphatics or vascular system by the time the diagnosis is made. It may spread along the rectovaginal septum to the pelvic nodes as well as to the groin nodes. At radical vulvectomy for Bartholin's gland carcinoma, an exploratory laparotomy should be performed because the disease may have extended beyond the pelvis. It is also important to remove portions of the vagina, levatores ani, and the ischiorectal fat as necessary. Frequently, posterior exenteration is required to ensure adequate extirpation. In the category of adenocarcinoma of Bartholin's gland there is an adenoid cystic carcinoma. This lesion is histologically similar to the corresponding tumor of the salivary glands. It tends to remain localized and seldom gives rise to widespread metastasis. Lymphatic spread does occur and lymphadenectomy should be included in the surgical treatment.

It should be noted that Bartholin's gland carcinoma may be of squamous or transitional cell origin. Indeed, we have seen one patient in whom the carcinoma showed squamous and adenocarcinomatous elements (Fig. 14). Usually these tumors arise from the duct of the gland and should be treated as are Bartholin's gland adenocarcinomas.

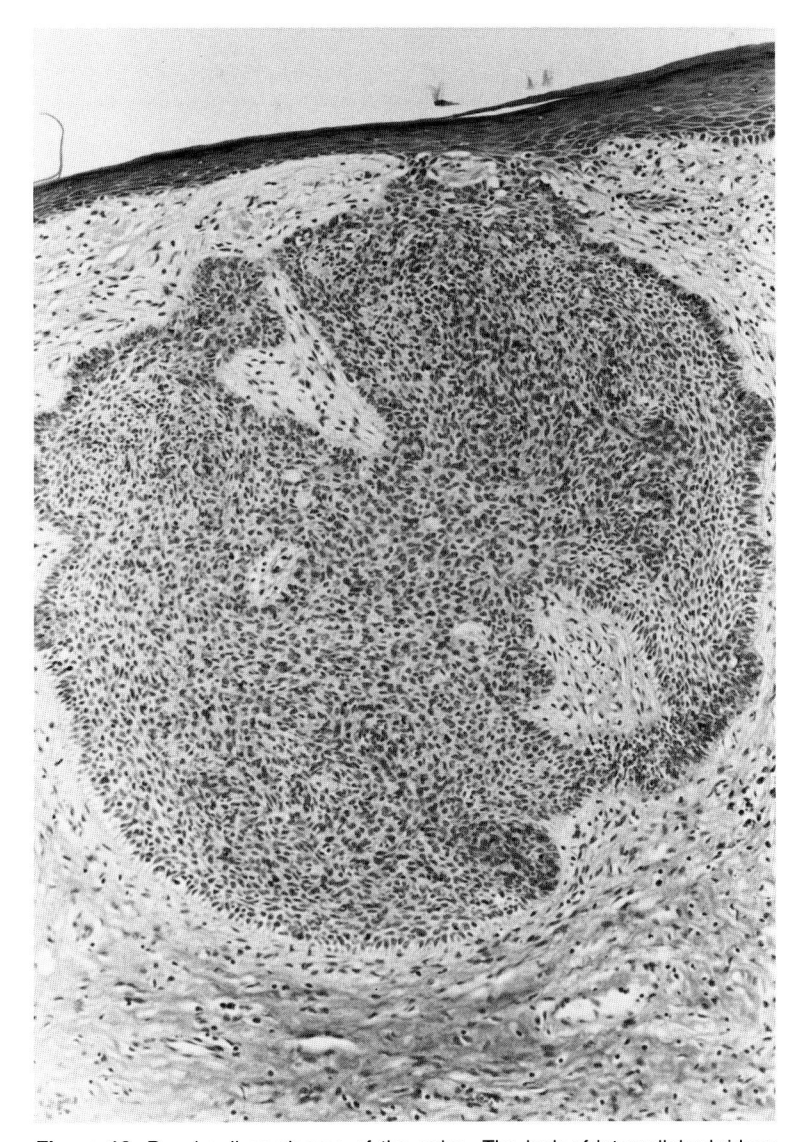

Figure 12. Basal cell carcinoma of the vulva. The lack of intercellular bridges, paucity of mitoses, and peripheral palisading of the cells are identical with the changes in basal cell carcinoma found commonly elsewhere on the skin.

MELANOMA OF THE VULVA

Melanoma of the vulva accounts for 3 to 7 percent of all melanomas in women and 5 to 10 percent of all vulvar carcinomas.[58–61] Less than 500 documented cases have been reported to date. All vulvar nevi are junctional nevi, which are the precursors of malignant melanomas.[62] The patient with melanoma of

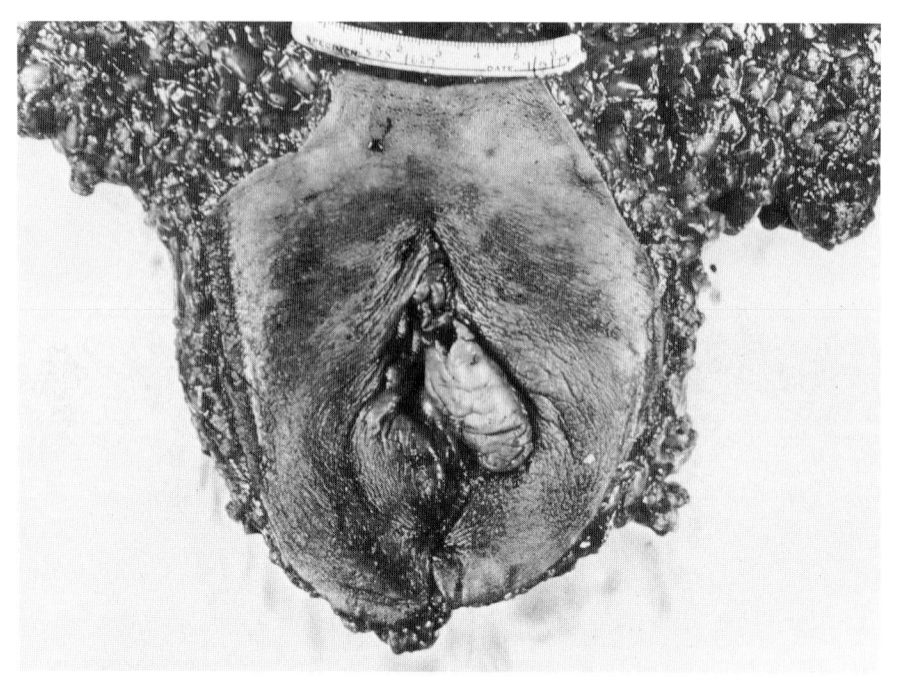

Figure 13. Carcinoma arising in the left Bartholin's gland that has dissected superiorly into the labium minus.

the vulva has an average age at the time of diagnosis of 55 years with a range of 15 to 84 years.[60] Thus, melanoma seems to develop at a younger age than does squamous cell carcinoma of the vulva. Melanomas of the skin are more common among whites,[63] but there was no evidence that the racial incidence of vulvar melanoma was increased in whites in the study by Morrow and DiSaia.[64] There is some evidence of a familial predisposition to melanomas and the familial melanoma tends to occur at a younger age. Thus, they have a better prognosis than melanomas in general.[65]

There was a high recurrence rate of malignant melanoma when associated with pregnancy.[59,66,67] Morrow suggests that pregnancy be postponed for several years after treatment even though pregnancy per se does not adversely affect prognosis.

Symptoms and Signs

The most common symptoms are the discovery of a vulvar tumor or enlarging mole, followed by pruritus and bleeding.[64] Some lesions are found incidentally during a routine gynecologic examination.[59-61] Delay in diagnosis is a frequent problem in vulvar melanoma, with an average patient delay of 13.5 months,[60] and the physician delay in diagnosis averaged 2.8 months.[61]

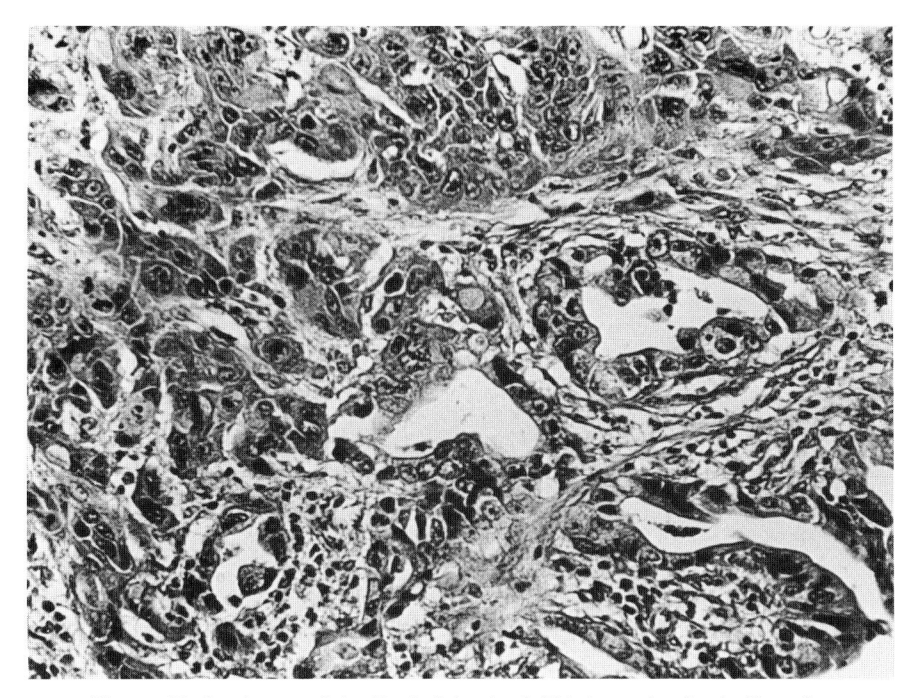

Figure 14. Carcinoma of the Bartholin's gland. This tumor is mixed with a glandular component (adenocarcinoma) in the lower right field and squamous carcinoma in the left upper field.

Site

Melanoma can arise anywhere in the vulva, but the labia minora and clitoris are the most common sites (Fig. 15). This is different from squamous cell carcinoma of the vulva, which most commonly involves the labia majora. At the labia minora and the clitoris the melanomas tend to spread superficially toward the urethra and the vaginal mucosa.[64] The extent of the disease at the time of diagnosis seems to correlate with the prognosis,[61] but the specific location of the primary tumor does not seem to alter the outcome unless the vagina or urethra is involved.

The amount of melanin production is widely variable, ranging from totally amelanotic lesions to black tumors. The amount of pigmentation has no effect on prognosis,[68] but the complete absence of pigment tends to delay the diagnosis of malignant melanoma.

Staging of malignant melanoma of the skin depends mainly on the depth of invasion as defined by Clark and associates.[69]

Level I. In situ, limited to the epidermis
Level II. Superficial, limited to the papillary dermis

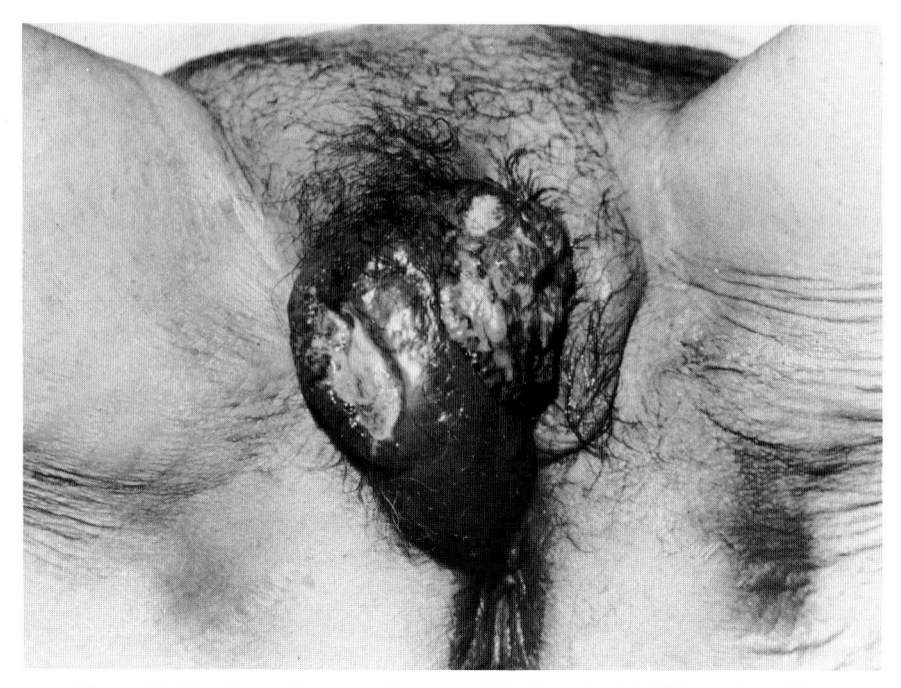

Figure 15. Massive malignant melanoma arising from the left labium minus. The patient had a lesion of the vulva for 4 years before seeking medical advice.

Level III. Intradermal, extending to the reticular dermis
Level IV.   Intradermal, extending into the reticular dermis
Level V.   Subcutaneous, involvement of the subcutaneous fat

Very superficial invasion does improve the generally poor prognosis of the vulvar melanoma.[62] However, the prognosis is bad when it involves the urethra or vagina.[64] The presence of satellite lesions is definitely correlated with a poor prognosis.[60] Clinical staging of melanoma of the vulva is similar to that of squamous cell carcinoma of the vulva. Inguinal lymph node metastases are found in approximately 33 percent of cases and distant metastases in 2.6 percent.[64]

Treatment

Nevi are common on the vulva, but they are almost invariably junctional nevi, and they should be removed prophylactically.[60,62] Excisional biopsy should be performed if the lesion is small. When a large lesion is found, adequate incisional biopsy should be done at the edge of the lesion including an adequate sample of pathologic tissue and normal tissue. Although the idea that incisional biopsy worsens the prognosis in melanoma has not been completely documented, we believe that an excisional biopsy should be performed if possible.

The minimal treatment for melanoma of the vulva is radical vulvectomy with bilateral inguinofemoral lymphadenectomy; bilateral pelvic lymphadenectomy is included when the groin nodes are positive for metastatic tumor. Symmonds and associates[59] suggest that pelvic lymphadenectomy should be a routine procedure because they believe that the additional surgery does not increase the morbidity postoperatively. They suggest that when melanoma of the vulva is diagnosed after adequate preoperative evaluation to rule out distant metastases, the patient should be explored for the detection of metastases in the upper abdomen and the para-aortic nodes. Total abdominal hysterectomy, bilateral salpingo-oophorectomy, and bilateral pelvic lymphadenectomy should then be performed. The treatment is completed by radical vulvectomy and bilateral groin dissection. The most common mistake in treating vulvar melanoma is inadequate local excision. The melanoma tends to grow outwards. This requires a wide excision from the margins of the lesion to ensure adequate resection. If the lesion involves the vagina, total vaginectomy is usually necessary. When the lesion involves the urethra, the vagina, or the rectum, pelvic exenteration should be considered.

Prognosis

For Stages I and II there is approximately a 75 percent 5-year survival. For Stages III and IV there is approximately a 15 percent 5-year survival. When the nodes are negative, the survival is approximately 56 percent, but it is approximately 14 percent when the nodes are positive.[64] As emphasized by Chung and associates,[70] survival is directly related to the depth of invasion. These authors found that no patient with a Level II lesion or less succumbed to the disease, whereas with Levels III, IV, and V lesions, prognosis becomes progressively worse. After careful study of 44 patients with malignant melanoma of the vulva, they concluded that minimal therapy should be radical vulvectomy with bilateral groin lymphadenectomy. It is our belief that an exploratory laparotomy should be done first to ensure that this extensive procedure is not being done on a patient who already has metastatic disease in the pelvis or upper abdomen. The report by Karlen and associates[71] of the poor results of conservative surgery supports this view, and these authors advise that adjunctive chemotherapy, immunotherapy, or radiotherapy be used if this course is followed. They also suggest that patients with positive nodes should receive such therapy, but no controlled studies are available for adequate assessment at this time.

In some patients with melanoma elsewhere, regression has been reported with dimethyltriazenoimidazole carboxamide (DTIC) and dactinomycin.[72] Immunotherapy with *C. parvum* or BCG may be useful and Gutterman and associates have achieved long disease-free intervals with the

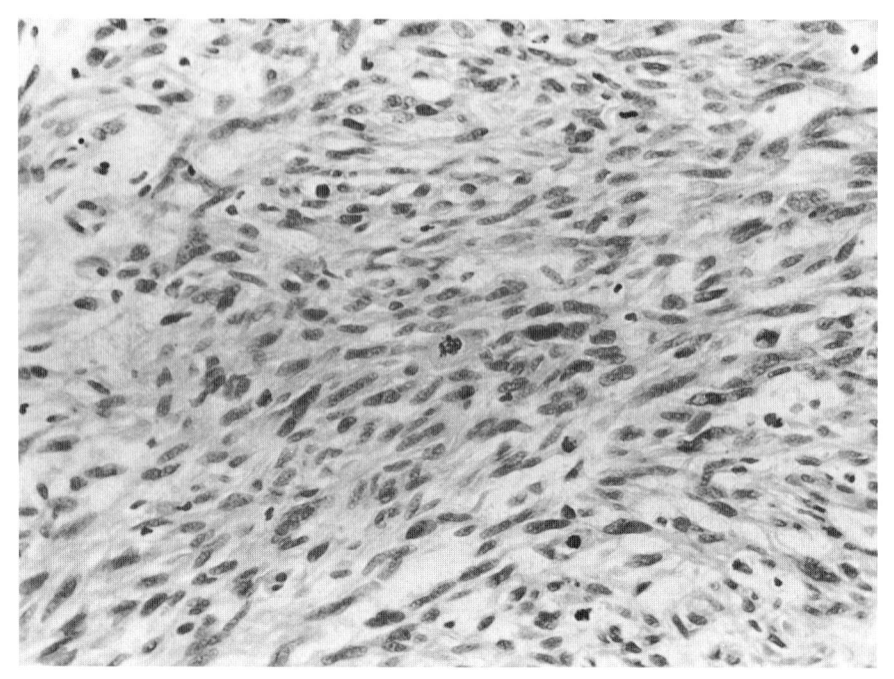

Figure 16. Leiomyosarcoma of the vulva. The presence of numerous mitoses differentiates this from its benign counterpart, the leiomyoma. Note the abnormal mitotic figure in the center of the field.

use of BCG scarification.[73] Immunotherapy has the potential for killing the last cancer cell, and thus may ultimately prove very useful in this disease. Radiation therapy has not proved to be effective in the primary treatment of vulvar melanoma.[74]

SARCOMA OF THE VULVA

This lesion is very rare as compared with carcinoma of the vulva. DiSaia and associates[75] reported a review of 12 patients. They found that sarcoma occurred at an earlier age than did carcinoma of the vulva, the mean age of their patients being 38 years. In patients with a poorly differentiated rhabdomyosarcoma, the tumors grow rapidly and metastasize early. However, leiomyosarcomas may be localized for long periods of time and usually metastasize slowly (Fig. 16). The treatment of choice will usually be radical vulvectomy with bilateral groin lymphadenectomy, but obviously blood-borne metastases will bypass the lymph nodes. In selected cases wide excision of the tumor may be more appropriate. The risk of local recurrence is great, and repeated excision is often necessary.

REFERENCES

1. Silverberg E: Statistical and epidemiological information on gynecologic cancer. Am Cancer Soc Prof Ed Pub, September, 1980
2. Green TH, Ulfelder H, Meigs JV: Epidermoid carcinoma of the vulva: An analysis of 238 cases. Am J Obstet Gynecol 75:834, 1958
3. Way S: Carcinoma of the vulva. Am J Obstet Gynecol 79:692, 1960
4. Morley GW: Infiltrative carcinoma of the vulva: Results of surgical treatment. Am J Obstet Gynecol 124:874, 1976
5. Morris JM: A formula for selective lymphadenectomy: Its application to cancer of the vulva. Obstet Gynecol 50:152, 1977
6. Magrina JF, Webb MJ, Gaffey TA, et al: Stage I squamous cell cancer of the vulva. Am J Obstet Gynecol 134:453, 1979
7. Cavanagh D, Shepherd JH, Praphat H, et al: Invasive carcinoma of the vulva. Some changing trends in surgical management. J Fla Med Assoc 69:447, 1982
8. Henson D, Tarone R: An epidemiologic study of cancer of the cervix, vagina, and vulva based on the Third National Cancer Survey in the United States. Am J Obstet Gynecol 129:525, 1977
9. Franklin EW, Rutledge FN: Epidemiology of epidermoid carcinoma of the vulva. Obstet Gynecol 39:165, 1972
10. Biometry Branch, National Cancer Institute: Cancer patient survival report 5. DHEW Publ 76-992. Washington, DC. US Govt Printing Office, 1977
11. Jeffcoate TNA: Chronic vulvar dystrophies. Am J Obstet Gynecol 95:51, 1966
12. Woodruff JD, Julian C, Puray T, et al: The contemporary challenge of carcinoma in situ of the vulva. Am J Obstet Gynecol 115:677, 1973
13. Buscema J, Stern J, Woodruff JD: The significance of the histologic alterations adjacent to invasive vulvar carcinoma. Am J Obstet Gynecol 137:902, 1980
14. International Society for the Study of Vulvar Disease: New nomenclature of vulvar disease. Obstet Gynecol 47:122, 1976
15. Friedrich EG Jr, Wilkinson EJ, Fu YS: Carcinoma in situ of the vulva: A continuing challenge. Am J Obstet Gynecol 136:830, 1980
16. Rutledge F, Sinclair M: Treatment of intraepithelial carcinoma of the vulva by skin excision and graft. Am J Obstet Gynecol 102:806, 1968
17. Forney JP, Morrow CP, Townsend DE, DiSaia PJ: Management of carcinoma in situ of the vulva. Am J Obstet Gynecol 127:801, 1977
18. Lobraico RV: Use of CO_2 laser in vulvar dystrophy. In Proceedings of the 5th International Congress International Society for the Study of Vulvar Disease. Maui, Hawaii, Oct 21 1979
19. Boehm J, Morris JM: Paget's disease and apocrine carcinoma of the vulva. Obstet Gynecol 38:185, 1971
20. Creasman WT, Gallager HS, Rutledge F: Paget's disease of the vulva. Gynecol Oncol 3:133, 1975
21. Franklin EW III, Rutledge F: Prognosis factors in epidermoid carcinoma of the vulva. Obstet Gynecol 37:892, 1971
22. Parker RT, Duncan L, Rampone J, et al: Operative management of early invasive epidermoid carcinoma of the vulva. Am J Obstet Gynecol 123:349, 1975
23. Wharton JT, Gallager S, Rutledge FN: Microinvasive carcinoma of the vulva. Am J Obstet Gynecol 118:159, 1974

24. Yazigi R, Piver MS, Tsukada Y: Microinvasive carcinoma of the vulva. Obstet Gynecol 51:368, 1978
25. DiSaia P, Creasman WT, Rich WM: An alternative approach to early cancer of the vulva. Am J Obstet Gynecol 133:825, 1979
26. Iversen T, Abeler V, Aalders J: Individualized treatment of Stage I carcinoma of the vulva. Obstet Gynecol 57:85, 1981
27. Friedrich EG, Wilkinson EJ: The vulva. In Blaustein A (ed): Pathology of the Female Genital Tract, 2nd ed. New York: Springer–Verlag, 1981, p. 13
28. Kabulski Z, Frankman O: Histologic malignancy grading in invasive squamous cell carcinoma of the vulva. Int J Gynaecol Obstet 16:233, 1978
29. Jakobsson PA, Encroth CM, Killander D, et al: Histologic classification and grading of malignancy of carcinoma of the larynx. Acta Radiol Ther Phys Biol 12:1, 1973
30. Barnes AE, Crissman JD, Schellhas HF, et al: Microinvasive carcinoma of the vulva. A clinicopathologic evaluation. Obstet Gynecol 56:234, 1980
31. International Society for the Study of Vulvar Disease Task Force and Subcommittee on Microinvasive Cancer of the Vulva. Gynecol Oncol 18:136, 1984
32. Rutledge F, Smith JP, Franklin EW III: Carcinoma of the vulva. Am J Obstet Gynecol 106:1117, 1970
33. Jimerson GK, Merrill JA: Multicentric squamous malignancy involving both cervix and vulva. Cancer 26:150, 1950
34. Marcus SL: Multiple squamous cell carcinomas involving the cervix, vagina and vulva: The theory of multicentric origin. Am J Obstet Gynecol 80:802, 1960
35. Franklin EW III: Clinical staging of carcinoma of the vulva. Obstet Gynecol 40:277, 1972
36. Krupp PJ, Lee FY, Bohm JW, et al: Prognostic parameters and clinical staging criteria in epidermoid carcinoma of the vulva. Obstet Gynecol 46:84, 1975
37. Boutselis JG: Radical vulvectomy for invasive squamous cell carcinoma of the vulva. Obstet Gynecol 39:827, 1972
38. Garcia C, Boronow RC: Carcinoma of the vulva: Anatomic and histologic prognostic facts. South Med J 65:237, 1972
39. Collins CG, Collins JH, Barclay DL, et al: Cancer involving the vulva. Am J Obstet Gynecol 87:762, 1963
40. Cavanagh D, Hovadhanakul P, Taylor H: Carcinoma of the vulva. Missouri Med 73:129, 1976
41. Cavanagh D, Beasley J, Ostapowicz F: Radical operation for carcinoma of the vulva: A new approach to wound healing. J Obstet Gynaecol Br Cwlth 77:1037, 1970
42. Shingleton HM, Fowler WC Jr, Palumbo L, Koch GG: Carcinoma of the vulva. Influence of radical operation on cure rate. Obstet Gynecol 35:1, 1970
43. Cavanagh D, Hovadhanakul P, Comas MR: Regional chemotherapy—a comparison of pelvic perfusion and intraarterial infusion in patients with advanced gynecologic cancer. Am J Obstet Gynecol 123:435, 1975
44. Frischbier HJ, Thomsen K: Treatment of cancer of the vulva with high energy electrons. Am J Obstet Gynecol 11:431, 1971
45. Daly JW, Million RR: Radical vulvectomy combined with elective node irradiation for T-X-N-O squamous carcinoma of the vulva. Cancer 34:161, 1974
46. Buschke A: Neisser's Stereoskopischer Atlas, 1896

47. Buschke A, Löwenstein L: Uber carcinomaähnliche Condylomata acuminata des Penis. Klin Wschr 4:1726, 1925
48. Ackerman LV: Verrucous carcinoma of the oral cavity. Surgery 23:670, 1948
49. Goethals PL, Harrison EG, Devine KD: Verrucous squamous carcinoma of the oral cavity. Amer J Surg 106:845, 1963
50. Kraus FT, Perez-Mesa C: Verrucous carcinoma—clinical and pathologic study of 105 cases involving oral cavity, larynx and genitalia. Cancer 19:26, 1966
51. Judge JR: Giant condyloma acuminatum involving vulva and rectum. Arch Path 88:46, 1969
52. Foye G, March MR, Minkowitz S: Verrucous carcinoma of the vulva. Obstet Gynecol 34:484, 1969
53. Sonck CE: Condylomata acuminata mit Vebergang in Karzinom. Z Haut Geschl Kr 46:273, 1971
54. Gallousis S: Verrucous carcinoma—Report of three vulvar cases and review of the literature. Obstet Gynecol 40:502, 1972
55. Lucas WE, Benirschke K, Lebherz T: Verrucous carcinoma of the female genital tract. Am J Obstet Gynecol 119:435, 1974
56. Isaacs JH: Verrucous carcinoma of the female genital tract. Gynec Oncol 4:259, 1976
57. Kneblich R, Failing JF: Giant condyloma acuminatum (Buschke–Löwenstein tumor) of the rectum. Am J Clin Path 48:389, 1967
58. Smith FR, Pollack RS: Carcinoma of the vulva. Surg Gynecol Obstet 84:78, 1947
59. Symmonds RE, Pratt JH, Dockerty MB: Melanoma of the vulva. Obstet Gynecol 15:543, 1960
60. Pack GT, Oropeza R: A comparative study of melanomas and epidermoid carcinomas of the vulva: A review of 44 melanomas and 58 epidermoid carcinomas 1930–1965. Rev Surg (Philadelphia) 24:305, 1967
61. Morrow CP, Rutledge FN: Melanoma of the vulva. Obstet Gynecol 39:745, 1972
62. Allen AC, Spitz S: Malignant melanoma: A clinicopathological analysis of the criteria for diagnosis and prognosis. Cancer 61:1, 1953
63. Pack GT, Davis J, Oppenheim A: The relation of race and complexion to the incidence of moles and melanomas. Ann NY Acad Sci 100:719, 1963
64. Morrow CP, DiSaia PJ: Malignant melanoma of the female genitalia: A clinical analysis. Obstet Gynecol Survey 31:233, 1976
65. Anderson DE: Clinical characteristics of the genetic variety of cutaneous melanoma in man. Cancer 28:721, 1971
66. Clayton SG: Melanoma of the vulva with pregnancy. Proc R Soc Med 39:578, 1946
67. Janovski NA, Marshall D, Taki I: Malignant melanoma of the vulva. Am J Obstet Gynecol 84:523, 1962
68. Mehnert JH, Heard JL: Staging of malignant melanomas by depth of invasion. Am J Surg 110:168, 1965
69. Clark WH Jr, From L, Bernardino EA, et al: The histogenesis and biologic behavior of primary human malignant melanoma of the skin. Cancer Res 29:705, 1969
70. Chung AF, Woodruff JM, Lewis JL: Malignant melanoma of the vulva—A report of 44 cases. Obstet Gynecol 45:638, 1975
71. Karlen JR, Piver MS, Barlow JJ: Melanoma of the vulva. Obstet Gynecol 45:181, 1975

72. Gerner RE, Moore GE, Didolkar MS: Chemotherapy of disseminated malignant melanoma with dimethyl triazeno imidazole carboxamide and dactinomycin. Cancer 32:756, 1973
73. Gutterman J, Mavligit G, McBride C, et al: BCG stimulation of immune responsiveness in patients with malignant melanoma. Cancer 32:321, 1973
74. Yackel DB, Symmonds RE, Kempers RD: Melanoma of the vulva. Obstet Gynecol 35:625, 1970
75. DiSaia PJ, Rutledge FN, Smith JP: Sarcoma of the vulva. Obstet Gynecol 127:8, 1977

CHAPTER 2
Cancer of the Vagina

Primary cancer of the vagina was first described by Cruveilhier[1] before the Anatomical Society of Paris in 1826. Primary carcinoma of the vagina is rare as compared with secondary involvement of the vagina from malignancies of the cervix, endometrium, and ovaries.[2,3] It accounts for between 1 and 2 percent of all primary gynecologic malignancies.[4-6] The disease was extensively reviewed by Way[7] in 1948. The 5-year survival rate was not improved until the last decade. This improvement has resulted from the better understanding of the modes of spread of the disease and a marked improvement in radiotherapy techniques. Over 90 percent of vaginal cancers are of squamous cell origin.[6,8,9] The remaining tumors are clear cell carcinomas, other adenocarcinomas, sarcomas, and melanomas.

In the past it was very difficult to compare the results of treatment methods used in different centers because the number of patients in each series was small, and because there was no universal staging system for the disease. In 1962 Whelton and Kottmeier[10] proposed a clinical classification for carcinoma of the vagina. Essentially this was the staging system adopted by the International Federation of Gynecology and Obstetrics (FIGO). In 1973, Perez and associates[5] suggested dividing Stage II into II A and II B, and using this modification there is even better correlation with prognosis than with the original FIGO classification. The modified FIGO classification is shown in Table 1.

TABLE 1. MALIGNANT TUMORS OF THE VAGINA—CLINICAL STAGING (FIGO)

Stage 0	Carcinoma in situ; intraepithelial neoplasia
Stage I	Invasive carcinoma confined to the vaginal mucosa
Stage II	Submucosal infiltration and into the parametrium but not extending to the pelvic wall
Stage II A	Subvaginal infiltration, not extending into the parametrium
Stage II B	Parametrial infiltration, not extending to the pelvic wall
Stage III	Tumor extending to the pelvic wall
Stage IV	Tumor extending to the bladder or rectum or metastasis outside of the true pelvis
Stage IV A	Extension to adjacent organs
Stage IV B	Spread to distant organs

SQUAMOUS CELL CARCINOMA OF THE VAGINA

This is the most common type of primary cancer of the vagina. To establish the diagnosis of primary vaginal cancer the following criteria are required:[11]

1. The primary site of growth is in the vagina.
2. The uterine cervix must not be involved.
3. There must be no clinical evidence of metastatic disease.

According to Murad and colleagues,[9] primary vaginal carcinoma is defined as a neoplasm that is discovered in the vaginal wall of patients who have exhibited neither concurrent nor antecedent genital cancer. Vaginal lesions discovered in patients in association with, or subsequent to, the diagnosis of other genital cancers are regarded as secondary. Underwood and Smith[12] are of the opinion that as the survival rate for patients with cervical carcinoma improves, primary vaginal malignancy will be more commonly recognized. As they point out, this is not illogical because both of these lesions are exposed to and influenced by essentially the same carcinogens.

INTRAEPITHELIAL CARCINOMA OF THE VAGINA

In 1952 Graham and Meigs[13] reported on two patients with intraepithelial neoplasia of the vagina and one with invasive carcinoma of the vagina, detected 6, 7, and 10 years after total hysterectomy for carcinoma in situ of the cervix. Multiple primary cancers of the vagina, cervix, and vulva have been reported by Ostergard and Morton,[14] and this suggests a field response to a common carcinogenic agent such as the herpes or papilloma viruses.

Vaginal intraepithelial neoplasia (VAIN) is much less common than cervical intraepithelial neoplasia. Stuart and associates[15] reported that the recurrence rate of carcinoma in situ of the vagina following treatment for in situ disease of the cervix is from 0.7 to 6.6 percent. However, these same authors remind us that 12 of their 29 patients with squamous cell carcinoma of the vagina had hysterectomies for benign disease. Thus, although it is especially important to follow patients who have had cervical intraepithelial neoplasia, it is also important to be aware that carcinoma in situ of the vagina can arise de novo.

In most cases, intraepithelial neoplasia of the vagina is first suspected by the use of the Papanicolaou smear.[16] Colposcopic examination will usually show areas of white epithelium, mosaicism, or punctation after the application of 2 percent acetic acid. Alternatively, the lesion may be outlined using Lugol's iodine with the nonstaining areas of the vagina being biopsied. It is more difficult to biopsy the vagina than the cervix, but this can usually be accomplished by raising the vaginal skin with a skin-hook, or Allis forceps, prior to the use of a Kevorkian-Young biopsy forceps. It should be kept in mind that vaginal intraepithelial neoplasia is multifocal in about 50 percent of the cases and may be associated with invasive carcinoma. Thus, it is essential to get adequate biopsies of all colposcopically abnormal areas.

Pathology

VAIN 1 (Mild Dysplasia). In this there is minimal loss of stratification and polarity of the cells. The nuclei are enlarged and often irregular and pyknotic. Atypia is confined to the lower third of the epithelium.

VAIN 2 (Moderate Dysplasia). Here the degree of epithelial abnormality extends into the middle third of the epithelium and is intermediate between VAIN 1 and VAIN 3.

VAIN 3 (Severe Dysplasia and Carcinoma in Situ). Here there is loss of polarity and stratification through almost all layers with only the superficial cells showing maturation. Atypia is pronounced and extends into the upper third of the epithelium. Carcinoma in situ involves extension of atypical cells to the surface with complete loss of stratification. It is included with severe dysplasia in VAIN 3 because, as in the cervix, the prognosis for severe dysplasia and carcinoma in situ is the same.

Management

1. Local excisional biopsy of the multiple areas involved may be therapeutic as well as diagnostic.
2. *5-fluorouracil cream (5-FU cream)*. This cream, in the form of 5 percent Efudex, may be applied in a vaginal applicator one-third full, or in a diaphragm, or in an impregnated tampon, depending upon the site of the lesion. 5-FU cream is usually best applied at night for a period of 5 to 10 days depending upon the patient's tolerance of the vaginal irritation. The vulva is protected with zinc-oxide ointment or Vaseline. The course can be repeated every 2 weeks, for a total of two to three courses, and the patient followed with cytology and colposcopy. The results of this treatment have been very satisfactory.[17-21]

3. *Cryosurgery.* This has been considered a safe and effective way of treating women with vaginal intraepithelial neoplasia. However, it is now giving way to laser treatment. Its attractiveness lies in its simplicity, but it must be kept in mind that all methods of treatment carry some hazard, and an ileovaginal fistula has been reported following cryosurgery for vaginal dysplasia.[22]
4. *Laser therapy.* The carbon dioxide laser is being used with increasing frequency to treat vaginal intraepithelial neoplasia. Jobson and Homesley[23] have reported that 20 of 24 patients with vaginal intraepithelial neoplasia had the disease ablated following a single operation. Of the four who failed, these were retreated successfully with the laser. Similar results have been reported by other authors.[24,25]
5. *Radiotherapy* has been used in the form of a local radium application for some years. The type of applicator depends upon the site of the intraepithelial neoplasia, and so careful colposcopic examination of the vagina is important prior to the application. Some workers have reported considerable success with this method.[26]
6. *Vaginectomy.* For many years this was the treatment of choice with or without the placement of a skin graft. In patients resistant to other types of treatment, operative treatment is still necessary. However, even after the removal of the entire vagina, the patient should continue to be followed with cytology and colposcopy, because recurrence in a neovagina is presently unknown.[27]

INVASIVE CARCINOMA OF THE VAGINA

Age
The average age of patients with primary carcinoma of the vagina is approximately 65 years with over two-thirds being over the age of 50.[5-7,10] This is a completely different age group from that of patients affected by clear cell adenocarcinoma of the vagina, but is similar to that of patients with other adenocarcinomas of the vagina.

Race
There is some disagreement as to the racial incidence of this disease. In the series by Perez and associates,[5] 92 percent of the patients were white and 8 percent were black. Prempree and colleagues[6] reported that 85 percent of their patients were white and 15 percent were black. Marcus[28] also suggested a higher incidence of vaginal carcinoma in whites than in blacks, but Underwood and Smith[12] found no difference in the racial incidence among their patients.

Parity
There is no definite relationship between parity and the development of vaginal carcinoma.[4,7,10,29]

Predisposing Factors
Many possible predisposing factors have been suggested. Way[7] reported that 4 of his 44 patients had either procidentia or were wearing pessaries at the time of diagnosis. In Rutledge's[30] series, 6 of 101 patients had histories of long-term use of pessaries. Herbst, Green, and Ulfelder[31] reported that 3 of their 68 patients were wearing pessaries for procidentia. Previous pelvic irradiation has been suggested as a cause of some types of malignancy, such as uterine sarcoma. There is considerable question whether this plays any part in the pathogenesis of vaginal carcinoma. In 1977 Pride and Buchler[32] reviewed 16 patients who developed neoplasia in the cervix or vagina 10 or more years following pelvic irradiation, and they concluded that the risk of developing radiation induced carcinoma in the upper vagina or cervix was remote.

Signs and Symptoms
The most common sign in vaginal cancer is bleeding, this being the main complaint in 50 to 83.7 percent of series collected from the literature.[4,7,10,12,29,33] In premenopausal women postcoital bleeding is a common complaint. Approximately 20 percent of the patients with vaginal carcinoma complain of vaginal discharge. Other complaints are of pelvic pain, urinary symptoms, rectal bleeding, and awareness of a growth developing in the vagina. It is interesting that patients are sometimes asymptomatic, this being noted in up to 21 percent of reported series.[33] The diagnosis in these cases is usually made during a routine pelvic examination for the taking of a Papanicolaou smear. These patients usually have the diagnosis made at an early stage of the disease, and their prognosis is good. The fact that these patients are not uncommonly asymptomatic gives further support to the idea that routine pelvic examinations and Papanicolaou smears should be done in posthysterectomy patients. Needless to say, these annual pelvic examinations are all the more important if a patient's ovaries have been preserved at the time of hysterectomy.

Site of Lesion
According to the lymphatic drainage, the vagina is divided into the upper third, middle third, and lower third. The upper third is the most common site for squamous carcinoma, and the middle third is the least common site. Posterior wall lesions are most common in the upper third, and anterior wall lesions are most common in the lower third of the vagina.[4,7,10,33] It is common to see a lesion on the lateral wall of the vagina. Often it is not possible to see precisely the point of origin, and so this information tends to be inaccurate unless great care is taken when inspecting the vagina. A vaginal speculum with adequate lighting is essential for this procedure.

Routes of Spread
The primary mode of spread for vaginal carcinoma is by direct invasion. Spread is also common by the lymphatic route, rarely by the bloodstream, and possibly by the interstitial route. The lymphatic drainage from the upper third of the vagina is similar to that of the cervix. The lymphatic drainage from the lower

third of the vagina is essentially that for the vulva. A lesion in the middle third of the vagina may spread by either of these lymphatic routes. Generally, lymphatic spread from the anterior wall of the vagina drains to the nodes in the lateral pelvic wall, especially to the internal iliac lymph nodes. Posterior vaginal wall lesions usually drain to the deep pelvic nodes, such as the inferior gluteal, sacral, and rectal nodes.[34] Although these generalizations can be made, it should be realized that there is a free anastamosis between lymphatics and veins, and between the lymphatics of the upper and lower halves of the vagina, as well as between those of the right and left walls of the vagina. When tumor involves the lower third of the vagina, 6 to 7 percent of patients have metastasis to the inguinal lymph nodes.[10,35] Although cross-drainage occurs, it is important to try to establish the site of the lesion as accurately as possible. This applies whether surgery or radiotherapy is to be used in treatment, but it is more obviously pertinent with regard to a surgical approach.

Histopathology

Squamous cell carcinoma accounts for approximately 92 percent of all vaginal cancers. When all tumors are assigned for a histologic grade 1 to 4 in the Broders' classification,[36] most of the patients are in grades 2 or 3[33] (Fig. 1). There is apparently no correlation between the grade of this tumor and either the prognosis following treatment, or the distribution of tumor grades by clinical stage.

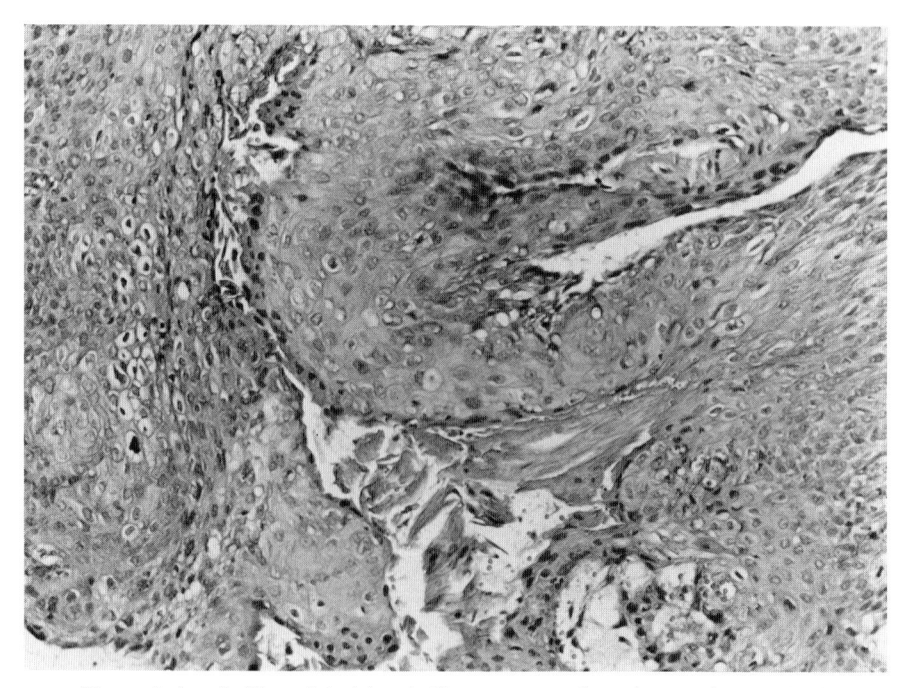

Figure 1. A well-differentiated (grade 2) squamous cell carcinoma, characterized by prominent cell borders, intercellular bridges, and keratin production. H&E. x160.

Clinical Staging

Review of large series demonstrates that vaginal carcinoma is generally distributed evenly in different stages (Table 2), although the majority of patients are in Stages I to II B. The detection rate for carcinoma in situ of the vagina is low when compared with carcinoma in situ of the cervix. This reflects the tendency toward the late diagnosis of vaginal cancer, as opposed to cervical cancer.

Treatment

The clinical staging and the location of the vaginal lesions are of prime importance in choosing proper therapy. The age, the necessity of maintaining a functional vagina, and the medical status of the patient must be considered. Gynecologic oncologists and radiotherapists agree that the management of vaginal carcinoma is difficult because of the close proximity of the vagina to the bladder and the rectum. It requires far more planning and individualization of treatment than do most other gynecologic cancers.

Radiotherapy. With the improvement of radiotherapy in the last decade, it has become the treatment of choice for most patients with vaginal cancer. A properly planned program integrating external irradiation with brachytherapy to fit the vaginal lesion will provide the best tumor control, as well as minimize the tendency to cystitis and proctitis, and maintain a functional vagina.

Patients with carcinoma in situ of the vagina are treated with brachytherapy only, and this treatment will deliver 6000 to 8000 rads to the vaginal mucosa.[6,8] Invasive carcinoma should be treated with a combination of brachytherapy (intracavitary and interstitial), and external beam therapy. The aim of brachytherapy is to deliver a minimum of 5000 rads to the mucosa. External radiation therapy consists of from 1000 to 2000 rads tumor dose to the whole pelvis for the early lesions, and from 2000 to 4000 rads for more advanced tumors. A supplemental parametrial dose is usually given with a midline block, to deliver a total of from 4000 to 5000 rads for early lesions, and 5000 to 6000 rads for the advanced lesions.[8]

Major complications occur in 6 to 8 percent of cases.[6,8] These consist of vesicovaginal fistula, rectovaginal fistula, pelvic abscess, and rectal stricture. It

TABLE 2. CARCINOMA OF THE VAGINA—NUMBER OF PATIENTS AND CLINICAL STAGING

Stage of Disease	Pride[32,33]	Prempree[6]	Perez[5]	Total
0	—	7	10	17
I	9	6	21	36
II A	6	20	22	48
II B	16	11	14	41
III	4	20	3	27
IV	8	7	6	21
Totals	43	71	76	190

appears that major complications occur mainly in the patients with more advanced disease, and it is almost always associated with progression of tumor rather than with radiation alone. Minor complications are radiation cystitis, radiation proctitis, urethral stenosis, and vaginal fibrosis. These usually occur in patients receiving a combination of brachytherapy and external beam therapy. It must be kept in mind throughout radiotherapy that the most serious complication of the treatment for cancer is recurrence. Unfortunately, this is frequently forgotten in carcinoma of the vagina and patients are often undertreated.

Surgery. Underwood and Smith[12] have suggested that surgery is the treatment of choice for carcinoma in situ of the vagina. The decision as to whether a patient is to have a simple vaginectomy, with or without a skin graft, depends on the need for a functional vagina. A Stage I lesion in the upper third of the vagina can be adequately treated with a radical vaginectomy, radical hysterectomy, and pelvic lymphadenectomy. For the advanced lesions, an exenterative procedure is required for complete surgery, because of the close proximity of the vagina to the bladder and the rectum. For a lesion at the lower third of the vagina, radical vulvectomy and bilateral groin dissection must be included in the surgical procedure. Surgery has disadvantages, as when the vagina has to be removed, partially or totally, and so radiotherapy combined with radical surgery should be considered in advanced vaginal lesions. Recurrent carcinoma of the vagina following radiation therapy should be evaluated with a view to further surgical therapy. Chemotherapy is only palliative at this time.

Prognosis

In the past the survival rate of women with vaginal carcinoma has been very poor. In 1950 Livingstone[37] reported 970 cases with a 5-year survival rate of 12 percent. In 1962 Whelton and Kottmeier[10] reported 129 cases with a 5-year survival rate of 24 percent. In the last decade, the survival rate for vaginal cancer has improved (Table 3). The improvement has been due to the proper integration of radiotherapy techniques, combining interstitial and intracavi-

TABLE 3. CARCINOMA OF THE VAGINA–FIVE-YEAR SURVIVAL RATE

Stage of Disease	Perez[5] No.	%	Prempree[6] No.	%
0	7/9	77	7/7	100
I	24/29	82	5/6	83
II A	17/32	53	13/20	65
II B	4/19	21	7/11	63
III	2/7	28	8/20	40
IV	1/7	14	0/7	0

tary radium with external supervoltage radiation. Only careful follow-up for postradiation patients will make the diagnosis of early recurrence possible. The proper use of exenterative surgery will further increase the 5-year survival rate for patients with carcinoma of the vagina.

CLEAR CELL ADENOCARCINOMA

Prior to 1976 this lesion was rarely reported. When it was reported, it was usually described as "mesonephric adenocarcinoma," although it is now evident that the lesion is of Müllerian rather than Wolffian origin. In 1971 the U.S. Food and Drug Administration issued a warning regarding synthetic, nonsteroidal estrogens such as diethylstilbestrol (DES). In the same year a "Registry of Clear Cell Adenocarcinoma of the Genital Tract" was established by Herbst, Scully, and Ulfelder. More recently the Registry has been renamed the "Registry for the Research on Transplacental Carcinogenesis" and 346 patients with clear cell adenocarcinoma of the vagina and cervix have been accessioned up to January 1979.[38] These cancers reached a peak incidence in the early 1970s and this has continued on the same level up to the present time. The facts appear to be as follows:

1. Two-thirds of the patients who have been reported as having clear cell adenocarcinoma have had a history of intrauterine exposure to a nonsteroidal estrogen, such as DES, hexestrol, or dienestrol.[39-41] It must be kept in mind, however, that adenocarcinoma may develop in the absence of the prenatal administration of estrogens even when this is combined with estrogen deficiency postnatally.[42]
2. If these hormones are carcinogenic, the problem is not entirely dose related because the dose has ranged from 150 to 15,000 mg according to the maternal histories, although the risk increases with the dose.[43]
3. In almost all cases the mothers of the offspring had taken the drug before the eighteenth week of pregnancy.[28] The extent of the problem will be realized when it is considered that from one-half million to two million women are estimated to have taken nonsteroidal estrogens, with from 34 to 90 percent of their female offspring showing evidence of DES syndrome.[43,44]
4. The most common manifestation of DES syndrome is the presence of glandular epithelium or its mucinous products in the vagina (adenosis)[45] (Fig. 2). In addition, these patients usually show evidence of squamous metaplasia.[46]
5. Although adenosis is seen with clear cell adenocarcinoma, there is only one case in the literature with apparent progression from adenosis to adenocarcinoma.[47]
6. Although adenosis is common after DES exposure, clear cell adenocarcinoma remains extremely rare.[38]
7. Anatomic defects are also manifestations of the DES syndrome. Ex-

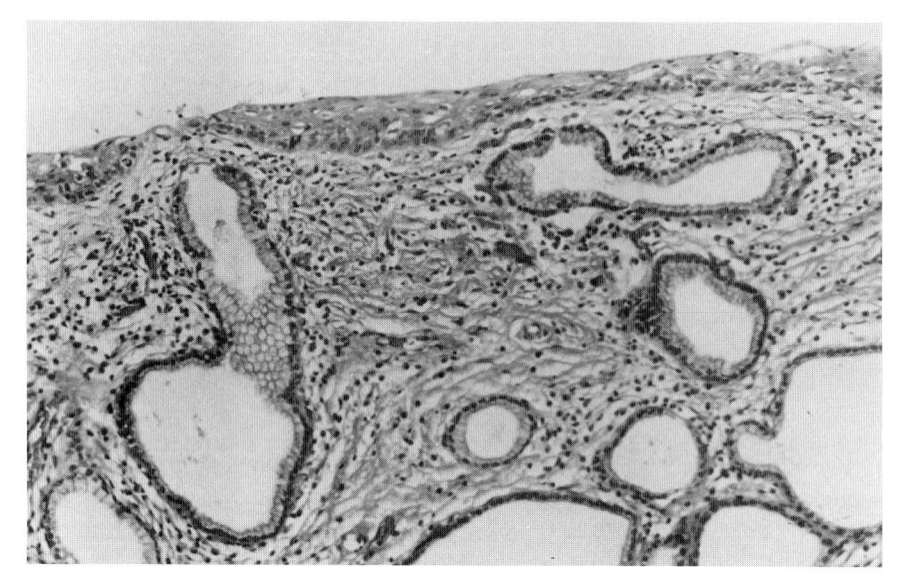

Figure 2. Vaginal adenosis. Underlying the benign squamous epithelium of the vagina are endocervical-like glands lined by mucus-producing epithelium. H&E. x80.

amples of these are the presence of a cervical "cockscomb," a cervical collar or transverse ridges located either on the cervix or in the vagina,[48-50] and the typical T-shaped uterus.[51]

8. The exact risk of clear cell adenocarcinoma developing in a patient whose mother was exposed to DES or a similar substance during pregnancy has not been ascertained at this time. As already mentioned, from one-half million to two million women probably took these agents in the late 1940s and 1950s, so that the vast majority of the exposed population is under the age of 30 years at the present time.

Screening of Women for DES Syndrome

Although it is not absolutely established that adenosis will progress to clear cell adenocarcinoma, it would seem prudent to establish screening examinations for women exposed to DES. These examinations should probably begin once the patient begins to menstruate or by the age of 14 years. As already mentioned, up to 90 percent of these women show evidence of adenosis and approximately 20 percent have abnormalities of the upper vagina and cervix in the form of a "cockscomb," vaginal hood, transverse vaginal and cervical ridges, or a cervical collar. The uterus is frequently hypoplastic.

Adenosis is sometimes accompanied by squamous metaplasia, this probably being the mechanism by which spontaneous healing occurs. The metaplasia frequently is immature and may be confused with dysplasia or carcinoma in situ. At this time it has not been established that there is an increased frequency of dysplasia or carcinoma in situ in patients with DES exposure,

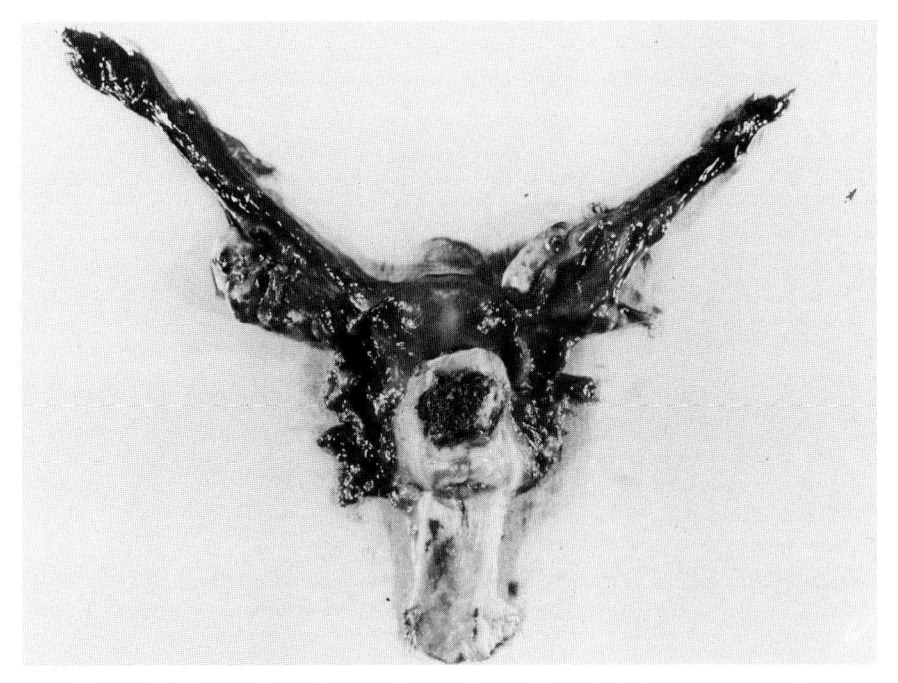

Figure 3. Clear cell carcinoma. A granular, erythematous tumor mass on the reflected anterior vaginal wall.

but this gives one more reason for careful follow-up of these patients. At the present time it seems reasonable that these patients should be seen every 6 months to a year and their examination should include the following:

1. *Cytology*. Cytologic examination remains a useful screening method, although Papanicolaou vaginal smears have been successful in detecting only 73 percent of known clear cell adenocarcinomas.[52]
2. *Colposcopy*. If not available, the Schiller test using Lugol's iodine should be employed.[44]
3. Selective *biopsies* on the basis of colposcopy, or a positive Schiller test should be performed, to rule out carcinoma.
4. *Hysterosalpingography* if the patient plans pregnancy, because an immature T-shaped uterus is frequently found.
5. Treatment in the form of excision or cryosurgery of these lesions is not indicated unless there is evidence of a premalignant or malignant lesion. If an invasive malignancy is found, it is probably best treated by radical surgery.

Clinical Picture in Clear Cell Adenocarcinoma

Approximately 20 percent of patients are asymptomatic when a diagnosis of clear cell adenocarcinoma is made. In this group the lesions are small, and the 5-year survival rate is over 90 percent.

In symptomatic patients the results are not so good. There may be a delay in diagnosis because the patients are young and the vaginal spotting is ignored. A careful examination will reveal a vaginal lesion, usually in the upper third of the vagina on the anterior wall (Fig. 3) or on the cervix. There is a significant risk of invasion when the tumor area exceeds 6 square centimeters, or if the depth of invasion is greater than 3 mm.[53] When the tumor involves the cervix, there is a high incidence of nodal metastasis. Thus, careful inspection of the cervix with endocervical and ectocervical biopsies is useful in treatment planning. Microscopically (Fig. 4) the lesion has a "hobnail" cell and generally shows less papillation than the vaginal adenocarcinomas sometimes seen in older women. Electron microscopy provides clarification with regard to cell type.[42]

Both surgery and radiotherapy have been used effectively in the treatment of clear cell carcinoma of the vagina. However, the generally accepted treatment of choice is a radical hysterectomy, vaginectomy, and pelvic lymphadenectomy. For recurrences, surgery is usually the treatment of choice with the operation being tailored to the needs of the individual patient.

Radiotherapy is effective for lesions less than 2 cm in diameter, and a surface dose of as low as 5000 rads has proved effective in the control of these

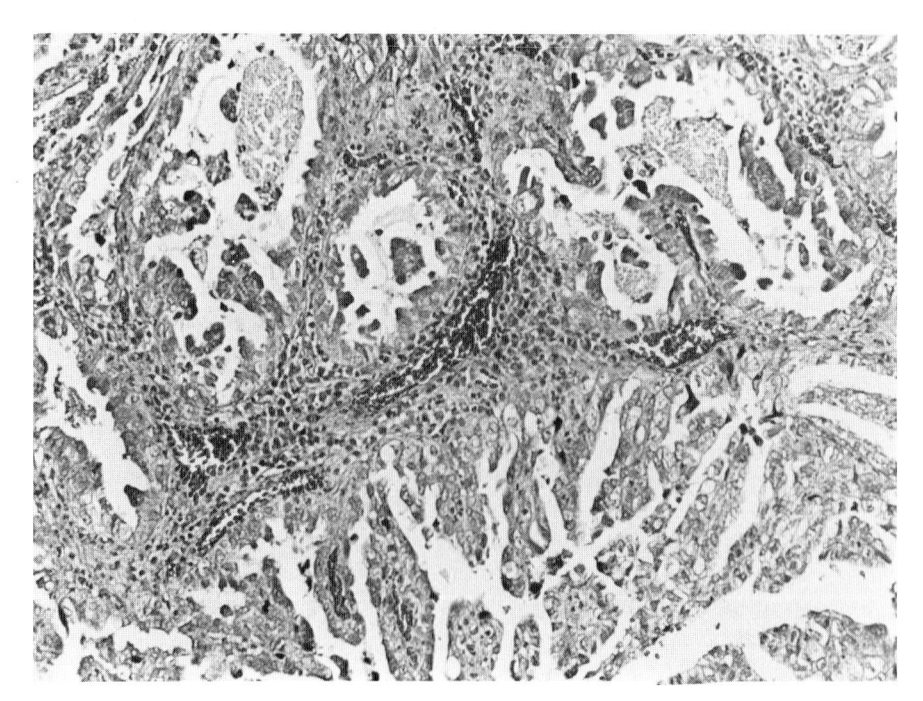

Figure 4. Clear cell carcinoma, with both glandular and papillary components, lined by cells with clear and eosinophilic cytoplasm, and presence of "hob-nail" cells protruding into lumen. H&E. x160.

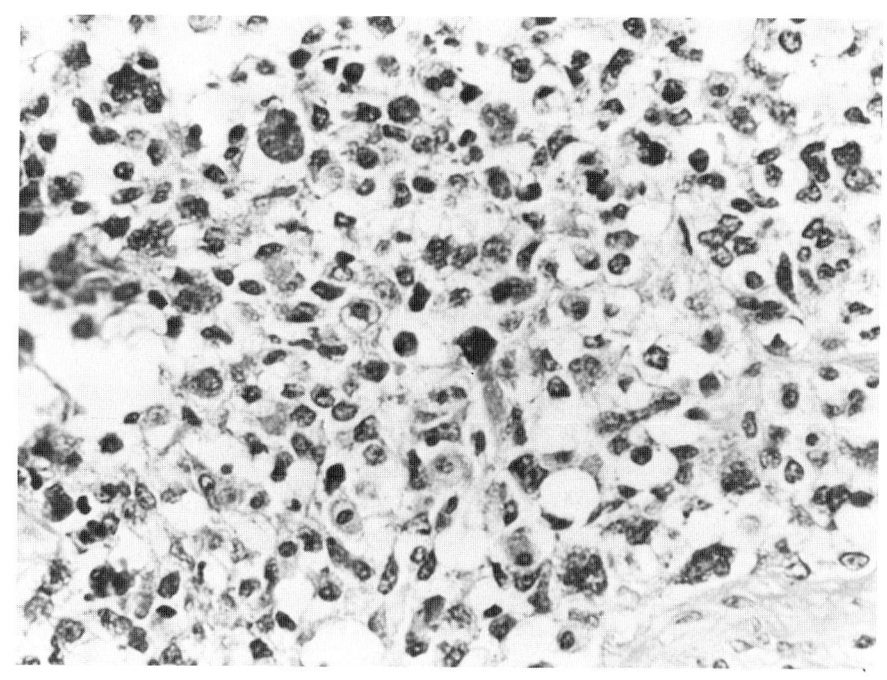

Figure 5. Rhabdomyosarcoma (Sarcoma botryoides). Extremely primitive malignant cells. Differentiation characterized by granular eosinophilic cytoplasm, at times forming "strap cells" (center), identifies the rhabdomyoblast. Cross-striations may be demonstrated with the aid of special stains. H&E. x400.

small vaginal lesions. When the lesion is larger, and the cervix is involved, larger doses of radiation will be required to effect cure.

Results

In January 1979, Herbst[38] presented the experience to date with clear cell adenocarcinoma to the Society of Gynecologic Oncologists. Follow-up periods ranged to 15.3 years (mean 4 years) and yielded an actuarial 5-year survival rate of 78 percent. The survival figures in patients with Stage I adenocarcinomas of the vagina and cervix are 87 percent and 91 percent respectively. Local excision of Stage I lesions appears to carry an increased risk of recurrence. The overall rate of recurrence for all cases was 23 percent at 5 years. Recurrences were most frequent in the pelvis, with the most common site of distant metastasis being the lungs. Thus, an x-ray examination of the chest every 6 months to 1 year is an important part of the follow-up in patients treated for clear cell adenocarcinoma. Surgical treatment, less often radiotherapy, resulted in the survival of 12 to 58 patients with recurrent tumor for 3 or more years. Chemotherapy was used in 34 patients but only 4 showed evidence of objective response, and none showed total remission of the disease.

CANCER OF THE VAGINA IN CHILDREN

These tumors are fortunately very rare.

Rhabdomyosarcoma (Sarcoma Botryoides)

Ninety percent of the patients with this condition are under 5 years of age. Their main complaint is of vaginal bleeding with a grape-like mass sometimes protruding from the vagina. The tumor may spread by the bloodstream or the lymphatic system and spread is early. Microscopically, the cancer is identified by the presence of rhabdomyoblasts ("strap cells") (Fig. 5). These are readily recognized by their cross-striations. Because of the rarity of this tumor, the best method of treatment has not yet been decided. Radical surgery, in the form of radical hysterectomy with vaginectomy and exenteration, has been used with success. Cures have also been reported with radiotherapy. Combined therapy with radical surgery, radiotherapy, and chemotherapy has also been used,[54] and chemotherapy with methotrexate alone has been successful in some cases.[55] It is important to differentiate sarcoma botryoides from pseudosarcoma botryoides, which may appear in infants and in pregnant as well as nonpregnant women.[56] Although the latter tumor is grossly similar, on microscopic examination no sarcomatous elements are evident.

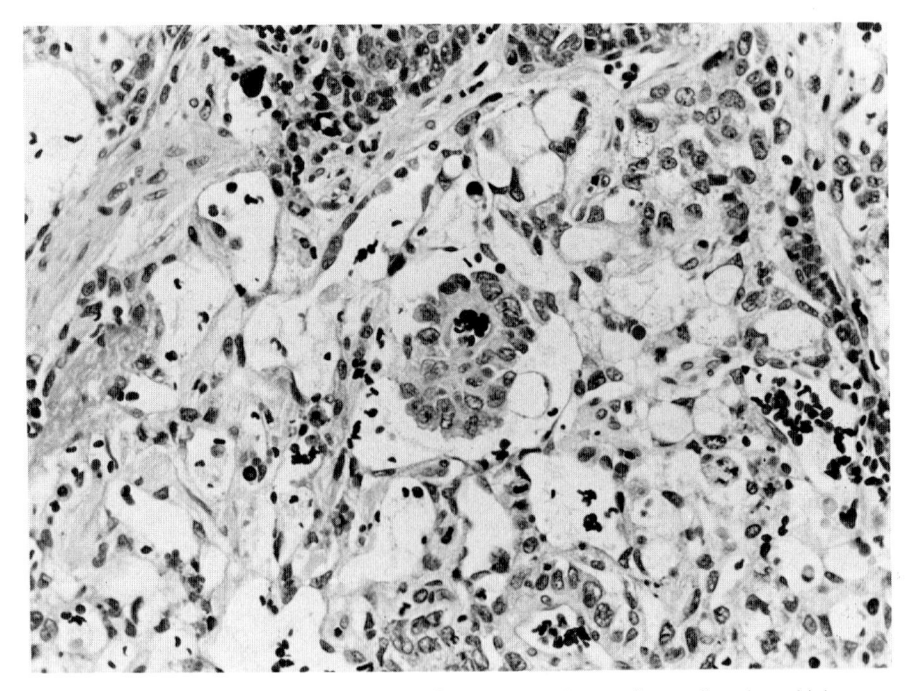

Figure 6. Endodermal sinus tumor. In a myxomatous, microcystic, sinusoidal background is a perivascular structure, "glomeruloid body," "Schiller-Duval" body, superficially resembling the endodermal sinus as seen in the rat placenta. H&E. x250.

Endodermal Sinus Tumor of the Vagina

This tumor may resemble sarcoma botryoides in gross appearance but microscopic examination reveals it to be an adenocarcinoma of a primitive type (Fig. 6). Most of the patients are under 2 years of age. The disease has been treated with a combination of surgery and radiotherapy but very few patients survive for 5 years.

MALIGNANT MELANOMA OF THE VAGINA

This lesion is extremely rare in the vagina and the possibility that the lesion is metastatic must be ruled out by demonstrating junctional changes in the overlying vaginal epithelium as described by Norris and Taylor.[57] These authors illustrate the difficulties in making a diagnosis because of the relative absence of melanin and the presence of a small cell, undifferentiated pattern (Fig. 7), and a sarcoma-like pattern. Nearly all pigmented lesions of the vulva are malignant, and nevi similar to those found in the skin have not been described.

Melanoma of the vagina is treated surgically. This is done in a similar manner to that for carcinoma of the vagina, but the outlook is very much worse because of the propensity of this lesion to metastasize by the blood-

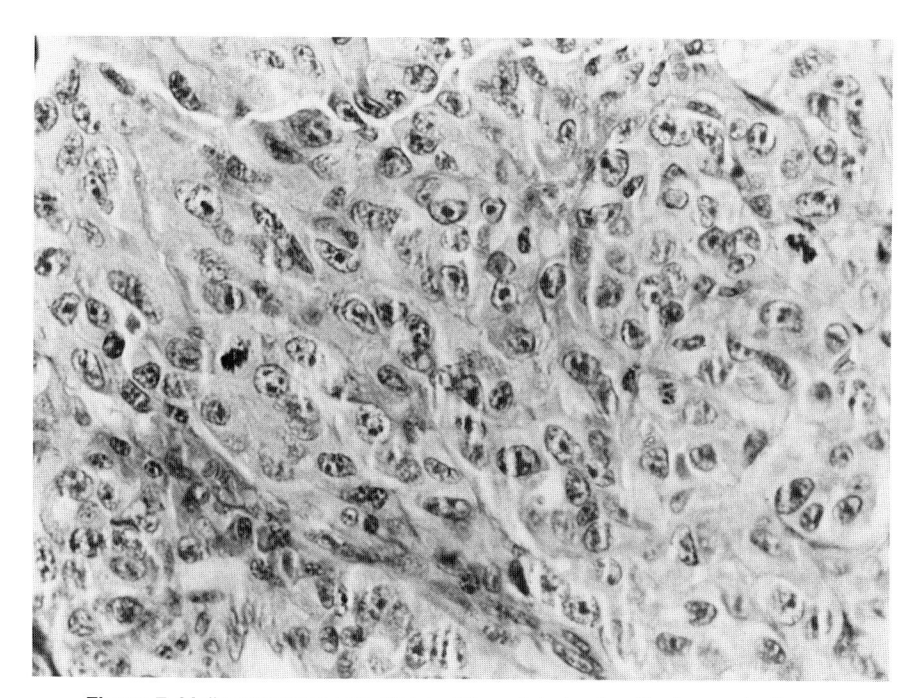

Figure 7. Malignant melanoma. Poorly differentiated cells with abnormal mitoses, abundant cytoplasm, minimal amount of dust-like particles of pigment, lack of intercellular bridges. H&E. x400.

stream, as well as by the lymphatic system. Metastases can be massive from a very small lesion. Hepatic and pulmonary metastases are common in association with this disease. Radiotherapy probably has no place in management.[58] Chemotherapy of combination type, including dimethyltriazenoimidazole carboxamide (DTIC), appears promising. Immunotherapy is experimental at this time.

METASTATIC CANCER OF THE VAGINA

Whereas primary cancer of the vagina is rare, metastatic cancer is common. Metastatic lesions are usually associated with primary cancer of the cervix, ovary, bladder, or rectum. Metastases from uterine adenocarcinoma, choriocarcinoma, and even upper abdominal malignancies sometimes recur at the vaginal vault. The treatment is essentially the treatment of the primary disease.

REFERENCES

1. Cruveilhier J: Bull Soc Anat Paris 1:199, 1826
2. Koss LG, Melamed MR, Daniel WW: In situ epidermoid carcinoma of the cervix and vagina following radiotherapy for cervical cancer. Cancer 14:353, 1961
3. May HC: Carcinoma in situ of the vagina subsequent to hysterectomy for carcinoma in situ of cervix. Am J Obstet Gynecol 76:807, 1958
4. Daw E: Primary carcinoma of the vagina. J Obstet Gynaecol Br Commonw 78:853, 1971
5. Perez CA, Arneson AN, Galakatos A, et al: Malignant tumors of the vagina. Cancer 31:36, 1973
6. Prempree T, Viravathana T, Slawson RG, et al: Radiation management of primary carcinoma of the vagina. Cancer 40:109, 1977
7. Way SJ: Primary carcinoma of the vagina. J Obstet Gynaecol Br Emp 55:739, 1948
8. Perez CA, Arneson AN, Dehner LP, et al: Radiation therapy in carcinoma of the vagina. Obstet Gynecol 44:862, 1974
9. Murad TM, Durant JR, Maddox WA, et al: The pathologic behavior of primary vaginal carcinoma and its relationship to cervical cancer. Cancer 35:787, 1975
10. Whelton J, Kottmeier HL: Primary carcinoma of the vagina. Acta Obstet Gynecol Scand 41:22, 1962
11. Annual report on the results of treatment in carcinoma of the uterus and vagina. International Federation of Gynaecology and Obstetrics. 1963, vol 13, pp 25–27
12. Underwood PB, Smith RT: Carcinoma of the vagina. JAMA 217:46, 1971
13. Graham GB, Meigs JV: Recurrence of tumor after total hysterectomy for carcinoma in situ. Am J Obstet Gynecol 64:1159, 1952
14. Ostergard DR, Morton DG: Multifocal carcinoma of the female genitals. Am J Obstet Gynecol 99:1006, 1967
15. Stuart GCE, Allen HH, Anderson RJ: Squamous cell carcinoma of the vagina following hysterectomy. Am J Obstet Gynecol 139:311, 1981
16. Oliver JA Jr: Severe dysplasia and carcinoma in situ of the vagina. Am J Obstet Gynecol 134:133, 1979

17. Daley JW, Ellis GF: Treatment of vaginal dysplasia and carcinoma in situ with topical 5-fluorouracil. Obstet Gynecol 55:350, 1980
18. Piver MS, Barlow JJ, Tsukada Y, et al: Postirradiation squamous cell carcinoma in situ of the vagina: Treatment by topical 20% 5-fluorouracil cream. Am J Obstet Gynecol 135:377, 1979
19. Sillman FH, Boyce JG, Macasaet MA, et al: 5-Fluouracil/chemosurgery for intraepithelial neoplasia of the lower genital tract. Obstet Gynecol 58:356, 1981
20. Caglar H, Hertzog RW, Hreshchyshyn MM: Topical 5-fluorouracil treatment of vaginal intraepithelial neoplasia. Obstet Gynecol 58:580, 1981
21. Pride GL, Chuprevich TW: Topical 5-fluorouracil treatment of transformation zone intraepithelial neoplasia of cervix and vagina. Obstet Gynecol 60:467, 1982
22. Dini MM, Jafari K: Ileovaginal fistula following cryosurgery for vaginal dysplasia. Am J Obstet Gynecol 136:692, 1980
23. Jobson VW, Homesley HD: Treatment of vaginal intraepithelial neoplasia with a carbon dioxide laser. Obstet Gynecol 62:90, 1983
24. Capen CV, Masterson BJ, Magrina JF, et al: Laser therapy of vaginal intraepithelial neoplasia. Am J Obstet Gynecol 142:973, 1982
25. Stanhope CR, Phibbs GD, Stuart GCE, et al: Carbon dioxide laser surgery. Obstet Gynecol 61:624, 1983
26. Hernandez-Linares W, Puthawala A, Nolan JF, et al: Carcinoma in situ of the vagina: Past and present management. Obstet Gynecol 56:356, 1980
27. Rotmensch J, Rosenshein N, Dillon M, et al: Carcinoma arising in the neovagina: Case report and review of the literature. Obstet Gynecol 61:534, 1983
28. Marcus SL: Primary carcinoma of the vagina. Obstet Gynecol 15:673, 1960
29. Perticucci S: Diagnostic, prognostic and therapeutic considerations in invasive carcinoma of the vagina. Obstet Gynecol 40:843, 1972
30. Rutledge FN: Cancer of the vagina. Am J Obstet Gynecol 97:635, 1967
31. Herbst AL, Green TH, Ulfelder H: Primary carcinoma of the vagina. Am J Obstet Gynecol 106:201, 1970
32. Pride GL, Buchler DA: Carcinoma of vagina 10 years following prior pelvic irradiation. Am J Obstet Gynecol 127:513, 1977
33. Pride GL, Schultz AE, Chuprevich TW, et al: Primary invasive squamous carcinoma of the vagina. Obstet Gynecol 53:218, 1979
34. Plentl AA, Friedman EA: Lymphatic System of the Female Genital Tract, chap 5. Philadelphia: Saunders, 1971
35. Brown GR, Fletcher GH, Rutledge FN: Irradiation of in situ and invasive squamous cell carcinomas of the vagina. Cancer 28:1278, 1971
36. Broders AC: Microscopic grading of cancer. Surg Clin North Am 21:947, 1941
37. Livingstone RG: Primary Carcinoma of the Vagina. Springfield, Ill: Charles C. Thomas, 1950
38. Herbst AL: Presentation to Society of Gynecologic Oncologists, Marco Island, Fla, January, 1979
39. Herbst AL, Ulfelder H, Poskanzer DC: Adenocarcinoma of the vagina: Association of material stilbestrol therapy with tumor appearance in young women. N Engl J Med 284:878, 1971
40. Herbst AL, Robboy SJ, Scully RE, et al: Clear-cell adenocarcinoma of the vagina and cervix in girls: An analysis of 170 registry cases. Am J Obstet Gynecol 119:713, 1974
41. Herbst AL, Poskanzer DC, Robboy SJ, et al: Prenatal exposure to stilbestrol: A

prospective comparison of exposed female offspring with unexposed controls. N Engl J Med 292:334, 1975
42. Shingleton HM, Younger JB, Beasley WE, et al: Adenocarcinoma of the vagina in a patient with gonadal dysgenesis. Obstet Gynecol 53:92S, 1979
43. O'Brien PC, Noller KL, Robboy SJ, et al: Vaginal epithelial changes in young women enrolled in the national cooperative diethylstilbestrol adenosis (DESAD) project. Obstet Gynecol 53:300, 1979
44. Sherman AL, Goldrath M, Berlin A, et al: Cervical-vaginal adenosis after in utero exposure to synthetic estrogens. Obstet Gynecol 44:531, 1974
45. Stafl A, Mattingly RF, Foley DV, et al: Clinical diagnosis of vaginal adenosis. Obstet Gynecol 43:118, 1974
46. Robboy SJ, Kaufman RH, Prat J, et al: Pathologic findings in young women enrolled in the national cooperative diethylstilbestrol adenosis (DESAD) project. Obstet Gynecol 53:309, 1979
47. Anderson B, Watring WG, Edinger DD, et al: Development of DES-associated clear-cell carcinoma: The importance of regular screening. Obstet Gynecol 53:293, 1979
48. Herbst AL, Kurman RJ, Scully RE: Vaginal and cervical abnormalities following exposure to stilbestrol in utero. Obstet Gynecol 40:287, 1972
49. Scully RE, Robboy SJ, Herbst AL: Vaginal and cervical abnormalities including clear cell adenocarcinoma, related to premature exposure to stilbestrol. Ann Clin Lab Sci 4:222, 1974
50. Sonek M, Bibbo M, Wied GL: Colposcopic findings in offspring of DES-treated mothers as related to onset of therapy. J Reprod Med 16:65, 1976
51. Kaufman RH, Binder GL, Gray PM Jr, et al: Upper genital tract changes associated with exposure in utero to diethylstilbestrol. Am J Obstet Gynecol 128:51, 1977
52. Taft PD, Robboy SJ, Herbst AL, et al: Cytology of clear cell adenocarcinoma of genital tract in young females: Review of 95 cases from the registry. Acta Cytol 18:279, 1974
53. Scully RE, Robboy SJ, Welch WR: Pathology and pathogenesis of diethylstilbestrol-related disorders of the female genital tract. In Herbst AL (ed): Intrauterine Exposure to Diethylstilbestrol in the Human. Chicago: Am Coll Obstet Gynecol, 1978, p 8
54. Piver MS, Barlow JJ, Wang JJ, et al: Combined radical surgery, radiation therapy and chemotherapy in infants with vulvovaginal embryonal rhabdomyosarcoma. Obstet Gynecol 42:522, 1973
55. Dewhurst CJ: Personal communication
56. Norris HJ, Taylor HB: Polyps of the vagina. A benign lesion resembling sarcoma botryoides. Cancer 19:227, 1966
57. Norris HJ, Taylor HB: Melanomas of the vagina. Am J Clin Pathol 46:426, 1966
58. Chung AF, Casey MJ, Flannery JT, et al: Malignant melanoma of the vagina. Report of 19 cases. Obstet Gynecol 55: 720, 1980

CHAPTER 3
Cancer of the Cervix

One hundred years ago cervical cancer was rapidly fatal, regardless of treatment. In 1883, Jackson[1] described the contemporary surgical approaches as "little more than antemortem examinations." Operative mortality was 70 percent and most patients who survived surgery died, "as though no operation had been performed." The following year, Munde[2] sounded a prophetic note, expressing the belief that "the inculcation of a wholesome fear" of cervical cancer might lead to earlier, more effective treatment. His hope, modest by modern standards, to allow "one quarter of the cases . . . to be healthy after two years," underscores the dismal survival statistics of his time. But despite advances in surgical technique and the development of radiotherapy, the plight of the patient with cervical cancer had improved little when, in 1926, Ewing[3] commented:

> Since early cervical cancer gives no specific symptoms . . . . examinations must be made at least every six months in suspicious cases, and once a year in others. The practical difficulties of instituting such measures for the general population are very great.

Even as Ewing spoke, the basic techniques of modern screening programs for cervical cancer were being developed. When asked to write a paper on cervical cancer in 1924, the German gynecologist Hans Hinselmann conceived the idea of examining the intact cervix under binocular magnification, and colposcopy was born.[4] At about the same time Schiller,[5,6] in Vienna, began using Lugol's iodine to stain the cervix and delineate abnormal areas for biopsy. In 1928, Babes[7] in Vienna, and Papanicolaou[8] in the United States, independently described methods for detecting cervical malignancy by exfoliative cytology. Although the name "Papanicolaou" is now synonymous with cervical cytology, it was Babes who arranged the first clinical trial of the technique, which was conducted by Viana[9] in Italy in 1928. It was not until 1941 that Papanicolaou and Traut[10] published their first paper on the clinical application of the technique. But despite the endorsement of such authorities as Meigs and associates[11] it was not until the late 1940s that large-scale screening programs were developed, and then only in the face of strong opposition from many leading pathologists.[12]

Emphasis on the early detection of cervical cancer was accompanied by an increasing interest in its origins. In 1886, Williams[13] described as "the earliest condition of cervical cancer" what we now term carcinoma in situ. Schauenstein,[14] in 1908, expressed the view that invasive cervical cancer was preceded by an intraepithelial phase of growth, and Rubin[15] published in support of this concept in 1910. Despite the interdependence of clinical and pathologic research, "there was no ready rapport between cytologist, histologist, and clinician" and "an increasing and often parochial subdivision of terminology" developed.[16] In the 1960s, Richart[17] integrated the different approaches into a simple terminology with both clinical and pathologic relevance. On the basis of a variety of complementary observations, he demonstrated that the precursors of cervical cancer formed a continuum, which he termed "cervical intraepithelial neoplasia" (CIN).[18]

The major treatment modalities used for invasive cervical cancer, radiotherapy, and radical surgery were largely developed independently and often in an atmosphere of intense competition. The first radical hysterectomies for cervical cancer were reported by Clark[19] in 1895, while he was a resident at Johns Hopkins Hospital. Wertheim,[20] by whose name the operation is still known, performed his first operation in 1898, and by 1905 was able to report 270 cases. The operative mortality rate was 30 percent in the first 100 cases, and in order to reduce this, Schauta[21] devised a radical vaginal hysterectomy which is still widely used today. X-rays were discovered in 1895 and radium in 1898. In the United States, radium was first used to treat cervical cancer in 1903 and the first long-term cure following its use was reported by Abbe in 1913.[22] By the 1920s, radiotherapy had largely replaced surgery in the treatment of cervical cancer in the United States because of the high mortality rates associated with surgery.

In 1944, Meigs[23] commented that it was apparent that "radiation is not the ideal method of treatment" because of a high incidence of severe morbidity and low cure rates. He conceded that the operative mortality rates reported by the proponents of surgery were unacceptable, but 1 year later he was able to report a series of 65 radical hysterectomies with no operative deaths, and he stated that "surgical removal of the early cervical cancer is as safe as radiation treatment."[24] Refinements of the techniques of both radiation and surgery, and a greater understanding of the benefits and limitations of each in specific clinical situations allow the modern oncologist to tailor a treatment plan to suit the specific needs of a particular patient.

These developments, together with a general improvement in socioeconomic conditions, appear to have resulted in a steady decline in both the incidence and mortality of invasive cervical cancer in the United States[25] and other developed countries.[26] The fact that the decrease in incidence of invasive disease was matched by an increasing incidence of preinvasive lesions (Fig. 1) gave support to the role of screening programs.[27]

There are, however, a number of areas for concern. The first is the markedly higher incidence rates observed among women in the lower socioeconomic groups and among black and hispanic Americans.[28] Moreover, although survival rates for blacks are improving, they trail well behind those for whites.[29] A further concern is that although screening programs appeared to be most effective in young women,[30] there is evidence of an increasing incidence and mortality for cervical cancer in women under 35 in Britain,[31] Australia,[32,33] New Zealand,[34] and the United States.[35] It is clear that there is a long way to go before this disease is eliminated.

CERVICAL INTRAEPITHELIAL NEOPLASIA

Richart[18] introduced the concept of cervical intraepithelial neoplasia (CIN) "as a generic term to designate the spectrum of intraepithelial disease that antedates invasive cancer." He believed that a rift had developed between "pathologists' diseases" and "patients' diseases" with the "subtle nuances" of the

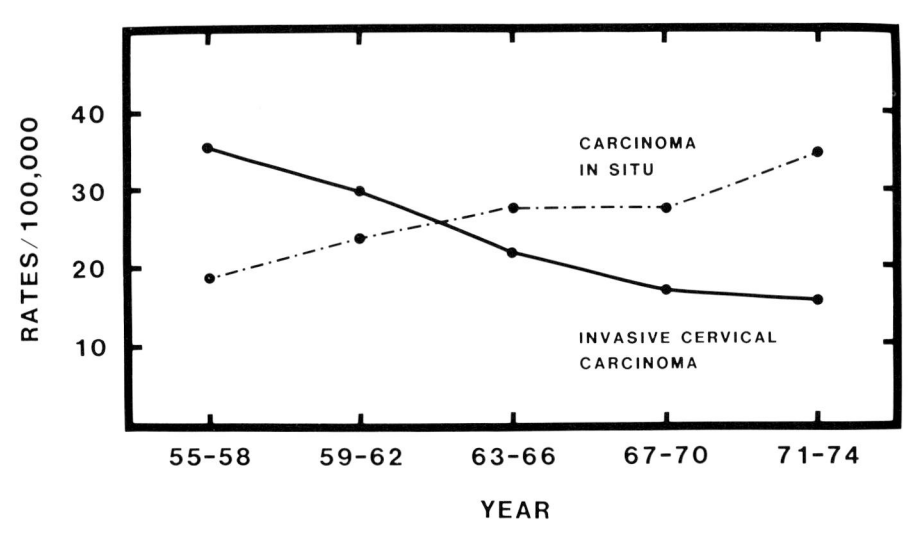

Figure 1. The changing proportions of intraepithelial and invasive cervical malignancy following the introduction of effective screening programs. (*From Kim K, et al: Cancer 42:2439, 1978, with permission.*)[27]

former interfering with the clinical management of the latter. The continuum of CIN replaced the two-tiered system of benign or premalignant dysplasias and preinvasive carcinoma in situ. As Stout[36] pointed out, the histologic differentiation between severe dysplasia and carcinoma in situ could often depend on the presence or absence of a single layer of partly differentiated cells on the surface of an otherwise totally anaplastic epithelium. To those who consider that the concept of CIN lacks the precision of the former classifications, Richart[37] replies that the clinical problem is not to define specific therapies for particular grades of the disease, but to exclude the presence of microinvasive or invasive cancer. Nevertheless, CIN is generally divided into CIN 1, corresponding to mild dysplasia, CIN 2 corresponding to moderate dysplasia, and CIN 3 which encompasses severe dysplasia and carcinoma in situ (Fig. 2).

The laboratory data supporting the concept of a continuum of CIN come from tissue culture studies, autoradiology, electron microscopy, chromosome

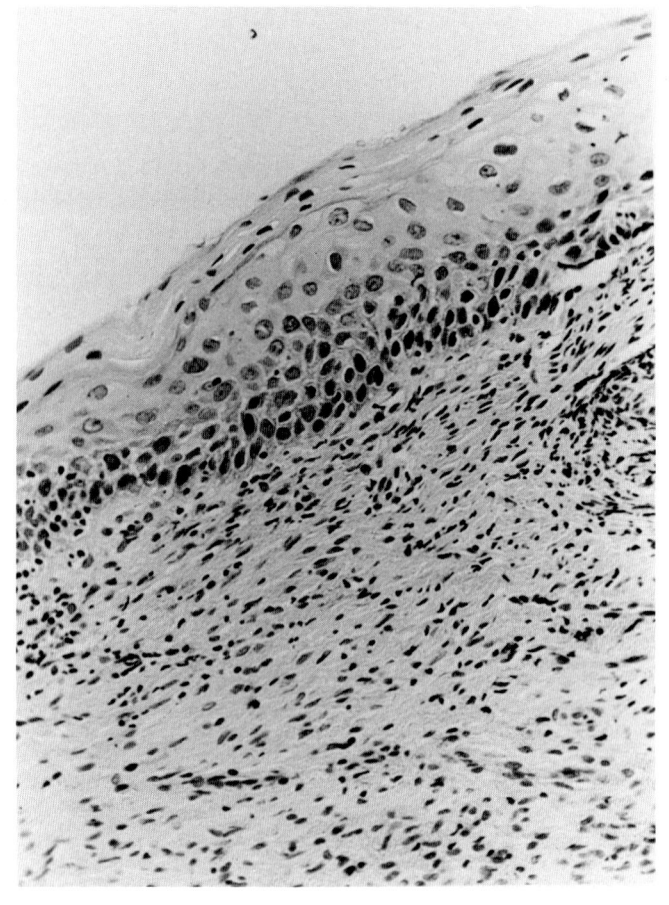

Figure 2A. CIN 1 (Mild dysplasia)—Cytologic changes characteristic of malignancy are present in the lower one-half of the epithelial thickness.

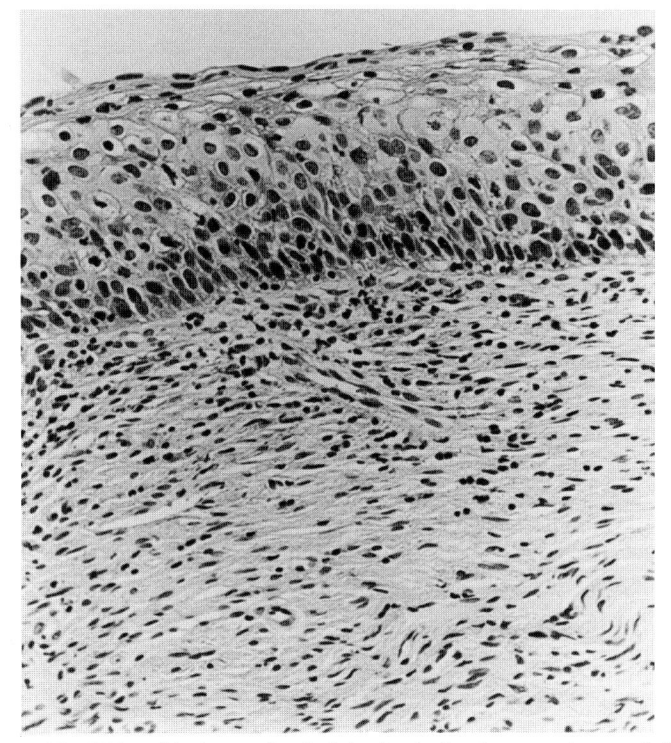

Figure 2B. CIN 2 (Moderate dysplasia)—Cytologic changes characteristic of malignancy extend to between one-half and three-quarters of the thickness of the epithelium.

analyses, and DNA microspectrophotometry.[18,38] From a clinical point of view, the question is "how often does CIN develop into invasive cancer, and over what period?" This question cannot be answered with precision because the definitive diagnostic method, biopsy, may be therapeutic in its own right.[38,39]

Stern and Neely[40] reported that, compared to the general population, women with a previous cytologic diagnosis of dysplasia were 20 times as likely to develop carcinoma in situ, and 7 times more likely to develop invasive cervical cancer. Koss[38] found that almost 40 percent of biopsy-proved dysplasias regressed, a fact he attributed to the biopsy, but that over 40 percent progressed to carcinoma in situ and 4 percent to invasive cancer. Fox[41] studied women following a single dysplastic smear and reported a 30 percent regression rate, but 60 percent progressed to a more serious lesion. Barron and Richart[42,43] used more stringent admission criteria for their study of the natural history of dysplasia, requiring three consecutive abnormal smears. About 50 percent of the cases of dysplasia progressed to carcinoma in situ, about 22 percent progressed to a higher grade of dysplasia and about 28 percent remained unchanged. Regression was uncommon and occurred only in patients with very mild dysplasia. More recently, Nasiell and colleagues[44]

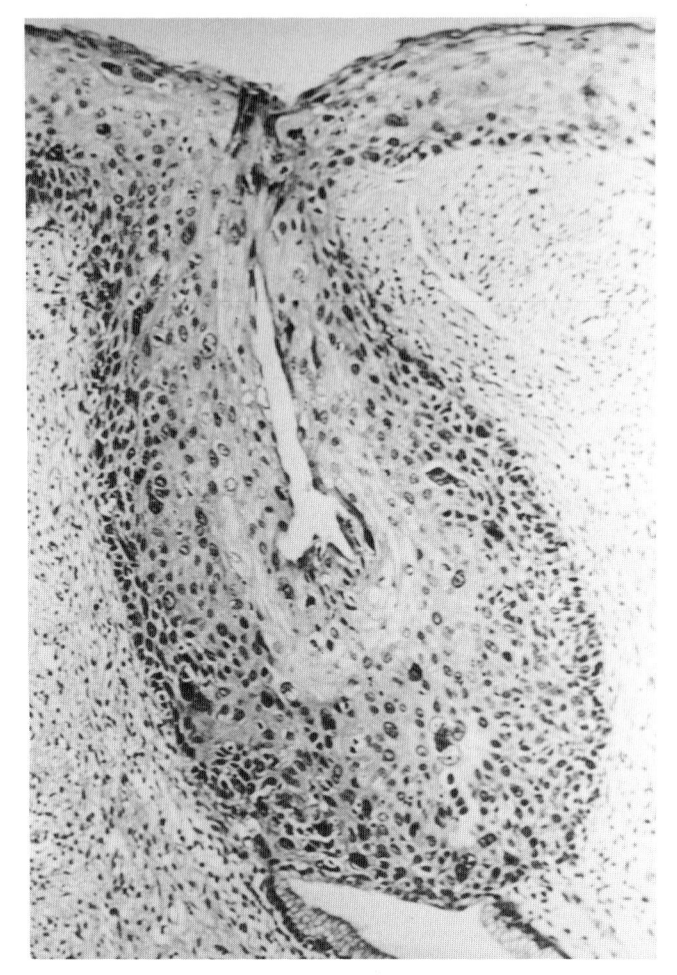

Figure 2C. CIN 3 (Severe dysplasia)—Cytologic changes characteristic of malignancy extend into the upper one-fourth of thickness of the epithelium. In this example the lesion extends into an endocervical gland.

reported the long-term follow-up of 894 women with moderate cervical dysplasia. In the entire sample, 54 percent regressed, 16 percent remained unchanged, and 30 percent progressed. Invasive cancer developed in three patients. Regression was significantly more common in patients who had punch biopsies. The authors were able to select a subgroup of patients who, like those studied by Richart and Barron,[43] had three consecutive abnormal smears and were not biopsied, and in this group only 28 percent regressed, while 50 percent progressed.

The proportion of patients with carcinoma in situ who subsequently develop invasive cancer is uncertain. Petersen[45] estimated that between 30 and 50 percent of patients with untreated carcinoma in situ would develop invasive

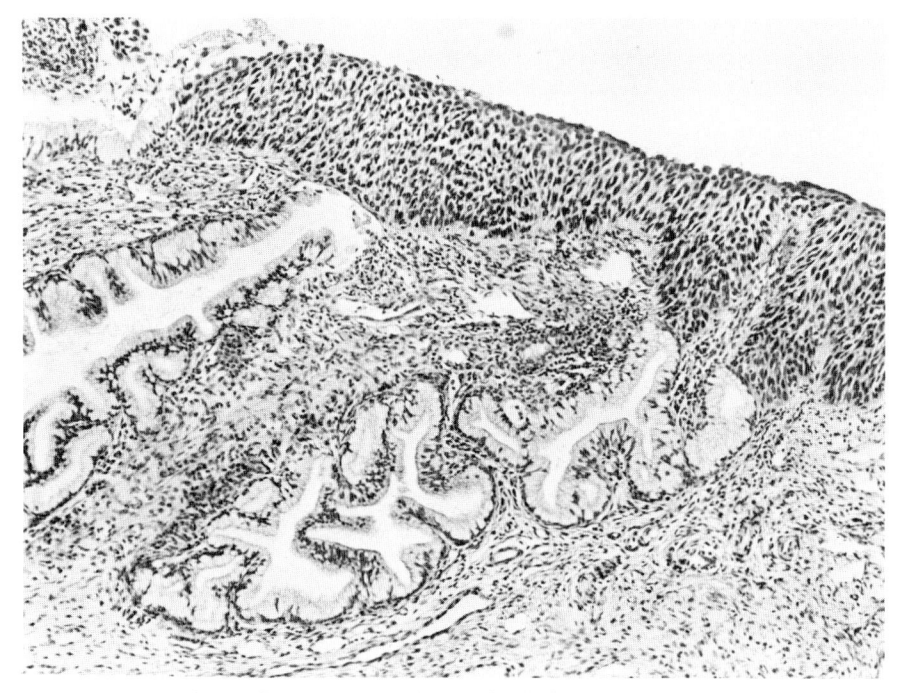

Figure 2D. CIN 3 (Carcinoma in situ)—The full thickness of the epithelium exhibits the cellular changes characteristic of malignancy. These are hyperchromatism, nuclei of irregular size and shape, loss of polarity, lack of maturation, and irregular chromatin distribution.

cancer within 10 years. The higher figure was derived by excluding any patients whose disease apparently regressed within the first year of study. Lange[46] studied 100 patients with untreated carcinoma in situ and found that 24 percent progressed to invasive cancer over a mean period of 7.5 years. When only women over age 35 were analyzed, 50 percent progressed to invasion. Gad[47] found that among 30 patients with severe dysplasia or carcinoma in situ diagnosed by biopsy, 9 developed invasive cancer, which was fatal in 2 cases. This figure does not take into account the fact that nine more of the patients had definitive treatment for CIN within 7 years of the original diagnosis.

It has been estimated that the median transit time to carcinoma in situ is 6 years for minimal dysplasia, 3 years for mild dysplasia, 2 years for moderate dysplasia, and 1 year for severe dysplasia.[43] The median time for carcinoma in situ to develop into invasive cancer has been estimated to be between 3 and 10 years.[48] Some authors have suggested that the transit time for carcinoma in situ is age dependent, falling from 17 years at age 25 to 4 years at age 70,[49] but the validity of this observation has been challenged.[48] In the study of Nasiell and associates,[44] the maximum rates of progression were seen in women between the age of 26 and 40 years. In a study of over 20,000 women attending a family planning clinic, Bamford and colleagues[50] found that the time interval between the first cytologic evidence of CIN and the development of CIN 3 was less than 2 years in over 80 percent of patients. This study utilized paired smears to minimize the false-negative smear rate.[51] Invasive cancer developed in three patients, two of whom had negative smears 2 to 4 years previously, and one of whom had only moderate to severe dysplasia 1 year earlier.

Epidemiologic observations of the natural history of CIN do not allow one to predict which patients with a given degree of CIN will develop invasive cancer in any particular time period. "Unfortunately, regardless of the name appended to the lesion the pathologist is unable to prognosticate the outcome of the disease."[38] Furthermore, "dysplasia cannot be dismissed as an innocuous lesion . . . as . . . invasive carcinoma can develop directly from a dysplasia of even mild or moderate grade, without transition to a carcinoma in situ."[39]

Epidemiology

CIN is predominantly a disease of younger women. In the United States, the mean age for carcinoma in situ is 35 years, which is about 15 years less than the mean age of diagnosis of invasive cancer.[52] The modal age is somewhat younger, in the range of 25 to 29 years,[53] and the modal age for dysplasia is somewhat lower.[54] In a screening program in St. Louis, we demonstrated that the modal age increased progressively for patients with dysplasia, carcinoma in situ, and invasive carcinoma (Table 1). CIN is being seen with increasing frequency among teenagers.[55] Although CIN is more common among blacks than whites, the difference disappears when correction is made for socioeconomic status.[56]

The incidence of cervical neoplasia is related to the early onset of coital activity,[57-59] and it is suggested that cytologic screening be initiated when a woman begins to have sexual intercourse.[60] Other risk factors include early age at first intercourse, early age at first pregnancy, multiparity, multiple sexual partners, low socioeconomic status, poor hygiene, and a history of sexually transmitted diseases such as syphilis, gonorrhea, and trichomoniasis.[58,59] After an exhaustive review of the literature, Rotkin[58] concluded that sexual intercourse before age 17 and multiple sexual partners "were the two most powerfully conditioning risks" for cervical neoplasia. Harris and col-

TABLE 1. DISTRIBUTION OF NEOPLASTIC LESIONS OF THE CERVIX BY AGE

Age	Dysplasia	Carcinoma in Situ	Carcinoma Invasive
15–29	517 (60%)	53 (31%)	2 (2%)
30–44	252 (30%)	86 (51%)	21 (24%)
45–59	57 (7%)	20 (12%)	33 (37%)
60 and over	28 (3%)	11 (6%)	33 (37%)
Total	854 (100%)	170 (100%)	89 (100%)

(From Cavanagh D, et al: unpublished data.)

leagues,[61] while confirming the importance of these two factors, found that CIN was related to the number of sexual partners, regardless of age at first intercourse, whereas when the number of sexual partners was controlled there was no significant relationship to age at first intercourse. Intercourse with uncircumcised men, once thought to be a risk factor,[62] is in fact not related.[63] Women whose sexual partners have in turn had multiple partners appear to be at greater risk.[64]

Etiology

It is apparent that cervical neoplasia is a venereal disease and that the causative agent is transmitted to a susceptible woman during intercourse. Carcinoma of the cervix is rare in virgins[65] and is relatively common in prostitutes.[66] There is an increasing body of evidence to suggest that herpes simplex virus type 2 (HSV-2) plays an important role in the pathogenesis of premalignant and malignant lesions of the cervix.[67] The epidemiology of cervical neoplasia and HSV-2 infections are similar,[68] and patients have a higher incidence of neutralizing antibodies to HSV-2 than do controls.[69] Exfoliated cells from some cervical cancers have been shown to contain herpes virus antigens,[70] and a recent study showed nonstructural herpesvirus proteins in cervical biopsies and explant cultures from patients with CIN or invasive cancer.[71] It was found that no viral capsid material was present, suggesting that part of the viral genome incorporated within the cell was producing its own proteins. The virus has oncogenic potential in animals,[72] and it is known that women with HSV-2 antibodies are seven times more likely to develop carcinoma in situ, and ten times more likely to develop invasive cervical cancer than women without antibodies.[73] In a prospective study, women with a history of genital herpes were found to have eight times the risk of carcinoma in situ, and twice the risk of invasive cervical cancer as matched controls.[74]

Another infectious agent that has been suggested as an etiologic agent for CIN is the human papillomavirus.[75] Between 20 and 25 percent of women with high-grade CIN have condylomata elsewhere on the cervix.[76] But the association is not evidence of causation. It has been suggested that up to 70 percent of lesions diagnosed as low-grade CIN are actually due to the effects of papillomavirus,[77] a fact which could explain the high regression rates for low-grade CIN reported in some studies. Of 620 cervical biopsy specimens from women with CIN or invasive cancer examined by Syrjanen,[78] over half had concomitant human papillomavirus infection. The association was significantly more frequent in younger women, and the so-called "flat" or "inverted" condylomata were associated with more severe lesions than the classic papillary wart. Interestingly, the incidence of demonstrable papillomavirus infection decreased as the severity of the CIN increased. A major difficulty in all studies is that even with the most modern techniques it may be difficult to differentiate accurately between papillomavirus infection and CIN.[79]

It has been postulated that CIN may develop, not from some infectious agent transferred during intercourse, but from some component of human sperm. Coppleson[80] originally proposed that the agent was sperm DNA incorporated into unstable cervical cells, but more recently he and his associates have suggested that it is one of the basic proteins of the sperm head, protamine.[81] Protamine interferes with the production and function of microfilaments on the surface of cells, and it is thought that the changes produced may inhibit the mechanisms which normally control cell replication, growth, and invasiveness. Men of the lower socioeconomic classes have higher concentrations of protamine in their sperm and their wives have a higher chance of developing cervical malignancy.[82]

It is entirely possible that a number of factors act either sequentially or in concert to lead to neoplastic changes in the cervix. Fish and colleagues[83] have shown that herpes virus can induce epithelial atypia in the cervices of rats, but they also found that, of a large range of irritants subsequently applied to the infected cervices, only human sperm led to increased atypicality.

The target tissue for whatever agent is responsible for the development of CIN appears to be the area around the junction of the original squamous epithelium of the cervix and the columnar epithelium of the endocervical canal. The eversion of the columnar epithelium onto the ectocervix, which occurs most frequently under hormonal stimulation, and is most common in adolescence, pregnancy, and the immediate postpartum period leads to a process of squamous metaplasia, in which columnar cells are transformed into squamous epithelium. The area of this change, termed the transformation zone, is believed to be particularly susceptible to carcinogens.

Diagnosis

Cytologic Screening. The best screening method for CIN is the Papanicolaou smear, because it is both accurate and simple. Although it is "widely assumed by lay groups and many physicians that cytology is 100 percent accurate,"[38] there is actually a false-negative rate on initial smearing of between 2 and 20 percent.[84] The technique of taking a smear is of great importance. First, the cervix must be visualized. This is essential because occasionally obvious carcinomas may give "negative" smears because blood, necrotic material, and leukocytes may obscure the often poorly preserved malignant cells.[85] Cervical cytology is primarily useful in asymptomatic patients and suspicious cervical lesions should be biopsied when first seen, rather than after the result of the Papanicolaou smear is reported. The optimal sampling technique combines an ectocervical scrape with a sample from the endocervical canal taken either by aspiration or with a moist cotton-tipped applicator. The vaginal pool technique carries an unacceptably high false-negative rate. The experienced cytologist will note on the report if endocervical cells are not present because this represents inadequate sampling. Combining endocervical sampling with the ectocervical scrape halves the false-negative rate,[86] and it can be further reduced by taking paired smears[51] or repeating the smear after a short period of time.[87] The specimen must be placed on the glass slide and fixed rapidly to avoid drying artefacts. When a cotton swab applicator is used it is possible to obtain 16 percent more cells on the glass slide when heavy pressure is exerted during smearing than when light pressure is used.[88]

Cost-benefit analyses notwithstanding, we believe that all women, who have at any time been sexually active, should have cytologic screening performed annually. A large retrospective study of women who developed invasive cervical carcinoma showed that 20 percent had at least two normal cytologic smears in the 3 years prior to the diagnosis of cancer.[89] The most common reason for these false-negative smears was sample error, and it is apparent that the longer the interval between smears the later the error will be detected. Furthermore, the patient who visits annually for cytology can be screened for breast cancer by palpation, for ovarian malignancy and other pelvic abnormalities by bimanual and rectovaginal examination, for vulvar neoplasia by careful inspection, and for anorectal carcinoma by rectal examination.

Colposcopy. In the United States, colposcopy is generally used as a technique to investigate patients with abnormal cervical cytology rather than as a primary screening tool. In experienced hands the diagnostic accuracy of this combination exceeds 95 percent.[90] The great advantage of colposcopy is that the source of abnormal cells found on cytologic examination can frequently be identified, the nature of the lesion assessed, and biopsies obtained, without resort to cone biopsy or other more radical measures. In performing colposcopic biopsies, care must be taken to ascertain that the area seen through the colposcope is actually biopsied. It is wise to take multiple biopsies to include both the area thought to be most abnormal and the surrounding transformation zone.

The major specific indication for colposcopy is a single abnormal Papanicolaou smear showing any degree of CIN, suspicious for malignancy, or reported as class 3, 4, or 5. Other indications include persistent abnormal benign cytology, persistent class II smears, and women exposed to diethylstilbestrol (DES) in utero. Colposcopy should also be performed in women who, despite a grossly normal cervix, complain of bleeding after intercourse or douching or who have an abnormal vaginal discharge. Another indication is a grossly abnormal cervix in the absence of obvious carcinoma. Regardless of the skill of the colposcopist any abnormalities detected should be biopsied to confirm and document the diagnosis. Endocervical curettage (ECC) should be performed as part of the examination in all patients. The endocervical canal must be thoroughly curetted with firm strokes and care taken to harvest all the tissue obtained onto a small piece of filter paper, or paper towel, prior to placing the specimen into fixative. These precautions will markedly reduce the false-negative rate. While this is most important when the entire transformation zone is not visualized colposcopically or when there is no visible cervical lesion despite abnormal cytology, we agree with Drescher and colleagues[91] that "the contribution of endocervical curettage to the outpatient work-up of abnormal cervical cytology is substantial and it should be performed in all patients in whom cone biopsy is not planned."

Diagnostic Conization. The need for diagnostic cone biopsy has been reduced at least 80 percent by the use of colposcopically directed biopsies[92,93] but it remains an important tool in many situations. In a prospective study by Praphat and associates[94] of 100 patients with abnormal cervical cytology, there was minimal disagreement between the diagnoses reached by colposcopically directed biopsies and conization (Table 2). It should be noted that such a good correlation is only possible with skilled colposcopists, and is dependent on the use of multiple biopsies of colposcopically abnormal areas and the surrounding tissue. When good colposcopy is not available, cone biopsy and fractional curettage is the best approach to exclude the presence of invasive carcinoma in patients with abnormal cytology and a grossly normal cervix. Other indications include failure to visualize the entire transformation zone or the entire lesion on colposcopy, the presence of abnormal endocervical curettings (unless they show invasive carcinoma), or cytologic smears indicating a more severe lesion than that determined by colposcopic biopsy. Cone biopsy should not be used where a lesser procedure could be reasonably expected to provide a diagnosis of invasive cancer; its use in the presence of an obvious invasive lesion is condemned.

Treatment of CIN

Many therapeutic options are available for patients with CIN. The abnormal transformation zone may be ablated by cryosurgery, electrocautery, or by

TABLE 2. CORRELATION OF HISTOPATHOLOGIC DIAGNOSIS ON COLPOSCOPICALLY DIRECTED PUNCH BIOPSY AND SUBSEQUENT COLD KNIFE CONIZATION

Diagnosis on Colposcopically Directed Biopsy	No. of Patients	Diagnosis on Subsequent Conization	No. of Patients
Chronic cervicitis	25	Chronic cervicitis	21
		Mild dysplasia	2
		Moderate dysplasia	2
Mild dysplasia	28	Mild dysplasia	21
		Moderate dysplasia	5
		Chronic cervicitis	2
Moderate dysplasia	26	Moderate dysplasia	17
		Mild dysplasia	4
		Severe dysplasia	2
		Chronic cervicitis	3
Severe dysplasia	12	Severe dysplasia	9
		Moderate dysplasia	2
		Chronic cervicitis	1
Carcinoma in situ	7	Carcinoma in situ	7
Invasive carcinoma	2	Invasive carcinoma, Cone biopsy not needed	2
Total	100		100

(From Praphat H, et al: Surg Gynecol Obstet 142:333, 1976, with permission.)[94]

laser vaporization, or it may be excised by conization or hysterectomy. A logical plan for investigation and management is shown in Figure 3.

Hysterectomy. Traditionally hysterectomy has been considered the definitive treatment for carcinoma in situ, and more recently for CIN 3, especially in the United States.[95-98] The main reason for this approach was fear of overlooking, and hence undertreating, invasive disease. The low rates of subsequent vaginal recurrence made the procedure especially appropriate for women with completed families and those considered unlikely to attend for regular follow-up.

Hysterectomy does not confer immunity from either recurrent CIN or even invasive carcinoma. In five studies,[98-102] involving over 4000 patients, carcinoma in situ recurred in the vaginal vault in 1 percent and invasive cancer in 0.4 percent (Table 3). Kolstad and Klem[101] emphasize that the length and completeness of follow-up rather than the mode of treatment determine the incidence of vaginal recurrences detected. They suggest a minimum follow-up of 10 years.

Vaginal hysterectomy has often been advocated, using either Schiller's test or colposcopy to enable an adequate vaginal cuff to be developed to clear all abnormal areas. Such an approach is logical, although Creasman and Rutledge[95] found no correlation between the size of the cuff and recurrence of the disease.

Despite a growing body of opinion favoring more conservative therapy for patients with CIN 3, we believe that hysterectomy is the treatment of choice for older or postmenopausal women, and for selected patients who have completed their families and desire sterilization, especially in the presence of other gynecologic conditions that could be treated by hysterec-

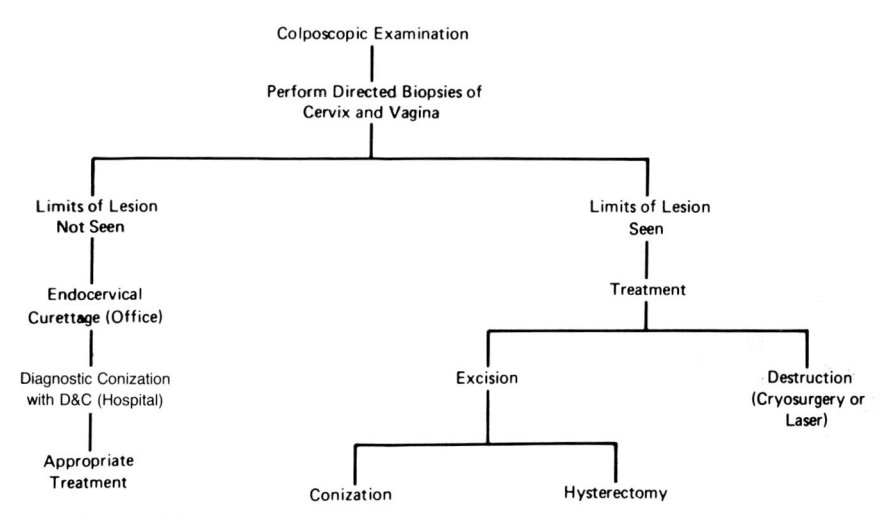

Figure 3. Diagram outlining a plan of management of a patient with a suspicious Papanicoloau smear. If a reliable cytopathologist reads a smear as abnormal, *do not* repeat the smear, but investigate the patient.

TABLE 3. INCIDENCE OF CARCINOMA IN SITU AND INVASIVE CARCINOMA OF THE VAGINAL CUFF AFTER HYSTERECTOMY FOR CARCINOMA IN SITU OF THE CERVIX

Authors	Patients	Recurrent CIS	Invasive Cancer
Boyes et al. (1970)[99]	2849	19	4
Creasman and Rutledge (1972)[95]	608	10	4
Brudenell et al. (1973)[100]	352	5	2
Kolstad and Klem (1976)[101]	238	3	5
Burghardt and Holzer (1980)[102]	166	4	2
Total	4213	41 (1%)	17 (0.45%)

tomy. In the younger woman the vaginal approach with ovarian conservation is appropriate. For the older woman total abdominal hysterectomy and bilateral salpingo-oophorectomy should be used. Patients must be warned that, despite the hysterectomy, regular follow-up including cytology is essential.

Therapeutic Conization. Cone biopsy can be both diagnostic and therapeutic for patients with CIN. As Table 4 shows, the overall results of conization in the treatment of carcinoma in situ compare favorably with those of hysterectomy.[99,101-104] When therapeutic conization has been performed, it is common to examine the margins of resection to ascertain whether or not they are clear of neoplasia. It is clear from a number of reports [102,103,105] that patients in whom the margins of resection are histologically involved have a significantly higher chance of persistent or recurrent disease, and of developing invasive cancer. Nevertheless, the presence of tumor-free margins on the excised cone is not a reliable indicator of the complete removal of the lesion (Table 5).[106-108]

Conization is not an innocuous procedure. The cold knife cone requires general or regional anesthesia and significant postoperative hemorrhage occurs in about 10 percent of cases.[103-105] In the long term, cervical stenosis may be seen in up to 7 percent of cases.[109] It is not known what proportion of women are involuntarily infertile after cone biopsy, but there is a high inci-

TABLE 4. INCIDENCE OF RECURRENT CARCINOMA IN SITU AND OF INVASIVE CARCINOMA OF THE CERVIX AFTER TREATMENT OF CARCINOMA IN SITU BY CONE BIOPSY

Authors	Patients	Recurrent CIS	Invasive Carcinoma
Boyes et al. (1979)[99]	808	28	3
Kolstad and Klem (1976)[101]	795	19	7
Bjerre et al. (1976)[103]	1671[a]	140	8
Burghardt and Holzer (1980)[102]	1158	34	7
Jones and Buller (1980)[104]	176[a]	3[a]	2
Total	4608	224 (5%)	27 (0.6%)

[a]CIN 3 (severe dysplasia + carcinoma in situ).

TABLE 5. ACCURACY OF PREDICTION OF RESIDUAL DISEASE IN THE HYSTERECTOMY SPECIMEN BASED ON HISTOLOGIC EXAMINATION OF THE CONE MARGINS

Residual CIN in Uterus	Patients
Predicted (cone margins involved)	25
Unpredicted (cone margins clear)	10
None present	65
Total	100

(From Schulman H, Cavanagh D: Cancer 14:795, 1961, with permission.)[106]

dence of unplanned and unwanted pregnancies after the procedure,[110] which may indicate that the incidence of infertility is overestimated by patients or their doctors. Comparison of a group of previously coned women with an age-matched control group failed to demonstrate any difference in the cumulative pregnancy rate from the time of commencing unprotected intercourse.[110]

The incidence of subsequent cervical incompetence is also difficult to ascertain. Several recent studies[110–112] fail to demonstrate any significant increase in the incidence of midtrimester abortions after conization, and in one the outcome of pregnancy was not improved by prophylactic cervical cerclage.[112] However, a case control study showed that women who had previously undergone cone biopsy were five times as likely to have a premature delivery, and twice as likely to have an infant under 2.5 kg.[113] Larsson and colleagues[112] demonstrated a sevenfold increase in the risk of premature delivery in women aged 21 to 25 but in no other age group. Leiman and associates[114] correlated the risk of both cervical incompetence and stenosis to the size of the cone, incompetence being more common after the larger cones, and stenosis after small cones. Labor may be either longer[110,113] or shorter[112] in women who have undergone conization. The size and shape of the excised cone must be individualized for each patient and the size and distribution of her lesion,[115] and these variations will clearly affect the complication rate.

In 1979, Dorsey and Diggs[116] described the technique of "microsurgical conization" in which the cone is excised using the carbon dioxide laser under direct colposcopic control. They concluded that this technique, in addition to providing a satisfactory specimen for pathologic examination, allowed precise control of the cone margins, minimized intraoperative and postoperative bleeding, and was followed by rapid healing with the squamocolumnar junction being readily visible on the ectocervix. They were able to perform the procedure on an outpatient basis using paracervical block anesthesia. Larsson and colleagues[117] compared the complication rates of cold knife and laser excisional cones and found that the former procedure had an overall complication rate of almost 24 percent while for the latter procedure it was approximately 5 percent. Hemorrhage, infection, and cervical stenosis were all significantly less common in the laser group. Our own experience with laser conization suggests that for equal size cones it has only slightly less complications and is somewhat slower than the cold knife technique.

Cryosurgery. In 1967, Crisp and associates[118] reported on the use of cryocautery for the treatment of CIN. The procedure requires no anesthesia, can be readily performed in the office using relatively inexpensive and simple equipment and has fewer complications than conization. Thus, it was soon in widespread use. When Charles and Savage[119] reviewed the literature in 1980, the reported "cure" rates for CIN ranged from a low of 27 percent to a high of 96 percent, with most series reporting rates in the 85 to 90 percent range. Table 6 summarizes the success rates reported from a number of centers since that time.[120–131] There is considerable variation in the selection of patients, techniques of treatment, definitions of success and failure, length of observation, and the number of patients lost to follow-up which may account for some of the variations in success rates.

Considering that a failure rate of about 10 percent is to be expected in even the best of hands, it is obvious that for this form of therapy to be safe, good follow-up is mandatory. Unfortunately, in most series a significant proportion of the patients are lost to follow-up within the 2-year observation period recommended by Figge and Creasman.[132] It has been stated that "the high percentage of patients lost to follow-up still makes this form of treatment unsatisfactory."[133]

Before using cryosurgery or any ablative method of therapy, it is essential that the nature and extent of the lesion be accurately determined. This is best

TABLE 6. RESULTS OF CRYOTHERAPY IN THE TREATMENT OF CERVICAL INTRAEPITHELIAL NEOPLASIA (CIN)[a]

	Recurrence/Patients Treated		
Authors	CIN 1	CIN 2	CIN 3
Ostergard (1980)[120]	13/205	9/53	4/22
Richart et al. (1980)[121]	11/898	3/977	8/964
Benedet et al. (1981)[122]	1/42	5/109	19/365
Charles et al. (1981)[123]	10/55	9/53	4/22
Hatch et al. (1981)[124]			33/246
Javaheri et al. (1981)[125]	3/73	10/49	2/50
Monaghan et al. (1982)[126]			16/109
Peckham et al. (1982)[127]	3/75	5/63	14/109
Stuart et al. (1982)[128]	2/29	5/56	11/51
Coney et al. (1983)[129]	26/240		
Van Lent et al. (1983)[130]			7/102
Creasman et al. (1984)[131]	15/276	17/235	46/259
Total	84/1893 (4.4%)	63/1595 (3.9%)	64/2299 (7.1%)

[a]These results represent recurrence rates. If persistent disease after cryotherapy is included the figures are often considerably higher.

achieved by the use of colposcopy with directed biopsies and endocervical curettage. The primary aim is to avoid inadvertently treating invasive cancer and the secondary aim to ensure that the entire lesion is obliterated. It is essential that even skilled colposcopists take multiple biopsies of abnormal areas[134] and that endocervical curettage be performed.[128,133,134] Treatment failures following cryotherapy are more common in patients with positive endocervical curettings[128,132,133,135,136] and failure to perform endocervical curettage has been implicated as an important factor in the subsequent discovery of invasive cancer after cryosurgery.[134,136] We believe that inadequate colposcopy or positive endocervical currettings mandates a cone biopsy.

The success rate of cryosurgery in eliminating CIN is related to both the histologic grade of the lesion and its physical extent.[126,128,131,133] While it is clear that cryosurgery is capable of eradicating all grades of CIN, "an objective assessment of the recent literature on cryotherapy would suggest that its use on CIN 3 must be supervised carefully and that its universal employment for these lesions should be avoided."[137]

Another important consideration is the technique of freezing. Most authors favor the so-called "double freeze" technique,[132] although others have produced excellent results with a single freeze.[123,128]

Although cryosurgery can be safe and effective treatment for CIN, "its use should be confined to patients desirous of further childbearing who are managed by physicians with the expertise and experience for proper evaluation. Only patients considered reliable and therefore amenable to long-term follow-up should be managed by this method."[119]

Electrocautery. Almost 40 years ago, Younge and colleagues[138] reported the successful eradication of carcinoma in situ of the cervix by electrocautery. Richart and Sciarra[139] later reported an 89 percent "cure" rate for CIN after one treatment with outpatient electrocautery and 97 percent after a second treatment. The technique has fallen from favor because it is no more effective than cryotherapy and is esthetically less acceptable.

Hollyock and Chanen[140] described a more radical approach. Only patients with adequate colposcopy and biopsy-proved CIN were treated. Under general or regional anesthesia, colposcopy, directed biopsies, and fractional curettage were performed. The cervix was then coagulated, initially by multiple punctures of a needle electrode to a depth of 1.5 cm into the cervical stroma, and then with a ball electrode to destroy the entire transformation zone. Their initial report showed that of 438 patients treated, almost half for CIN 3, 94 percent were cured with a single treatment. Chanen and Rome[141] reported on the results of this treatment on over 1800 patients, 64 percent of whom had CIN 3. The "cure" rate was 97 percent. Only 2.5 percent of patients had complications: 1.4 percent had secondary hemorrhage, 0.5 percent developed cervical stenosis, and 0.6 percent developed acute pelvic infection. In long-term follow-up, the procedure was found to have minimal adverse effects on fertility, pregnancy, labor, or menstrual function.[142]

This procedure, although not suitable for office use, appears to be as effective as cone biopsy but to have a lower complication rate. It does, however, suffer the same disadvantage as all ablative procedures do when compared to cone biopsy, namely, the absence of a complete specimen for histologic examination. It deserves serious consideration as therapy for selected patients, provided it is used with the same care as its protagonists exercise.

Laser Vaporization. The carbon dioxide laser was developed in 1966, and in 1972 Jako[143] reported on the use of this device, coupled to an operating microscope, for surgery of the vocal cords. In 1973, Kaplan and associates[144] used the laser to treat cervical erosions, and in 1977 Stafl and colleagues[145] reported on its use for CIN. Analysis of the results of laser therapy in 12 series show them to be broadly comparable to those of cryosurgery (Table 7).[145-156] In a controlled comparison of patients treated with either laser or cryosurgery, Townsend and Richart[155] showed no significant difference in cure rates between the two modalities. Cryotherapy was less painful but produced more discharge, while the laser-treated cervices healed more rapidly. A similar study by Wright and colleagues[156] found the laser to be more effective than cryosurgery in eradicating CIN. It is also claimed that laser vaporization "leads to a remodelled cervix in which the endocervical canal is accessible and where any recurrence can easily be seen colposcopically."[157]

Clearly, laser vaporization is a reasonable outpatient therapy for CIN but, like all ablative methods, must be used with caution, in order to avoid the inadvertent treatment of invasive disease. We would emphasize that adequate biopsy material, from both the lesion and the endocervical canal, is a critical part of the procedure.

TABLE 7. RESULTS OF LASER VAPORIZATION OF THE CERVIX FOR THE TREATMENT OF CIN, AS REPORTED IN 12 SERIES

Authors	Recurrences/Patients Treated		
	CIN 1	CIN 2	CIN 3
Stafl et al. (1977)[145]	0/9	1/14	4/23
Carter et al. (1978)[146]	2/16	1/17	4/16
Baggish (1980)[147]	5/25	13/43	15/47
Bellina and Seto (1980)[148]	2/45	4/147	3/55
Burke et al. (1980)[149]	6/21	11/19	5/20
Bellina et al. (1981)[150]	1/92	8/99	9/65
Benedet et al. (1981)[151]	0/12	5/29	12/43
Wright and Davies (1981)[152]	0/41	1/51	3/39
Anderson (1982)[153]	3/26	15/78	86/337
Popkin (1983)[154]	3/26	7/82	3/30
Townsend and Richart (1983)[155]	1/10	3/37	7/53
Wright et al. (1983)[156]	2/92	7/37	11/200
Total	25/415 (6%)	76/653 (12%)	162/928 (17%)

Other Approaches. The epidemiology of CIN, and the fact that it often appears to undergo spontaneous regression, has encouraged the search for alternative, more conservative treatments, some of which merit brief discussion.

On the assumption that a sexually transmitted factor initiates or promotes neoplastic changes in the cervix, Richardson and Lyon[158] investigated the effect of condom use on the course of proved CIN. This simple strategem was followed by regression of the lesion in a significant number of cases. The study was not controlled and the authors do not claim that this is a therapeutic method in its own right. They see it as a potential part of an overall regimen of investigation, treatment, and follow-up for women with CIN.

In 1969, Kitay and Wentz[159] reported abnormal cervical cytology among pregnant women with folate deficiency. These changes preceded the development of overt hematologic changes and were rapidly reversed by the administration of folic acid. The long-term use of oral contraceptives may be associated with reduced folate levels.[160] Butterworth and colleagues[161] carried out a study of the effects of oral folic acid or placebo on the course of CIN in oral contraceptive users. They found that the folate-supplemented group showed an improvement in cytology during treatment, when compared with the placebo group, and that the differences at the termination of the study, as indicated by biopsies, were highly significant. They comment that "either a reversible, localized derangement in folate metabolism may sometimes be misdiagnosed as cervical dysplasia, or such a derangement is an integral part of the dysplastic process that may be arrested, or in some cases reversed, by oral folic acid supplementation."[161]

Vitamin A and the retinoids have long been known to be involved in the modulation of cell division and differentiation in many tissues, including epithelia.[162] Topical retinoids have been successfully used in the treatment of a number of epithelial tumors in humans.[162,163] Romney and colleagues[164] conducted a case control nutritional and biochemical study on women with CIN. They showed that women with cervical dysplasia gave dietary histories showing significantly lower intakes of vitamin A, its precursors, and its analogs, than did control patients. Moreover, the level of retinol-binding proteins in cervical biopsy specimens was inversely related to the degree of dysplasia present. Bernstein and Harris[165] showed no significant difference in dietary profiles between a group of women with CIN and controls, but the former group had significantly lower serum levels of vitamin A. In a trial of topically applied transretinoic acid, Surwit and colleagues[166] showed regression of CIN in 6 of 18 patients and complete disappearance of the lesion in 2 patients.

Another agent that has been used for the topical treatment of CIN is human leukocyte interferon. This agent has been reported to produce regression of malignant melanoma, bladder papillomas, and breast cancer,[167] head and neck tumors,[168] and invasive cervical cancer.[169] Moller and his colleagues[170] used a hydrophilic gel containing interferon on the cervices of six women with previously stable CIN, and after 12 weeks of treatment all showed regression of the lesions, which was complete in three cases. There were no appreciable side effects.

While these observations are of great interest, they do not supplant the more traditional methods of treatment. They do, however, hold out the hope that with continued research it may become possible to prevent the development or progression of cervical neoplasia by simple measures.

MICROINVASIVE CARCINOMA

Both the definition and the optimal treatment of microinvasive carcinoma of the cervix have long been areas of controversy and confusion. The aim is to identify a group of patients with "early" invasive cancer who may safely be treated with procedures carrying lower morbidity and mortality than radical surgery or radiotherapy. The radical treatment of cervical cancer aims to remove or sterilize the primary tumor, the parametrium, and the pelvic lymphatics in order to minimize the risk of recurrence or metastasis. The concept of microinvasion arose when it was recognized that in some "early" lesions involvement of the parametrium or lymphatics was rare.

Microinvasion is generally defined in terms of the depth to which malignant cells penetrate into the cervical stroma. The term "microcarcinoma" was first used in 1947 by Mestwerdt[171] for tumors invading no more than 5 mm, and this definition has been used by many authors subsequently. While some have argued that a maximum of 1 mm of stromal invasion is a more appropriate limit,[172,173] in 1974 the Society of Gynecologic Oncologists defined a microinvasive lesion as "one in which neoplastic epithelium invades the stroma to a depth of 3 mm or less beneath the basement membrane . . . and in which lymphatic or blood vascular involvement is not demonstrated." Those attempting to review the literature face a "confusing dilemma,"[174] partly because over 18 different terms have been used to describe these lesions.[175] Furthermore, in a review of 41 publications reporting over 2100 cases, Benson and Norris[176] found only 4 reports, encompassing a total of 98 cases, which were free from factors which would markedly alter the apparent frequency of nodal metastases. The incidence of positive nodes will be higher if preclinical, rather than microinvasive, lesions are studied, if the diagnosis is by biopsy or a small cone, or if only the more advanced cases are selected for lymphadenectomy. On the other hand, lymph node involvement will be apparently less common if cases of questionable invasion are included, or if those with lymph-vascular space permeation or confluent growth patterns are excluded. Even when stringent criteria are specified the diagnosis is not necessarily reliable. Of 265 patients entered into a Gynecologic Oncology Group study after being diagnosed as having microinvasive carcinoma by pathologists at their own institution, 132 were rejected by the reviewing board on the grounds that they did not constitute microinvasion. Specifically, 99 cases showed no invasion and a smaller number had invasion greater than 5 mm.[177]

Van Nagell and associates[178] combined the cases considered suitable for evaluation by Benson and Norris[176] with their own experience and that of other authors, and estimated that the incidence of lymph node metastasis with stromal invasion of 3 mm or less is of the order of 0.25 percent, while for invasion between 3.1 mm and 5 mm it is about 8 percent (Table 8).

In addition to defining a maximum depth of invasion of 3 mm, the Society of Gynecologic Oncologists excluded cases with lymph-vascular space permeation from the category of microinvasion. The prognostic significance of lymph-vascular space involvement in frankly invasive cervical carcinoma was demonstrated by Barber and associates[187] who reported that the 5-year survival rate for Stage I B disease was 90 percent when no lymph-vascular space involvement was seen and 59 percent when it was present. The significance of this finding in microinvasive lesions is less clear. Roche and Norris[180] made multiple step sections of cone biopsy specimens from 30 cases of microinvasive carcinoma where radical hysterectomy had subsequently been performed. Lymph-vascular permeation had been reported in nine cases following the initial examination of the cones, but step sectioning demonstrated it in a further eight cases, bringing the total incidence to 57 percent, but in no case were positive lymph nodes found. Lymph-vascular permeation was found to be related to both the depth of invasion and the number of sites of invasion. Leman and associates[181] demonstrated lymph-vascular permeation in 24 percent of their patients, but none had lymph node involvement. While these and other authors[189] would minimize the significance of lymph-vascular space permeation, many consider the finding highly significant. Averette[190] describes a patient with only 0.2 mm invasion, but obvious lymph-vascular permeation, who had massive lymph node metastases. Seski and colleagues[182] found no positive nodes among 37 women without lymph-vascular permeation, but 1 of 4 patients with this feature had positive nodes. In a study of

TABLE 8. INCIDENCE OF PELVIC LYMPH NODE INVOLVEMENT IN RELATIONSHIP TO DEPTH OF STROMAL INVASION[a]

	\multicolumn{4}{c}{Depth of Stromal Invasion}			
	3 mm or Less		3.1 mm to 5 mm	
Authors	Cases	Positive Nodes	Cases	Positive Nodes
Foushee et al. (1969)[179]	16	0	13	1
Roche and Norris (1975)[180]	9	0	21	0
Leman et al. (1976)[181]	32	0	3	0
Seski et al. (1977)[182]	37	0	—	—
Taki et al. (1979)[183]	55	0	—	—
Yajima and Noda (1979)[184]	90	0	—	—
Hasumi et al. (1980)[185]	106	1	29	4
Van Nagell et al. (1983)[178]	52	0	32	3
Total	397	1	98	8

[a]As reported in a series thought to be without biasing factors.

lesions invading to a maximum of 5 mm, Iverson and associates[191] found a 38 percent recurrence rate for women with lymph-vascular permeation, and only 1 percent when this was absent. Larsson and colleagues[192] performed a multivariant analysis to determine the prognostic factors in 343 cases of early cervical cancer and concluded that lymph-vascular permeation was an important risk factor. Their results may be somewhat biased because 23 percent had invasion greater than 3 mm.

The pattern of invasion is often cited as an important prognostic factor. Fidler and Boyes[193] distinguish between "intraepithelial carcinoma with discrete microinvasive foci" and "occult carcinoma where there are confluent, frankly invasive foci" which they considered much more ominous. More recently, Lohe[194] has distinguished "early stromal invasion" from "microcarcinoma:" the former consists of isolated foci of invasion originating from a field of carcinoma in situ, while the latter is a confluent mass of microinvasive carcinoma. In a clinical study, Lohe and colleagues[195] showed that the latter lesion carried a poorer prognosis than did the former. On the other hand, Roche and Norris[180] dismiss the confluent pattern as "ill defined and vague" and of doubtful significance, as do Seski and colleagues.[182] In the multivariant analysis of Larsson and colleagues,[192] confluent invasive patterns carried no increased risk of recurrence or death. Leman and associates[181] found no correlation between confluence, depth of invasion, lymph-vascular permeation, or nodal metastases, but Sedlis and colleagues[177] found confluence to be more common with increasing depth of invasion.

The average thickness of the normal cervical epithelium is 0.26 mm in women with ovulatory cycles, and 0.41 mm in carcinoma in situ.[186] Lymph-vascular spaces are demonstrable within 0.5 mm of the basement membrane. Penetration of the stroma to a depth of only 1 mm represents between 66 and 88 cell layers depending on whether the tumor is of the small or large cell variety. Studies have shown that the depth and lateral extent of tumors are related,[177] so tumor volume will increase markedly with increasing depth of invasion. Burghardt and Holzer[188] used extensive step sectioning of cone biopsy specimens to calculate the volume of microinvasive cancers, and concluded that tumors with a volume of less than 500 μL were "in general, incapable of metastatic spread," although they caution that in the presence of lymph-vascular permeation rather smaller volumes may, on rare occasions, be associated with recurrence and even death.

"The diagnosis of microinvasive carcinoma should not be undertaken lightly."[177] Studies of patients initially diagnosed as having carcinoma in situ show that between 3 and 8 percent will actually prove to have microinvasion.[196] Creasman and Parker[197] reported that microinvasive disease accounted for 4 percent of all invasive cervical cancers at their institution. Although the presence of microinvasion may be suggested by cytology,[198,199] and its recognition aided by colposcopy,[200] the diagnosis must be based on the study of an adequate cone biopsy or the study of the excised uterus if the diagnosis was initially missed. Directed biopsy, even in the most experienced hands, is not adequate to exclude invasive disease elsewhere in the cervix. Larsson and colleagues[192] showed that the depth of invasion and the incidence of lymph-vascular permeation were both significantly underestimated when assessed from wedge biopsies rather than from cone biopsies or excised uteri. Proper histologic evaluation of the cone is essential. Cursory examination may over- or underestimate the depth of invasion and may miss lymph-vascular permeation. Burghardt and Holzer[188] believe that 60 to 70 sections are required for an adequate evaluation. Each section must be examined using a microscope with an ocular micrometer to accurately assess the depth of invasion.[178] It is important to assess the margins of excision of the cone, for if they are positive there is a high chance that residual disease, possibly more severe than that in the cone, remains behind. Residual disease in the uterus is more common when the cone margins are involved and in tumors with large surface areas.[181] Seski and colleagues[182] demonstrated that cone biopsy had a diagnostic accuracy of 83 percent for microinvasive carcinoma, but that the most significant area was not detected in 5 percent of cases and the presence of microinvasion was missed in 13 percent of cases in which it was subsequently found in the excised uterus. They also claimed that cone biopsy failed to eliminate all intraepithelial and microinvasive disease in 78 percent of cases. Burghardt and Holzer[188] found involved cone margins in almost half their cases, and of patients having a hysterectomy following a cone with involved margins, 38 percent had residual neoplasia, one-quarter of which was microinvasive or invasive carcinoma.

The treatment of microinvasive carcinoma must be based on a careful evaluation of the patient and her cone biopsy specimen. Clinical examination of the cervix, including bimanual rectovaginal examination, will help detect the enlarged, friable, or nodular cervix, or the shortening of the cardinal or uterosacral ligaments that may indicate the presence of unsuspected invasive disease. The importance of this clinical assessment is often overlooked but it is of great value, especially in experienced hands. The pathologist and the clinician should review the cone biopsy together, in the light of the clinical findings, and if necessary have more blocks cut. We believe that the maximum permissable depth of invasion for the diagnosis of microinvasion is 3 mm. It is essential to differentiate true microinvasion from occult invasive carcinoma. Boronow[201] demonstrated very clearly that while nodal metastasis is not common with true microinvasion, it is a frequent occurrence with occult invasive cancer.

Some authors have suggested that cone biopsy may be adequate therapy for selected patients with small microinvasive lesions without confluence or lymph-vascular permeation.[189] They emphasize the need for extremely thorough follow-up in such cases. We are reluctant to accept such an approach except in cases where a single focus of doubtful microinvasion is present, without confluence or lymph-vascular permeation, in a young woman willing to be followed-up fastidiously for many years. If a patient's lesion consists of a single, isolated tongue with minimal invasion, without confluence or lymph-vascular permeation (Fig. 4A), extrafascial abdominal or vaginal hysterectomy is reasonable. This group of tumors has been termed "borderline microinvasive carcinoma" by Wilkinson and Komorowski.[202] We favor the abdominal approach because it allows a better assessment of the nodal status. On the other hand, if confluent tongues of invasion or lymph-vascular permeation are present on the cone (Fig. 4B), radical abdominal hysterectomy and pelvic lymphadenectomy should be performed. Patients who undergo simple hyster-

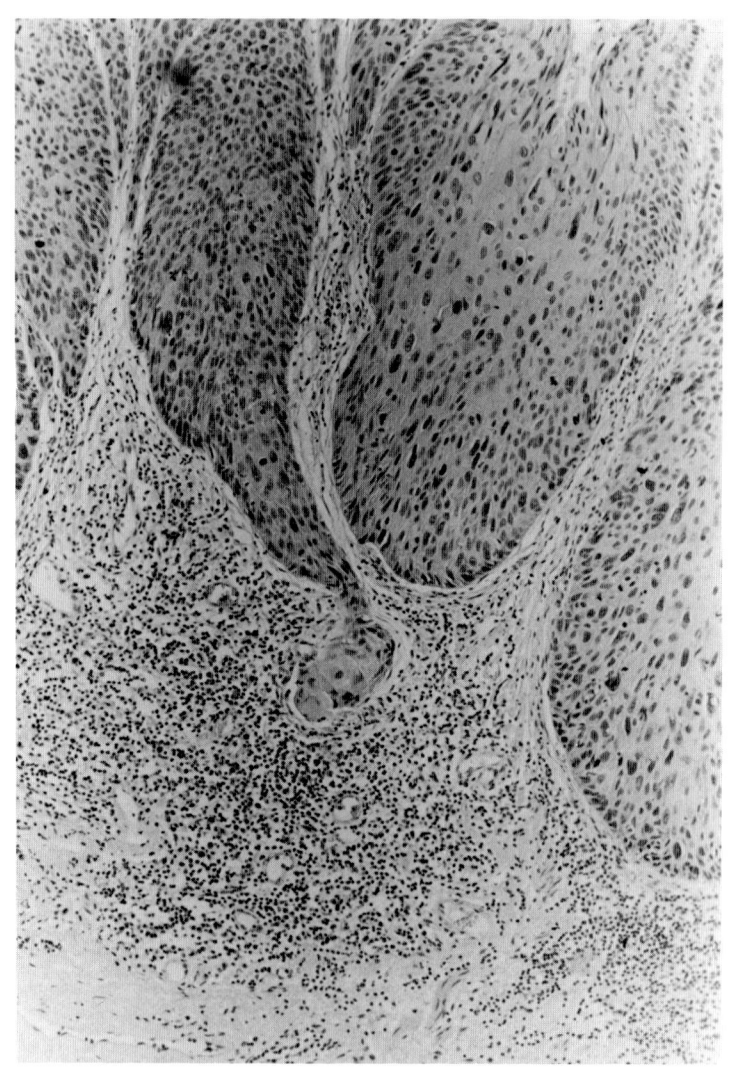

Figure 4A. Microinvasion (Early stromal invasion). An isolated tongue of tumor has penetrated the basement membrane, and is surrounded by a lymphocytic infiltrate.

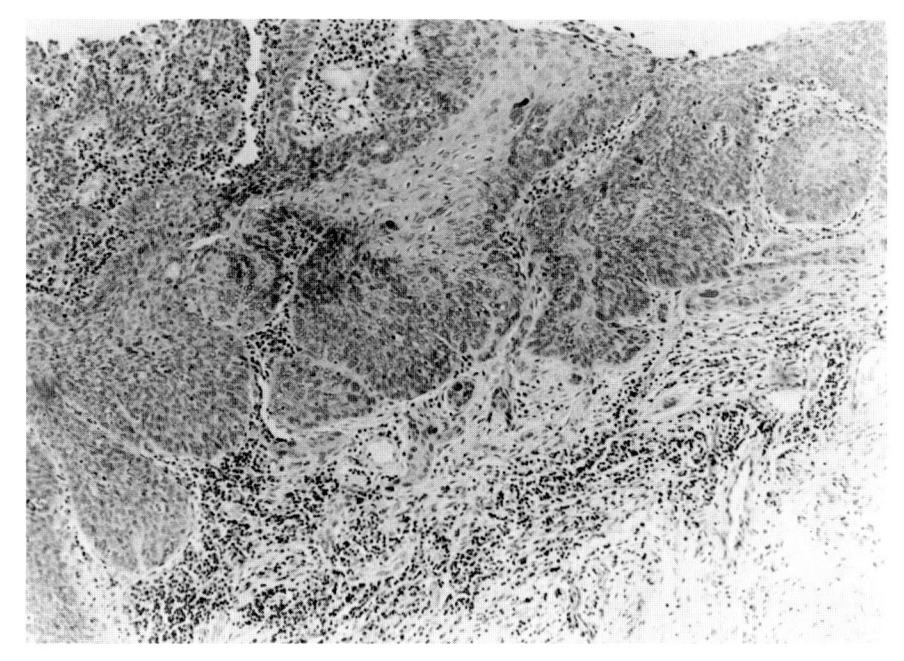

Figure 4B. Microinvasion of the diffuse or confluent type, with invasion limited to 3 mm maximum depth.

ectomy and are found to have residual microinvasion with either confluence or lymph-vascular permeation present in the specimen are advised to have pelvic radiotherapy.

The diagnosis and management of microinvasive carcinoma require the utmost in cooperation among the patient, the gynecologist, and the pathologist. The desire for conservatism must be tempered by the recognition that the literature abounds with anecdotal stories of tragedies attendant on well-intentioned under-treatment of this lesion, and most gynecologic oncologists could add cases from their own experience to the list.

INVASIVE CERVICAL CANCER

In the United States and other developed countries, the incidence and mortality from cervical cancer are on the decline.[29] However, it is still the most common malignancy of the female reproductive tract in most developing countries and a major public health problem.[203] Even in the United States, the higher incidence and mortality in the lower socioeconomic groups are cause for concern.[204] It is estimated that there will be 16,000 new cases of invasive cervical cancer diagnosed in the United States in 1984, and that 6800 women will die from the disease.[29] While these figures represent a significant improvement on past experience they are not grounds for complacency.

Gross Pathology

The gross appearance of invasive carcinoma of the cervix varies considerably and depends on the nature of its growth pattern and the mode of spread. Three main types of gross lesion are seen.

Exophytic Lesions. These originate on the portio vaginalis and may form large friable masses (Fig. 5A). They may exceed 8 cm in diameter and are particularly prone to contact bleeding.

Infiltrative Lesions. These generally present as an expanded, stony hard cervix, which to inspection often shows little sign of the presence of the tumor. They are endophytic lesions, which cause expansion of the cervix so that it becomes barrel-shaped (Fig. 5B). In extreme cases the tumor may almost fill the pelvis, making it almost impossible to estimate the extent of parametrial infiltration.

Ulcerative Lesions. These lesions excavate the cervix and often involve the vaginal fornices. They are often associated with infection and a foul-smelling vaginal discharge (Fig. 5C).

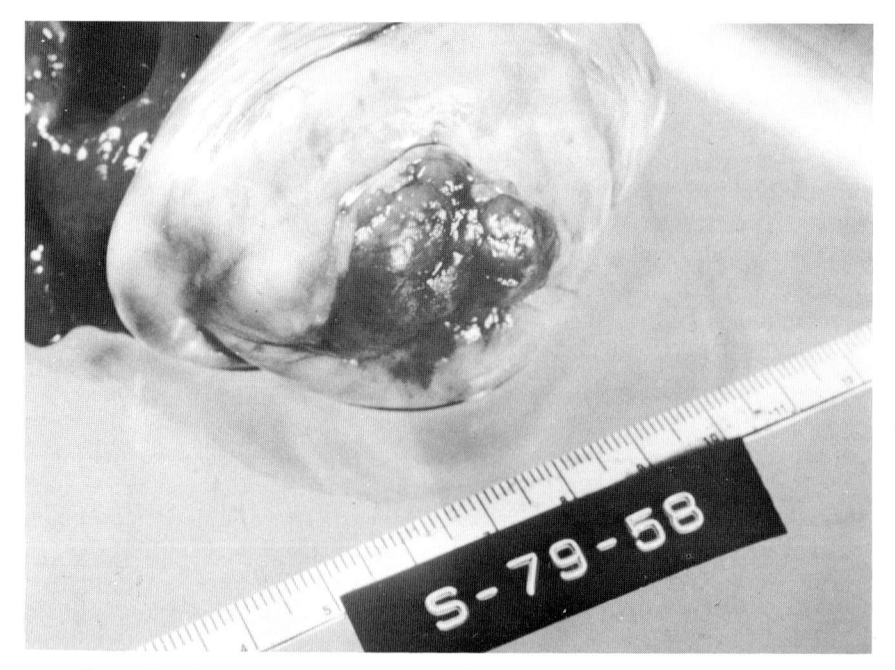

Figure 5A. Squamous cell carcinoma of the cervix, exophytic type. A friable, erythematous tumor protrudes from the anterior lip of the cervix.

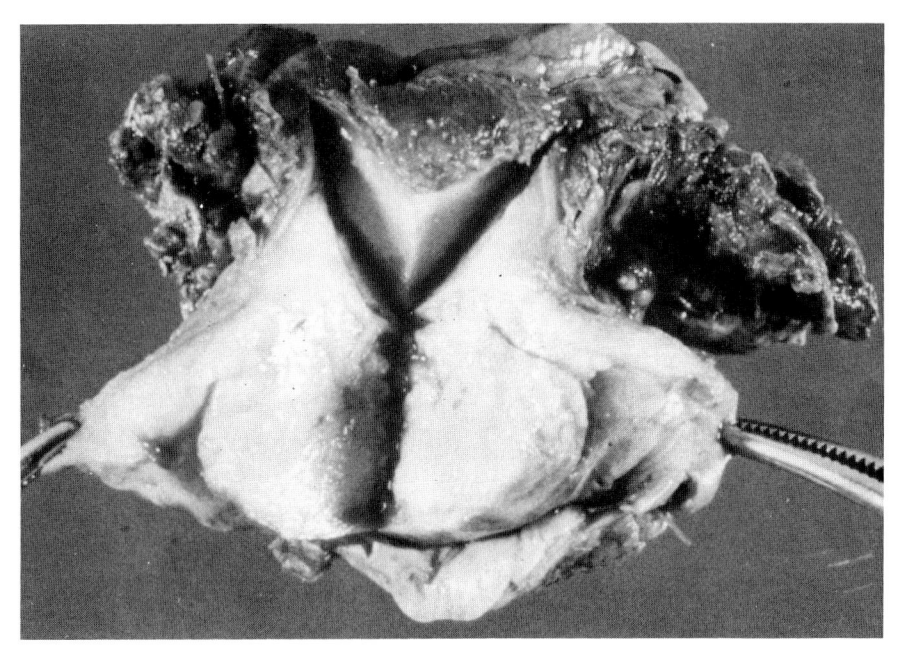

Figure 5B. Squamous cell carcinoma of the cervix, infiltrative type. The tumor has infiltrated and expanded the cervix to produce a "barrel-shaped" lesion.

Microscopic Pathology

Squamous Cell Carcinoma. Approximately 90 percent of cervical malignancies are of the squamous cell variety. Reagan and Wentz[205] proposed a subclassification of these tumors into large cell nonkeratinizing (Fig. 6A), large cell keratinizing (Fig. 6B), and small cell (Fig. 6C) varieties. For patients treated with radiotherapy, this classification was shown to have prognostic significance. For Stage I large cell nonkeratinizing tumors the 5-year survival rate was 78 percent, compared with 45 percent for large cell keratinizing tumors, and 17 percent for small cell tumors.[206] Swann and Roddick[207] found a correlation between survival and cell size in patients treated by radiotherapy, but not in those treated by surgery. On the other hand, Van Nagell and associates[208] found that the prognosis for small cell tumors was significantly worse, regardless of the mode of treatment. They attributed this to a propensity of small cell tumors for early extrapelvic lymphatic spread, and Nahhas and colleagues[209] supported this view. Despite this, Beecham and colleagues[210] could show no difference between small or large cell tumors in terms of lymphatic metastases or crude 2-year survival. Prempree and associates[211] investigated the apparently poorer prognosis of cervical cancer among younger women, and attributed it to a higher proportion of small cell tumors with more frequent lymph node metastasis. Overall, the relative proportion of large cell nonkeratinizing tumors appears to be increasing in recent years.[212]

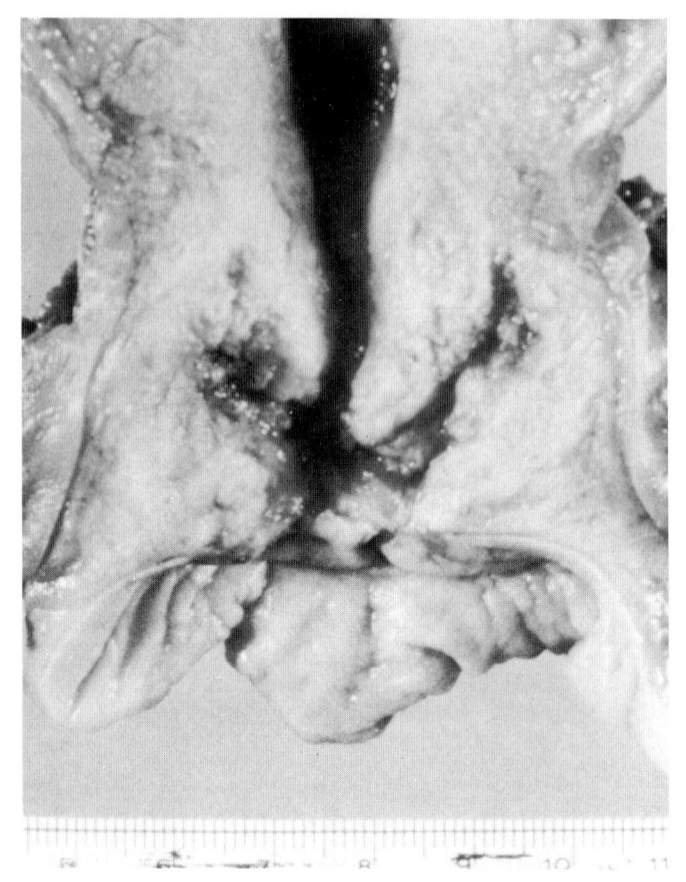

Figure 5C. Squamous cell carcinoma of the cervix, ulcerating and excavating type.

Tumor grading, in terms of the degree of cellular differentiation and anaplasia, appears to be of little prognostic significance, although Sedlacek and associates[213] found an increased incidence of lymph node metastasis in patients with the more poorly differentiated tumors.

Adenocarcinoma. Adenocarcinoma (Fig. 7) accounts for about 10 percent of cervical cancers. It is generally believed that this tumor requires a combination of surgery and radiotherapy for effective treatment, and this will be discussed later. Adenosquamous carcinoma (Fig. 8) is being seen more frequently, and as in the uterine corpus, it carries a poorer prognosis.

Sarcoma. Sarcomas of the cervix are rare, and despite a variety of therapies their prognosis is very poor.[214] It is sometimes difficult to distinguish sarcomas from poorly differentiated squamous carcinomas using light microscopy (Fig.

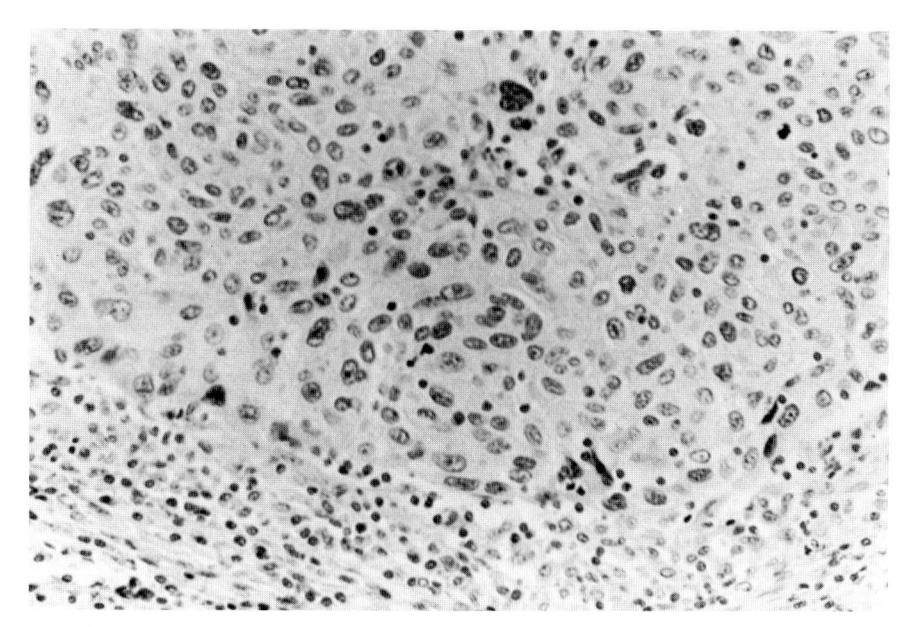

Figure 6A. Squamous cell carcinoma of the cervix, large cell, nonkeratinizing type. The nuclei are approximately three times the size of the surrounding lymphocytes. This is the most common histologic type.

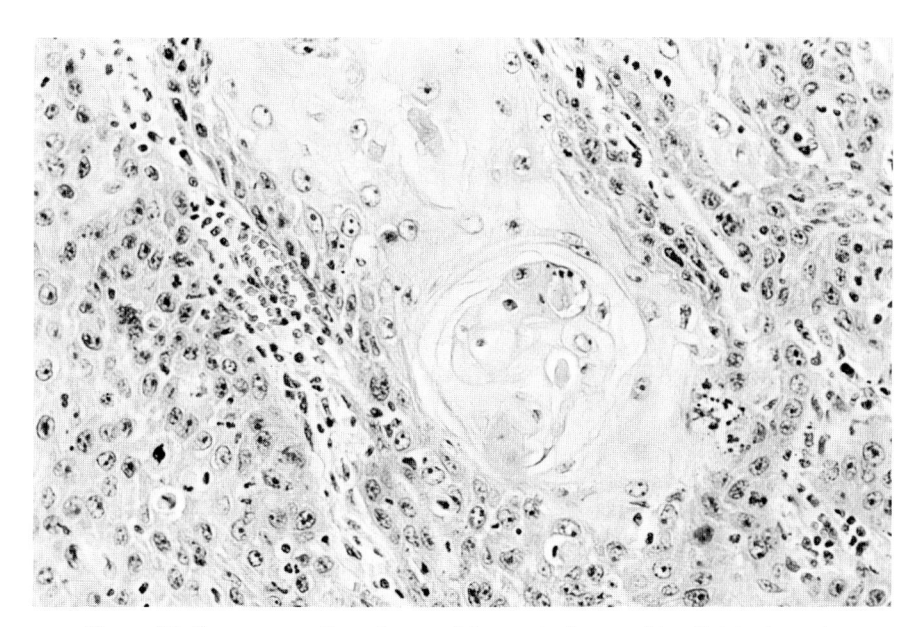

Figure 6B. Squamous cell carcinoma of the cervix, large cell keratinizing type. A glassy, eosinophilic pearl is present in the center field.

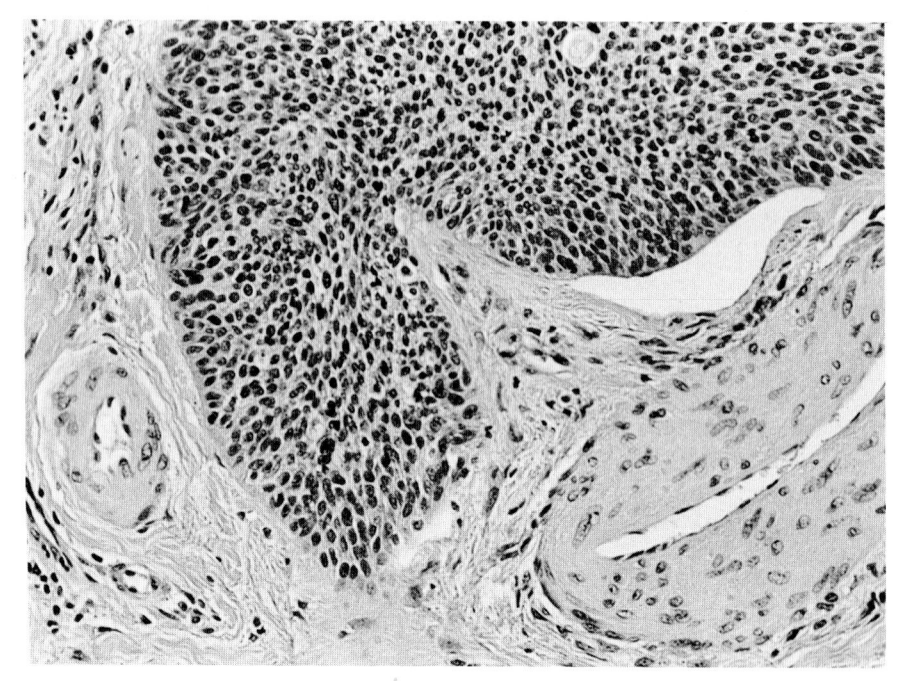

Figure 6C. Squamous cell carcinoma of the cervix, small cell type. The nuclei are only slightly larger than lymphocytes. This is the least common type.

9) and electron microscopy may be needed. Distinguishing between the two is important because the treatments are different.[215]

Routes of Spread

Carcinoma of the cervix spreads by direct extension, by lymphatic (Fig. 10) and vascular (Fig. 11) permeation, and probably also by interstitial spread (Fig. 12). The tissues first involved are usually the vaginal mucosa, the myometrium of the lower uterine corpus, and the parametrial tissues.

Lymphatic Spread. This is the best established method of spread for cervical cancer. The paracervical lymphatics drain to primary and secondary groups of nodes as described by Hendriksen[216] in 1949. The primary nodes are the parametrial nodes, the internal iliac nodes, the external iliac nodes, and the sacral nodes. The secondary nodes are the common iliac group, the inguinal nodes, and the para-aortic group. The distribution of lymph node metastases among women dying from untreated cervical cancer is shown in Figure 13. The presence of lymph node metastases has long been recognized as an adverse prognostic factor. The incidence of nodal involvement is related to the clinical stage of the disease, being present in approximately 15 percent of patients with Stage I disease, 30 percent with Stage II, and almost 50 percent with Stage III tumors.[217] Piver and Chung[218] have shown that within Stages

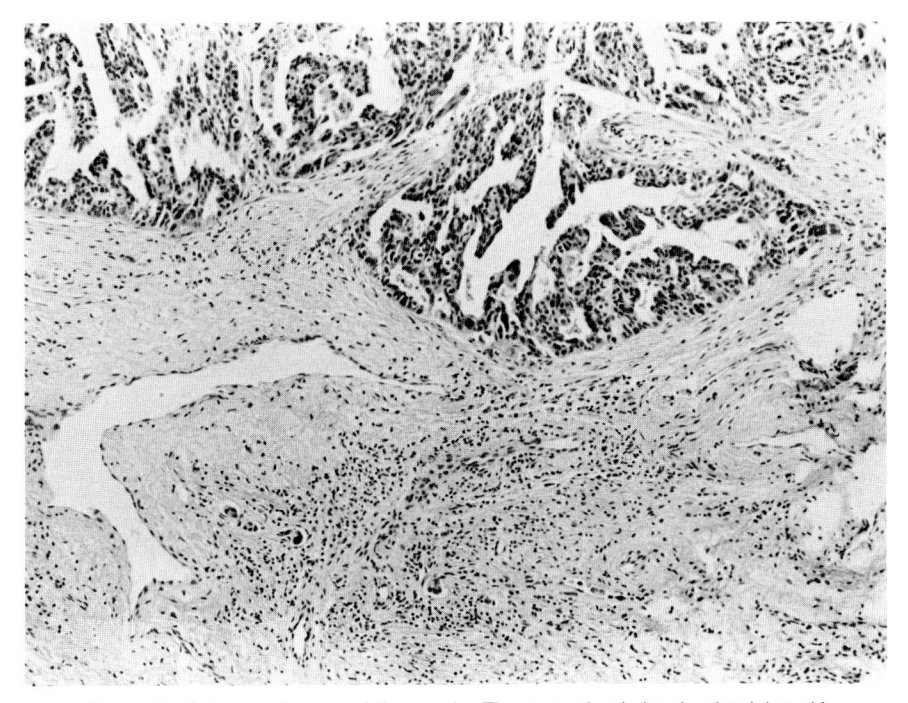

Figure 7. Adenocarcinoma of the cervix. The tumor is obviously glandular with papillary fronds.

I B and II A both the incidence of lymph node metastasis and the prognosis are related to the size of the tumor. Burghardt and Pickel[219] concluded that the incidence of lymph node involvement was closely related to the size of the tumor, as determined by giant frontal sections of excised uteri, than to the clinical stage. Bleker and colleagues[220] reported that for patients with Stages I B and II A tumors the presence of pelvic lymph node involvement reduced the 5-year survival from 90 to 62 percent. In a study of 562 patients with Stage I B cervical cancer treated by radical hysterectomy and pelvic lymphadenectomy, Martinbeau and associates[221] showed that the 5-year survival of patients with positive pelvic nodes was only 53 percent despite the use of adjunctive pelvic radiotherapy, whereas patients with no nodal metastases had a 92 percent 5-year survival. They also demonstrated that involvement of nodes above the bifurcation of the common iliac artery carried a poorer prognosis than when nodes below this level were involved. The presence of nodal metastasis rather than the number of nodes or groups involved was the important prognostic factor.

Hematogenous Spread. The presence of tumor cells in blood vessels generally carries a poorer prognosis for any tumor. In addition to direct spread into the vessels, the tumor may enter through the numerous lymphaticovenous

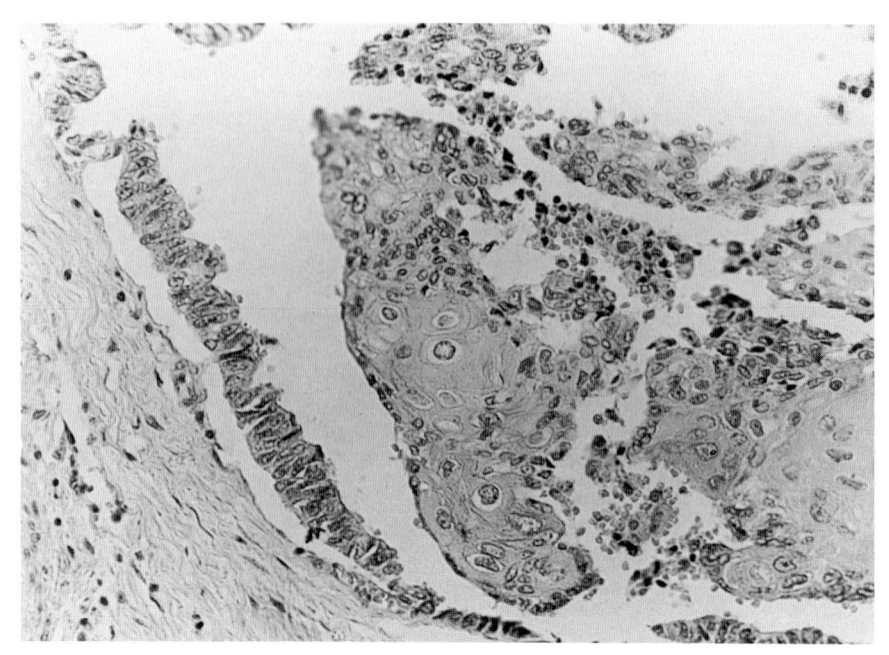

Figure 8. Adenosquamous carcinoma of the cervix. This is a well-differentiated tumor with a malignant squamous component in the center of the field, surrounded by adenocarcinoma.

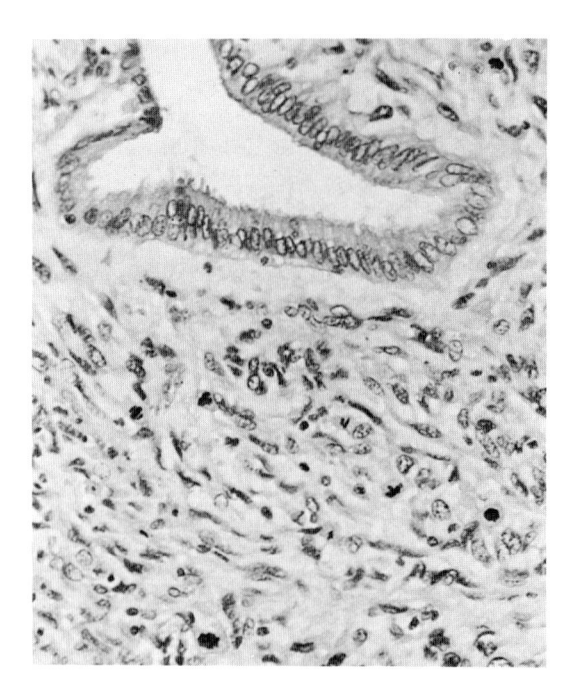

Figure 9. Squamous cell carcinoma of the cervix, spindle cell or "pseudosarcomatous" type. The abnormal cells which appear to be of stromal origin were identified by electron microscopy as squamous cells. A normal endocervical gland is present at the top of the field.

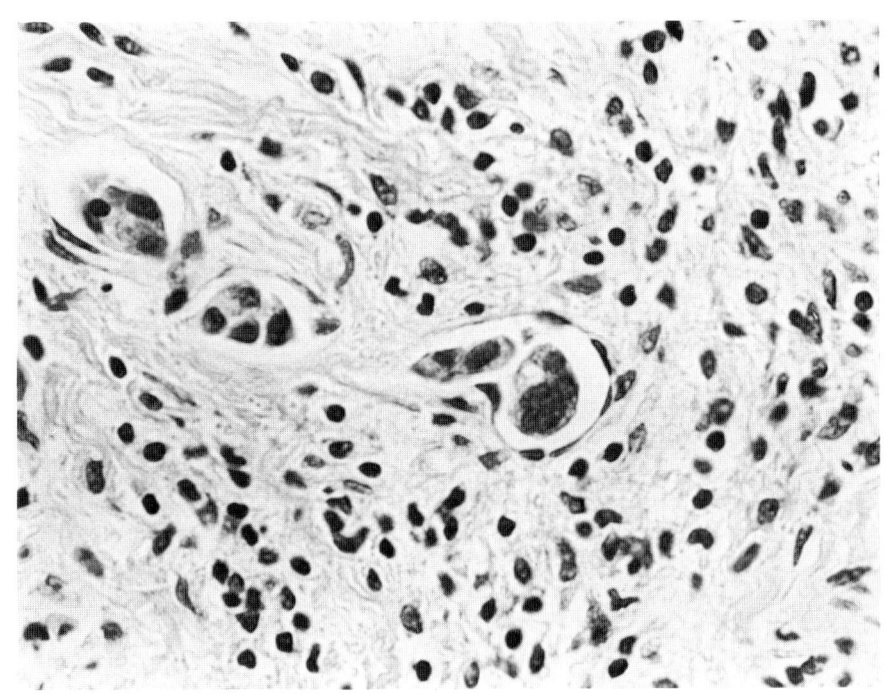

Figure 10. Lymph-vascular permeation of tumor. Tumor emboli are seen within endothelial lined lymphatic or "capillary-like" spaces.

anastomoses that are present. As pointed out by Van Nagell and associates[222] in a study of the hysterectomy specimens from 100 patients with Stage I B cervical cancer, vascular invasion is associated with a significant increase in nodal metastases and the recurrence of tumor in extrapelvic sites. They also noted that a marked lymphoplasmacytic infiltration around the tumor was associated with a reduced incidence of lymph node metastasis and tumor recurrence. Distant hematogenous spread generally occurs late in the course of the disease, with the lungs, liver, and bone being the most common sites of metastases.[217]

Interstitial Spread. This has received very little attention in gynecologic cancer, but it seems logical that the initial spread of tumor cells must be through interstitial fluid, with dissemination proceeding through tissue planes along the lines of least resistance, possibly in "capillary-like" spaces[177] or in perineural or perivascular spaces.

As shown by Ucmakli and associates,[223] nonlymphatic metastases increase with advanced stages of the disease and the parametrium and upper vagina are the most common sites.

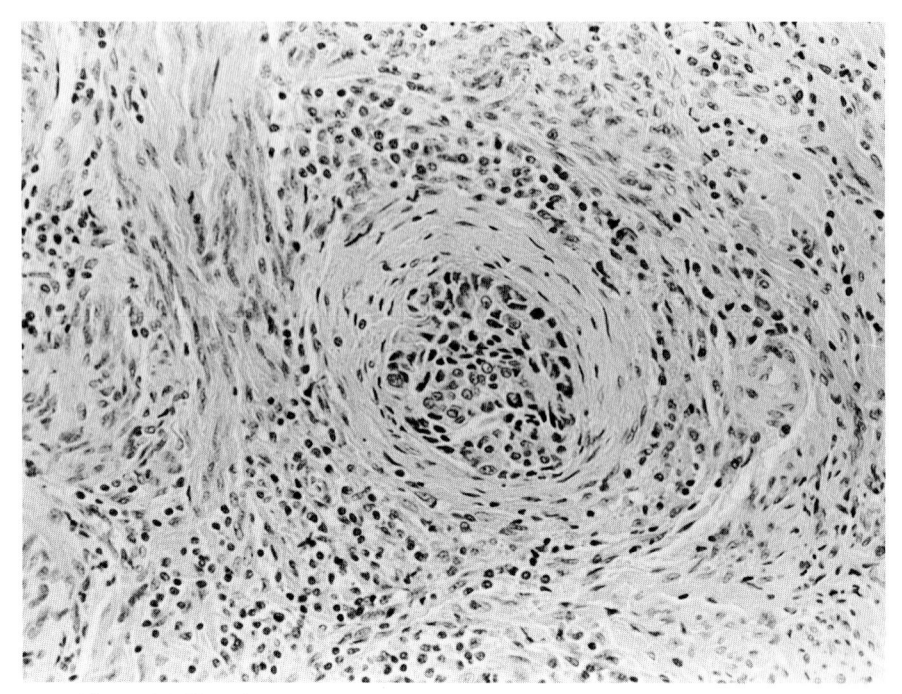

Figure 11. Vascular spread of tumor. Tumor cells are seen within a blood vessel which has a thick muscular wall.

PRETREATMENT EVALUATION

Clinical Staging and Pretreatment Investigations

The most commonly used staging system is that adopted by FIGO[224] (Table 9). The basis of this staging system is a fastidious clinical examination. This should include both inspection and palpation of the tumor. Careful bimanual vaginal and rectovaginal examination, with particular attention to the parametria and the cardinal and uterosacral ligaments, is mandatory. This examination is most accurate if performed by one experienced in the management of gynecologic cancer and may be carried out under anesthesia. Punch biopsies may be required, or even conization, although the latter is avoided if the diagnosis can be made by other means. Fractional curettage, hysteroscopy, cystoscopy, and sigmoidoscopy may be employed, although clinical experience indicates that in the absence of specific indications the yield of useful information is low. A chest x-ray and intravenous pyelogram are mandatory and a barium enema may be useful. Tests such as bone scans and liver scans are of little value unless specific indications are present. Although computerized tomography (CT) is widely used, we have not found it to be particularly

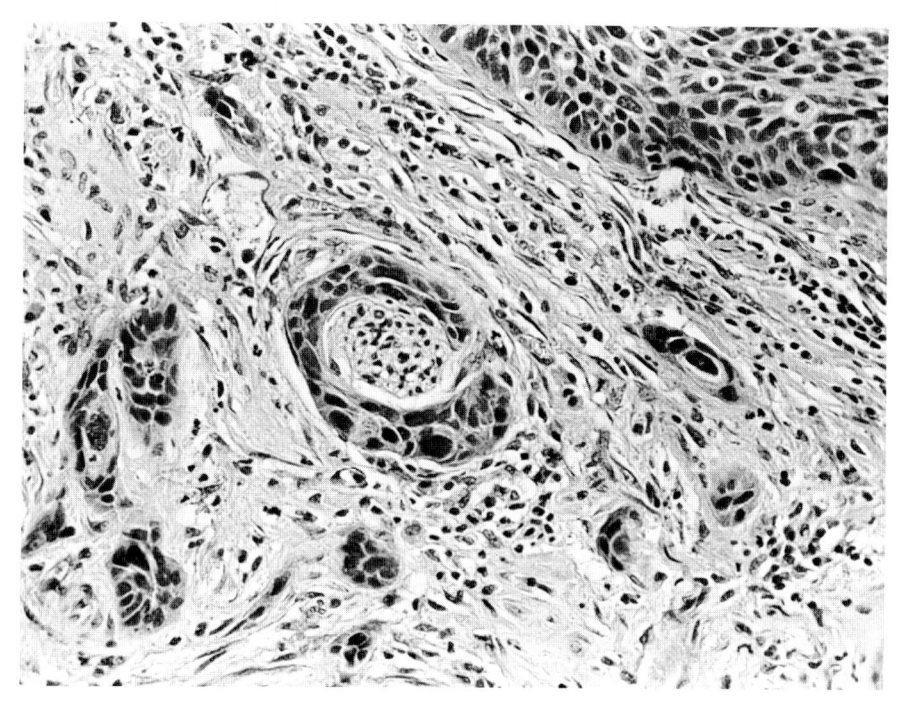

Figure 12. Intersitital spread of tumor. Tumor cells are seen in interstitial "planes of least resistance," including the perineural spaces (center).

useful, and have been given misleading information in a number of cases. In a recent study it was found to be no better than clinical examination in the assessment of Stages I and II disease, though it did provide useful information in more advanced lesions.[225] In this study CT scanning was about 80 percent accurate in predicting para-aortic nodal metastases. We believe that CT scanning adds little to the information obtained by careful clinical examination and intravenous pyelography. Nuclear magnetic resonance scanning may be useful in the future, but it is not yet of established value.

Lymphangiography has been used in a number of centers for the detection of para-aortic lymph node metastasis. Piver and Barlow[226] believe that the technique is of value in patients with clinical Stages III and IV disease, to enable extended field radiation to be performed with a lower morbidity than would follow lymphadenectomy. Our experience agrees more with that of Brown and colleagues[227] who concluded that "the specificity of lymphangiographic examinations is not accurate enough to be of clinical significance. . ." A combination of lymphangiography or CT scanning and fine needle aspiration of suspicious nodes may occasionally be of value in certain clinical situations.[228]

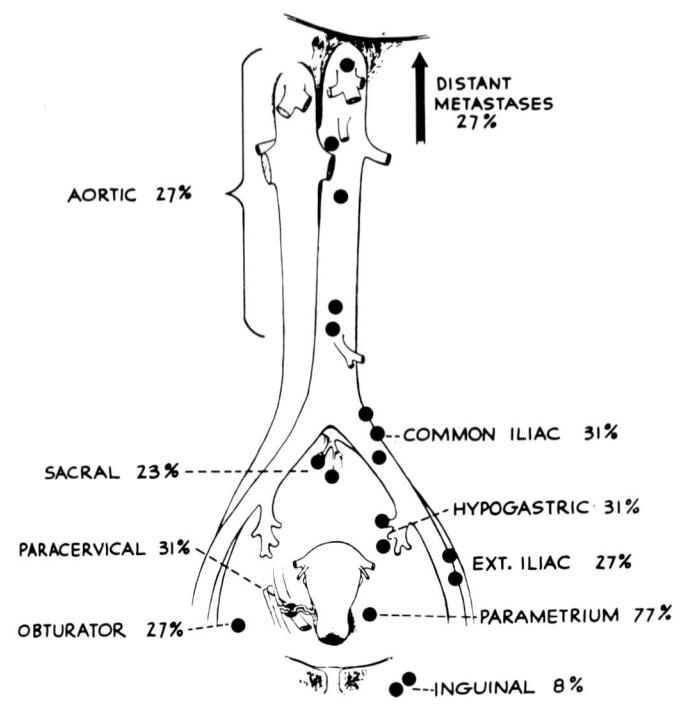

Figure 13. Distribution of lymph node metastasis in patients dying of untreated carcinoma of the cervix. (*From Hendriksen E: Am J Obstet Gynecol 58:924, 1949, with permission.*)[216]

Other tests that have been suggested as adjuncts to pretreatment evaluation include carcinoembryonic antigen,[229,230] pelvic arteriography,[231] transrectal ultrasonography,[232] and the assay of tumor antigen TA-4.[233]

Routine studies ordered on all patients with cervical cancer should include a complete blood count and platelet count, coagulation profile, serum electrolyte studies, and basic liver and renal function tests. In older women, an electrocardiogram should be obtained and for patients with respiratory or cardiovascular problems appropriate consultation should be obtained.

Surgical Staging

It is obvious that patients treated for cervical cancer by pelvic radiotherapy will have little hope for cure if extrapelvic spread is already present. "The potential benefits of operative evaluation, including pelvic and para-aortic lymphadenectomy . . . include modification of radiotherapy . . . a better understanding of the natural history of the disease process, and the possible improvement in cure rates of patients at high risk to fail therapy."[234] As shown in Table 10, the reported incidence of para-aortic lymph node metastasis in cervical cancer is significant, and especially in more advanced lesions.[235–239] The reports of Wharton and associates[240] and of Piver and Barlow[241] empha-

TABLE 9. THE FIGO CLINICAL STAGING FOR CARCINOMA OF THE CERVIX

Stage 0:	Carcinoma in situ
Stage I:	The carcinoma is confined to the cervix (Extension to the corpus is disregarded)
Stage I A:	Microinvasive carcinoma
Stage I B:	All other Stage I cases. Occult carcinoma should be marked "occ"
Stage II:	The carcinoma extends beyond the cervix, but not to the pelvic wall. The tumor involves the vagina, but not so far as the lower third
Stage II A:	No obvious parametrial involvement
Stage II B:	Obvious parametrial involvement
Stage III:	The carcinoma has extended onto the pelvic wall. On rectal examination there is no cancer-free space between the tumor and the pelvic wall. The tumor involves the lower third of the vagina. All cases with hydronephrosis or a nonfunctioning kidney are included
Stage III A:	No extension to the pelvic wall
Stage III B:	Extension to the pelvic wall and/or hydronephrosis or a nonfunctioning kidney
Stage IV:	The carcinoma has extended beyond the true pelvis or has clinically involved the mucosa of the bladder or rectum. Bullous edema as such does not permit the case to be alloted to Stage IV
Stage IV A:	Spread of growth to adjacent organs
Stage IV B:	Spread to distant organs

Notes: Stage I A, or microinvasive carcinoma, represents those cases of epithelial abnormalities in which histologic evidence of early stromal invasion is unequivocal. The diagnosis is based on microscopic examination of tissue removed by biopsy, conization, portio amputation, or removal of the uterus. Cases of early stromal invasion should be allocated to Stage I A

The remainder of Stage I cases are allocated to Stage I B. As a rule, these cases can be diagnosed by routine clinical examination

Occult cancer is a histologically invasive cancer that cannot be diagnosed by routine clinical examination. As a rule it is diagnosed on a cone biopsy, the amputated portio, or the removed uterus. Such cancers are classified as Stage I B, occ

(From ACOG Tech Bull No. 47, June 1977, with permission.)[224]

sized the high mortality rate of radiotherapy given after staging laparotomy. The former group reported severe complications in 27 percent of cases and deaths in 13 percent. On the other hand, Averette and colleagues[235] and Buchsbaum[236] report very low complication rates. If transperitoneal para-aortic lymphadenectomy is performed it is wise to confine the procedure to sampling only, rather than to perform a complete dissection, and to avoid extensive surgical exploration of the pelvic spaces.[239] One approach to reducing the rate of complications from radiation after surgical staging is to perform

TABLE 10. INCIDENCE OF PARA-AORTIC NODE INVOLVEMENT IN THE VARIOUS STAGES OF CERVICAL CARCINOMA

Authors	I	II	III	IV	Overall
Averette et al. (1972)[235]	3/40	4/18	2/20	1/2	10/80 (12%)
Buchsbaum (1972)[236]	0/23	1/12	7/20	1/2	9/57 (16%)
Nelson et al. (1977)[237]	—	9/63	15/39	0/2	24/104 (23%)
Sudasanam et al. (1978)[238]	11/53	7/43	5/19	0/3	23/218 (11%)
Lagasse et al. (1980)[239]	8/143	23/80	19/64	1/4	51/291 (18%)
Total	22/259 (8%)	44/216 (20%)	48/162 (30%)	3/13 (23%)	117/750 (16%)

an extraperitoneal lymphadenectomy. Berman and associates[234] compared this procedure to the transperitoneal approach and found that patients in the latter group had a 30 percent rate of intestinal morbidity and a 7 percent mortality rate, after radiotherapy, while those who had undergone extraperitoneal exploration had an enteric morbidity rate of only 2.5 percent with no deaths.

Another alternative is to perform a transperitoneal pelvic and para-aortic lymphadenectomy and, if frozen section reveals positive nodes, to give intraoperative external beam radiation to the involved areas. Initially described by Goldson and associates[242] for patients with positive para-aortic nodes, the technique has recently been expanded to cover both the para-aortic and pelvic node-bearing areas.[243] The bowel is packed aside and a linear accelerator is used to deliver a carefully calculated dose of radiation in the form of a high-energy electron beam. While the initial results of this approach are promising, further investigation is necessary to assess the long-term success and complication rates.

Another factor to be considered in assessing the role of staging laparotomy is the long-term survival of patients after treatment for positive para-aortic lymph nodes. Buchsbaum[244] reported a 35 percent incidence of supraclavicular lymph node metastasis in women with positive para-aortic nodes, and Nelson and associates[237] attributed the appearance of other distant metastases in over half of the patients treated for para-aortic spread to the fact that the tumor was more widely distributed at the time of treatment. Scalene node biopsy has been advocated prior to extended field treatment for patients with para-aortic node involvement to avoid this situation.[245] It does appear that a proportion of patients with positive para-aortic nodes can be cured by radiation, but the exact proportion is difficult to assess.[239,246]

We believe that a transperitoneal staging laparotomy should be performed on all patients who are fit for surgery. If positive para-aortic nodes are present, supraclavicular lymph node biopsy should be performed prior to extended field radiotherapy.

MANAGEMENT

Ideally the management of the patient with cervical cancer is a team approach. The gynecologist and radiation oncologist should see the patient together and review all biopsy specimens with a pathologist at the treating institution in the light of their clinical findings. There should be a plan of therapy for each stage of the disease with individualization depending on the general condition of the patient, the stage of the disease, and the surgical and radiotherapeutic facilities available.

Radiation Therapy

In the treatment of Stages I and II A cervical carcinoma, the prospects for cure following radiotherapy or radical surgery are equally good in the best centers and the choice of the primary therapeutic modality is based on the needs and condition of the patient and the facilities available. Following radical surgery, the presence of adverse prognostic factors in the excised material may indicate adjuvant radiotherapy. The majority of more advanced lesions are treated by primary radiotherapy and in fit patients the fields are guided by the findings of a "staging laparotomy."

Small lesions in Stages I and II A may be treated with intracavitary radium or cesium,[247] although this modality will not control disease in pelvic lymph nodes if it is present. For most I B or II B lesions the patient is treated initially with external therapy to a dose of 4000 to 5000 rads to the whole pelvis. This reduces the size of the primary lesion so that subsequent intracavitary radium or cesium will be more effective. The combination of external and intracavitary radiation provides doses that are generally tumoricidal for the central tumor and for microscopic disease on the pelvic side walls. The intracavitary applications are usually best fractionated, being given as two treatments approximately 2 weeks apart. In order to avoid excessive obliteration of the fornices and stenosis of the cervix and upper vagina from precluding a subsequent implant, it is essential that pelvic examinations be performed at weekly intervals and, if necessary, the implants performed before the completion of the course of teletherapy. In this case the external treatments are finished after the appropriate brachytherapy.

Intracavitary Applicators

We favor the use of the Fletcher-Suit afterloading applicators, as they allow the safe and unhurried positioning of the applicators without risk to the staff (Fig. 14). If possible both the gynecologist and radiation oncologist should cooperate in the insertion of the tandem and ovoids, as the examination under anesthesia offers an excellent opportunity to review the clinical regression of the disease. After placement of the tandem and ovoids, anteroposterior and lateral x-ray films are obtained (Fig. 15) to allow the calculation of isodose curves.

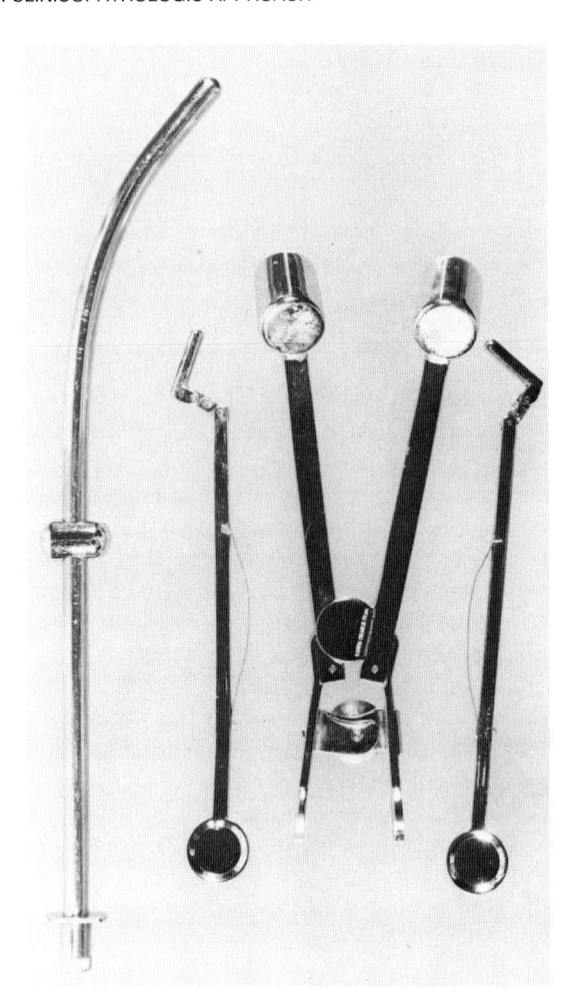

Figure 14. Fletcher-Suit radium applicators. The tandem (on the left) is inserted into the uterine cavity, and the ovoids (on the right) are placed in the vaginal fornices, on either side of the cervix. The applicators are inserted empty, and when a satisfactory placement has been assured, are loaded with radium or cesium (afterloading technique).

Whole Pelvis Radiotherapy

With modern equipment anterior and posterior portals with a surface size 15 cm × 15 cm are generally used, often with lateral portals with surface sizes of 15 cm × 9 cm. The dosage to the whole pelvis is generally of the order of 4000 to 5000 rads. While the height of the fields is always a minimum of 15 cm, it may be expanded in the midline to cover the para-aortic chain where these nodes are positive. In general the dose to the para-aortic nodes should not exceed 4500 rads.

Supplementary Parametrial Irradiation

This modality may be used to augment the dosage given by an intracavitary system and is aimed primarily at the parametrium and the regional lymphat-

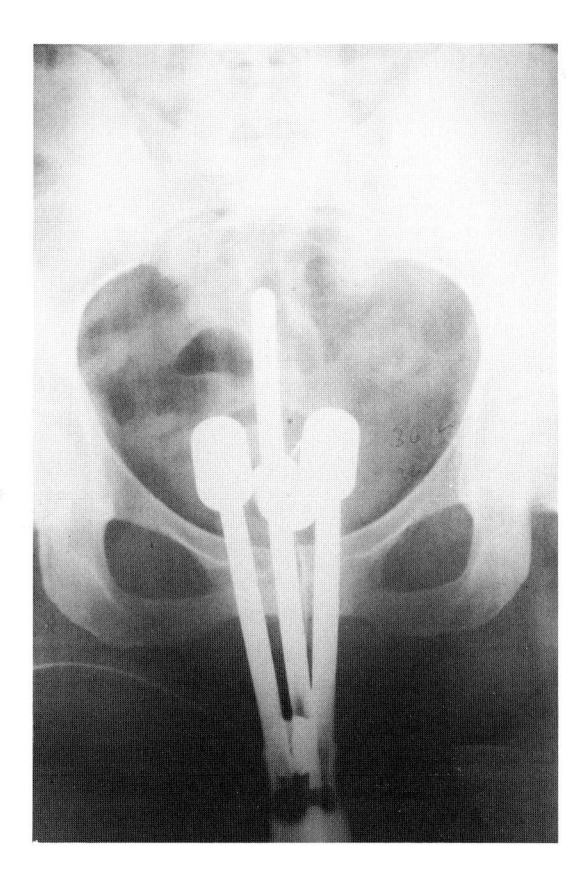

Figure 15A. Radiograph (anteroposterior view) of Fletcher-Suit applicators in a good position after insertion.

ics. Generally a 15 cm × 15 cm field is used with midline shielding of a size determined by the isodose curves constructed on the basis of the configuration and loading of the intracavitary system.

Transvaginal Cone Radiotherapy

This approach, utilizing 140 to 250 kV still has a role in halting hemorrhage from large exophytic lesions or shrinking such tumors before commencing whole pelvic radiation. Usually 1000 rads are given in two daily fractions of 500 rads. An alternative approach in the same situation is three fractions of 400 rads each, using megavoltage equipment, through 10 cm × 10 cm fields directed at the midline. While transvaginal cone radiation can be ignored in calculating rectal and vesical tolerance, the dose delivered through pelvic fields cannot.

The details of radiotherapeutic technique are beyond the scope of this book, but are admirably covered in Fletcher's text.[248] His suggested therapeutic regimes are outlined in Table 11.

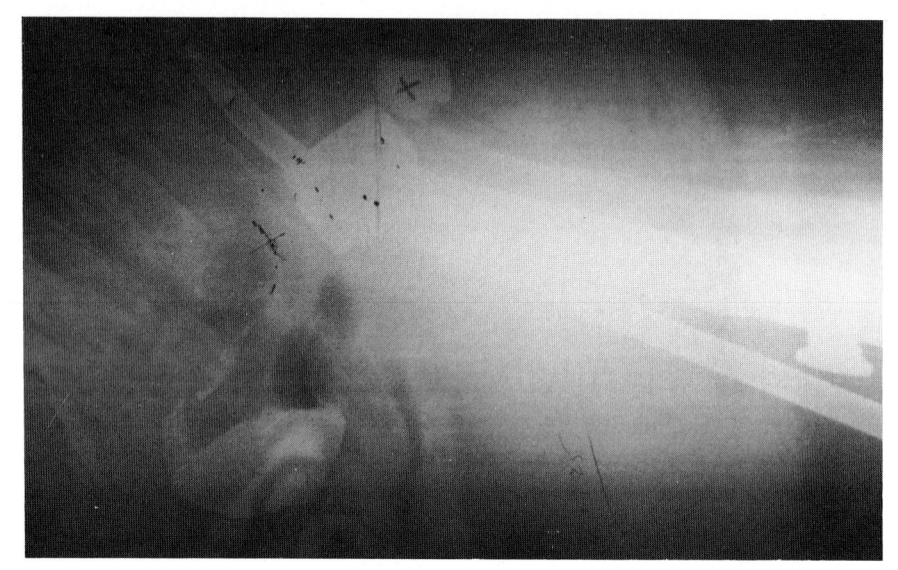

Figure 15B. Radiograph (lateral view) of Fletcher-Suit applicators in good position after insertion. There is radiopaque material present in the bulb of the Foley catheter in the bladder, and also in the rectum.

Results of Radiotherapy

The collected survival statistics for conventional radiotherapeutic techniques in patients with Stages I B and II A disease, as reported by Hoskins and associates[249] are shown in Table 12. It is apparent that there is considerable variation depending on the institution and the method of reporting used. The survival figures for over 61,000 patients treated by radiation worldwide is of the order of 80 percent for Stage I, 60 percent for Stage II, 30 percent for Stage III, and 10 percent for Stage IV.[257]

Immediate side effects of radiotherapy are usually mild, and include anorexia, nausea, and occasionally vomiting. Diarrhea and cystitis are common, but usually respond to simple medical therapy. The gastrointestinal symptoms will often lead to some weight loss. Vaginal stenosis, which may preclude proper examination, may occur unless intercourse or vaginal dilation is used. More major complications of radiotherapy include hemorrhagic cystitis, radiation proctosigmoiditis, bowel stricture and obstruction, vault necrosis, and vesicovaginal, rectovaginal, or enterovaginal fistula formation. Rarely obstructive uropathy may occur, especially following surgery and radiation, but it is essential to exclude recurrent tumor, which is present in 90 percent of such cases. The rate of major complications following radiotherapy has been reduced to less than 2 percent by modern techniques[249] (Table 13), but some radiotherapists remain blissfully unaware of the complications of their treatment as the patient often seeks help elsewhere (Fig. 16).

TABLE 11. RADIOTHERAPEUTIC REGIMENS FOR CERVICAL CARCINOMA[a]

Tumor Size (Stage Ignored)	Whole Pelvis	Radium mg/hr	Parametrial
Up to 1 cm	None	10,000	None
1 to 3 cm Minimal parametrial extension	1. None 2. 2000 rads 3. 4000 rads	9000 7500 5500	4000 rads 2000 rads None
3 to 6 cm Endocervical or bulky tumor	4000 rads	5500–6500 rads	None
Over 6 cm Barrel-shaped or endocervical	4000 rads	5000 rads	None
Over 6 cm Extending near pelvic side wall or to lower vagina	1. 4000 rads 2. 5000 rads 3. 6000 rads[b]	5500–6600 rads 4000–5000 rads 3000–4000 rads	May add up to 1000 rads to side of maximal involvement
Massive disease of bladder or rectum involved	Up to 7000 rads[b]	None	None

[a] The maximal recommended dosages are listed. This table is a guide only, to help the clinician understand the radiotherapeutic plans.
[b] Field size is reduced during therapy.
(From Fletcher GH: Textbook of Radiotherapy, 3rd ed. Lea & Febiger, Philadelphia, 1980, with permission.)[248]

Radiation Potentiators

A variety of chemotherapeutic agents including doxorubicin and cisplatin are known to potentiate the effects of radiation on various tissues. In 1974, Piver and his associates[263] showed a significant increase in the survival rate of patients with locally advanced cervical cancer treated with radiotherapy and hydroxyurea. More recently they reported a double-blind controlled study of the effects of hydroxyurea on the response of selected patients with Stage II B cervical cancer treated by radiation.[264] A staging laparotomy was used to exclude patients with para-aortic metastases. The life table survival for patients receiving hydroxyurea was 94 percent compared to 53 percent for the placebo group. The death rate from cervical cancer was 5 percent in the hydroxyurea group and 45 percent in the placebo group. There was no significant difference in the incidence of side effects in the hydroxyurea group. This work, if substantiated in larger trials, would represent a major breakthrough in the treatment of cervical cancer.

TABLE 12. SURVIVAL FIGURES FOR PATIENTS WITH STAGE I AND STAGE II CERVICAL CARCINOMA TREATED BY RADIOTHERAPY[a]

Authors	Stages	Patients	5-Year Survival
Blaikley et al. (1969)[250]	I	183	67%
	I & II	551	54%
Dickson (1972)[251]	I B	348	72%
	I B & II A	983	60%
Fletcher (1971)[252]	I B	549	92%[b]
	I B & II A	973	84%[b]
Kline et al. (1969)[253]	I B	45	81%
	I B & II A	64	71%
Kottmeier (1964)[254]	I B	611	90%
	I B & II A	1576	79%
Muirhead and Green (1968)[255]	I	194	78%
	I & II	208	68%
Wall et al. (1966)[256]	I	101	86%
	I & II	208	74%
Average	I		84%
	I & II		76%

[a]It should be noted that patients undergoing radiotherapy are often a selected group, as young and healthy patients will often be treated surgically.
[b]Actuarial survival.
(From Hoskins WJ, et al: Gynecol Oncol 4:278, 1976, with permission.)[249]

SURGICAL TREATMENT

While radiotherapy is undoubtedly an effective treatment for cervical cancer, surgery offers specific advantages in selected cases. The basic requirements, prior to considering patients for radical surgery, are that the lesion should be

TABLE 13. MORBIDITY OF RADIOTHERAPEUTIC MANAGEMENT OF STAGE I AND STAGE II CERVICAL CANCER[a]

Authors	Patients	Complications
Boronow & Rutledge (1971)[258]	975	0.8%[b]
Kottmeier (1964)[254]	1576	1.9%
Mickal et al. (1972)[259]	92	8.6%
Peckham et al. (1969)[260]	611	8.2%
Strockbine et al. (1970)[261]	126	4.0%[b]
Villasanta (1972)[262]	414	25%
Wall et al. (1966)[256]	217	3.8%
Average		6.1%

[a]Only complications requiring surgical intervention or producing permanent disability are included.
[b]Fistulas only: other complications not included.
(From Hoskins WJ, et al: Gynecol Oncol 4:278, 1976, with permission.)[249]

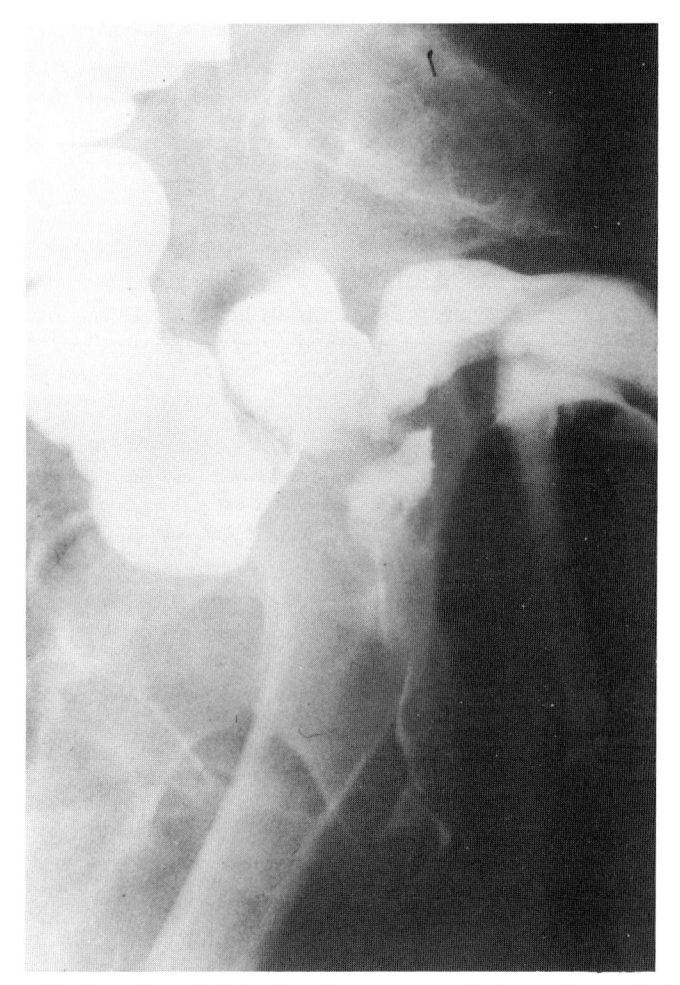

Figure 16. Sigmoidovaginal fistula subsequent to radiotherapy for cervical carcinoma. The tract is demonstrated on this lateral radiographic view.

surgically resectable, the patient in good condition, and that no other form of therapy offers a better hope for cure with less morbidity. The surgical team must have the technical skill to perform the operation and manage any complications, and be well acquainted with the natural history of cervical cancer and its mode of spread.

Radical Abdominal Hysterectomy

Radical abdominal hysterectomy is an appropriate method of treatment for the otherwise healthy younger woman with Stage I B or II A cervical carcinoma. Among the advantages of the surgical approach are a more thorough assessment of the spread and extent of the disease, the potential for retaining ovarian function, and a more functional vagina.

The operation is performed through a generous vertical incision extending from the symphysis pubis to just above the umbilicus. This incision allows optimal exposure of the upper abdomen, para-aortic nodal areas, and the pelvis. After thorough exploration of the upper abdomen and frozen section biopsy of any suspicious lesions, para-aortic lymphadenectomy is performed. Provided these nodes are negative on frozen section, attention is directed to the pelvis. The pelvic lymph nodes should be removed from the bifurcation of the aorta to the inguinal ligament. Thus the common iliac, internal and external iliac, sacral and obdurator groups will be removed. In addition, an adequate amount of parametrium and the upper one-third of the vagina should be removed (Fig. 17). In excising the parametrium, the ureter must be freed from its canal in the cardinal ligament, and one important reason for pyelography is to detect any abnormalities such as double ureters prior to surgery (Fig. 18). Ovarian conservation is feasible for younger patients undergoing radical hysterectomy[265] and ovarian function is normal in at least 50 percent of cases.[266] If the ovaries are to be saved, consideration should be given to suspending them outside the field of possible subsequent radiation. Metastasis to the ovaries is extremely rare in cervical cancer. The survival rates for patients with Stages I B and II A cervical cancer treated by radical hysterectomy and pelvic lymphadenectomy compare favorably with those achieved by radiotherapy[249] (Table 14).

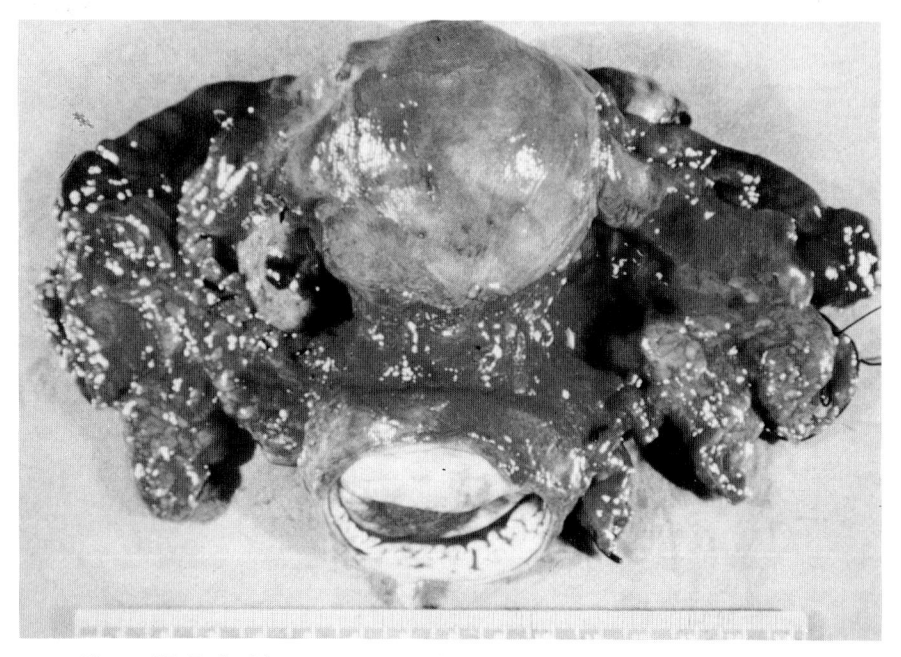

Figure 17. Radical hysterectomy specimen consisting of uterus, tubes, ovaries, parametrial tissues, and upper vagina. The pelvic lymph nodes were taken separately, and are not shown.

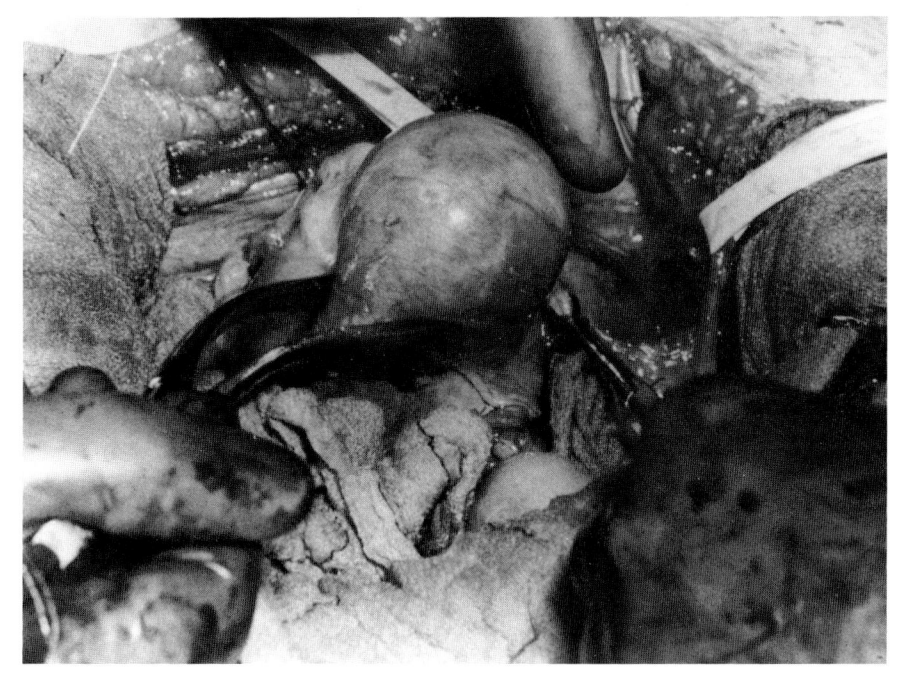

Figure 18. Double ureters demonstrated during radical hysterectomy in a patient with Stage I B (FIGO) carcinoma of the cervix, and a myomatous uterus. Penrose drains are placed around each ureter for demonstration purposes.

Webb and Symmonds[273] have provided a current appraisal of the role of radical hysterectomy and pelvic lymphadenectomy in the treatment of Stages I B and II A cervical carcinoma. Of 564 patients, 17 percent had positive nodes. In Stage I B the incidence of positive nodes was 14.5 percent and in Stage II A it was 27.7 percent. The operative mortality was 0.3 percent and the operative morbidity was also low. Obesity, though making the procedure more difficult, did not affect the morbidity. The authors advise prophylactic low-dose heparin to minimize the risk of thromboembolism and the use of postoperative suction drainage of the pelvis to reduce both the febrile morbidity and incidence of lymphocysts. The incidence of urinary and intestinal fistulas was less than 5 percent, although a subgroup of patients who had "extended" radical hysterectomies, which included the resection of bowel or bladder in patients following radiation, had a fistula rate of 30 percent. This latter finding suggests that exenteration would be more appropriate in this type of patient. Interestingly, the same authors could not demonstrate any increase in morbidity when radical hysterectomy followed cone biopsy.[274] This is in contrast to our own findings,[275] and we in general believe that radical hysterectomy should either be performed within 48 hours of cone biopsy or be delayed for 4 weeks. Under certain circumstances the slightly increased

TABLE 14. SURVIVAL RATES FOR PATIENTS WITH STAGE I B AND STAGE II A CERVICAL CARCINOMA TREATED BY RADICAL HYSTERECTOMY AND PELVIC LYMPHADENECTOMY[a]

Authors	Stages	Patients	5-Year Survival
Blaikley et al. (1969)[250]	I B	98	66%
	I B & II A	161	51%
Brunschwig and Barber (1966)[267]	I B	173	82%
	I B & II A	308	76%
Christensen et al. (1964)[268]	I B	168	83%
	I B & II A	219	77%
Ketcham et al. (1971)[269]	I B	28	86%[b]
	I B & II A	42	87%
Liu and Meigs (1955)[270]	I B	116	78%
	I B & II A	165	72%
Masterson (1967)[271]	I B	120	88%
	I B & II A	150	83%
Park et al. (1973)[272]	I B	126	91%
Average	I B		82%
	I B & II A		74%

[a]It should be noted that patients considered unfit for surgery will be treated by radiotherapy, and so direct comparisons are not strictly fair.
[b]Actuarial survival.
(From Hoskins WJ, et al: Gynecol Oncol 4:278, 1976, with permission.)[249]

risk of infection may be offset by such factors as a patient's extreme anxiety and the procedure done sooner.

As already stated, comparisons of the results of radical surgery and radiotherapy for the primary treatment of Stage I B carcinoma of the cervix show little difference in results.[276,277] Nevertheless, if recurrence does occur after radical surgery, radiotherapy may still offer a reasonable prospect for cure. Failure of radiotherapy is often more difficult to diagnose and there may ultimately be little opportunity for salvage by operation. The patient with a large necrotic cervix after radiation poses a particularly difficult problem, and often multiple biopsies of the cervix and parametrium, and sometimes even laparotomy, may be needed to demonstrate recurrence.

The operative mortality from radical hysterectomy is of the order of 1 percent (Table 15), most commonly related to thromboembolism, sepsis, or hemorrhage. The most serious source of morbidity is urinary fistula formation (Table 16). The incidence of urinary fistula formation in our last 100 patients is 1 percent, and we believe this low rate is due to suspension of the distal ureter to the hypogastric artery, suction drainage of the pelvis, and prolonged bladder drainage. We achieve long-term bladder drainage by the use of a Foley catheter with a leg bag for 6 weeks postoperatively, and in addition to helping reduce the fistula rate, we find bladder dysfunction only very rarely when it is removed.

TABLE 15. OPERATIVE MORTALITY FOR PATIENTS WITH STAGE I B AND STAGE II A CARCINOMA OF THE CERVIX TREATED BY RADICAL HYSTERECTOMY AND PELVIC LYMPHADENECTOMY

Authors	Patients	Operative Mortality
Blaikley et al. (1969)[250]	257	1.9%
Brunschwig and Barber (1966)[267]	438	1.1%
Christensen et al. (1964)[268]	394	0.5%
Ketcham et al. (1971)[269]	84	2.7%
Liu and Meigs (1955)[270]	473	1.7%
Masterson (1967)[271]	180	1.1%
Mickal et al. (1972)[258]	64	4.7%
Park et al. (1973)[272]	150	0.6%
Symmonds (1966)[298]	101	0.0%
Average		1.3%

(From Hoskins WJ, et al: Gynecol Oncol 4:278, 1976, with permission.)[249]

COMBINATIONS OF RADIATION AND SURGERY

It has already been mentioned that radiotherapy may be given after radical surgery for patients found to have such adverse prognostic factors as lymphvascular permeation, occult parametrial involvement, or positive pelvic lymph nodes, and for recurrent tumor after primary radical surgery. There are certain treatment plans which routinely involve various combinations of radiation and surgery.

One such approach combines the routine use of preoperative intracavitary radium or cesium with a subsequent radical hysterectomy for patients with Stages I B and II A cervical cancer. The rationale for this therapy is that the implant will devitalize the primary tumor and "seal" the paracervical lymphat-

TABLE 16. URETEROVAGINAL FISTULA RATE FOLLOWING PRIMARY SURGICAL TREATMENT OF STAGE I B AND II A CARCINOMA OF THE CERVIX

Authors	Patients	Fistula Rate
Blaikley et al. (1969)[250]	252	3.9%
Christensen et al. (1964)[268]	340	8.8%
Ketcham et al. (1971)[269]	42	7.1%
Masterson (1967)[271]	180	4.4%
Mickal et al. (1972)[258]	64	1.6%
Park et al. (1973)[272]	126	0.0%
Symmonds (1966)[298]	64	0.0%
Average		4.8%

(From Hoskins WJ, et al: Gynecol Oncol 4:278, 1976, with permission.)[249]

ics, and hence reduce the incidence of central recurrence. Surwit and colleagues[278] compared two groups of patients with Stage I B tumors—one group treated with radium and a subsequent radical hysterectomy with lymphadenectomy and the other group with radical surgery alone. There was no significant difference in morbidity between the groups, but the 5-year survival of the radium-treated group was 90 percent compared to 75 percent for those treated with surgery alone. One of the most prominent proponents of this approach is Stallworthy,[279] but a number of other authors have reported good results, utilizing either radical hysterectomy[280-282] or radical vaginal hysterectomy.[283] Despite the theoretic advantages of the combined approach, there is no good evidence that it improves the prognosis when compared to results in patients carefully selected for treatment by radiation or surgery alone.

Another approach to treatment was proposed by Quigley and associates[284] who used a three-stage protocol combining surgery and radiotherapy for treating 136 patients with Stage I B cervical cancer. Treatment consisted of two radium applications followed 6 weeks later by an extraperitoneal lymphadenectomy. If the nodes were negative, a simple hysterectomy was performed in 3 to 6 months, but if they were positive external radiation was given instead of the hysterectomy. The incidence of positive nodes was 10 percent, there were minimal complications, and the actuarial 5-year survival was 89 percent. Again this is comparable to the results achieved by radiation or surgery alone in the best centers.

A special problem is the patient with the large barrel-shaped lesion. The shape and size make optimal radiation dosage to the entire tumor difficult and central recurrence more likely.[285] Fletcher and colleagues[286] proposed that such patients be treated with a slightly reduced radiation dosage, followed by extrafascial hysterectomy. This approach appears to be effective in reducing recurrence rates in patients with large central lesions[287] and with Stage I B tumors over 5 cm in diameter,[208] and the morbidity is within acceptable limits.

PELVIC EXENTERATION

In patients with recurrent carcinoma of the cervix, who have already received a full course of radiation, pelvic exenteration offers the only hope for cure. Such patients have only about a 10 percent chance of surviving 1 year, and virtually no chance for 5-year survival.[288] In carefully selected patients with central recurrence and no evidence of metastatic spread, exenteration offers 5-year survival rates of about 30 percent (Table 17). Where exenteration is performed as a primary procedure, the survival rate is almost doubled. Only a small proportion of patients with recurrent tumors will be candidates for exenteration and the reported survival rates depend on the care with which patients are selected.

The operative mortality rate is of the order of 10 percent and the morbid-

TABLE 17. THE OPERATIVE MORTALITY RATES, AND 5-YEAR SURVIVAL RATES FOR PATIENTS TREATED FOR ADVANCED OR RECURRENT CERVICAL CANCER BY PELVIC EXENTERATION

Authors	Patients	Operative Mortality	5-Year Survivors
Douglas and Sweeney (1957)[289]	23	4%	22%
Parsons and Friedell (1964)[290]	112	21%	21%
Brunschwig (1965)[291]	535	16%	20%
Kiselow et al. (1967)[292]	153	10%	35%
Krieger and Embree (1969)[293]	35	11%	37%
Ketcham et al. (1970)[294]	162	7%	38%
Symmonds et al. (1975)[295]	198	8%	32%
Morley and Lindenauer (1976)[297]	34	3%	62%
Rutledge et al. (1977)[296]	296	14%	33%
Average	1548	13%	29%

ity is high, especially after radiotherapy. Exenteration should be performed only by individuals with adequate experience, who are willing to accept responsibility for the prolonged postoperative care and rehabilitation required by patients after such radical surgery. The patients and their families should be fully informed of the nature of the procedure so they may be psychologically, as well as physically prepared for it.[298]

While an anterior exenteration, with preservation of the rectum, or a posterior exenteration, with preservation of the bladder, are occasionally possible, it is generally wiser to perform a total exenteration in patients who have a recurrence after radiation. In this procedure the patient has both a colostomy and a urinary conduit constructed. In many cases a supralevator procedure is feasible, with preservation of the vulva. This will facilitate the production of a functional vagina using the safe and relatively simple Williams' procedure.[299,300]

CHEMOTHERAPY

Overall, the results of chemotherapy for cervical cancer have been disappointing. For patients with nonresectable Stages III and IV disease, regional chemotherapy appeared to have great promise, but this was not borne out, even when a closed technique was used.[301] A comparison of regional perfusion with the simpler technique of intra-arterial perfusion revealed that the simpler technique was equally effective, but with significantly less side effects.[302] The value of these techniques appears to be very limited.[303]

Reports of systemic chemotherapy, utilizing many different regimens, show disappointing results in terms of survival times. The most commonly evaluated agents are bleomycin, doxorubicin, mitomycin C, and cisplatin, in various combinations. While response rates are encouraging, survival times are still short and toxicity is often severe.[304–309] We have used a combination of cyclophosphamide, doxorubicin, and cisplatin in the treatment of 26 patients with advanced and recurrent cervical cancer. The actuarial survival rates were 38 percent at 1 year and 25 percent at 2 years, although the median survival time was only 8 months. We consider these results sufficiently encouraging to continue with this type of therapy at the present time.

ADENOCARCINOMA OF THE CERVIX

Primary adenocarcinoma accounts for less than 10 percent of invasive carcinomas of the cervix.[310] Although the mean age of patients with these tumors is generally said to be younger than that of patients with squamous carcinoma, two recent reports found no difference.[311,312] The disease is significantly more common in nulliparous women, those with hypertension, and those from rural areas, and appears to be epidemiologically closer to endometrial cancer than squamous carcinoma of the cervix.[311] Areas of adenosquamous carcinoma may be present in one-third of patients.[313] It is generally stated that adenocarcinoma has a significantly higher recurrence rate and a poorer prognosis than squamous carcinoma.[312] This may be due to the fact that there is sometimes very deep invasion into the lower uterine segment, so that the tumors are not adequately treated by the techniques used for squamous cell carcinoma. Patients with endometrial extension have a high incidence of intrauterine residual disease after radiation. Adenocarcinoma has generally been considered more radioresistant, probably because of the endophytic nature of the lesion, rather than the cell type itself. For the primary treatment of adenocarcinoma of the cervix, there are proponents of radiation alone[314,315] and those who advocate a combination of radiation and surgery.[310,316,317] We agree with Shingleton and associates[313] that treatment should be individualized.

For patients with small Stage I lesions, we believe radical hysterectomy and pelvic lymphadenectomy is the best treatment, provided the patient is suitable for surgery. Otherwise radiotherapy is used. Postradiation hysterectomy is probably not required unless the tumor appears to respond poorly to radiation.

For large or barrel-shaped Stage I B lesions and Stage II disease, external radiation and intracavitary radium or cesium should be followed by an extrafascial hysterectomy and bilateral salpingo-ophorectomy.

Stage III tumors are treated with radiation. Surgery is not routinely used and is only indicated for a central residual tumor with the pelvic wall free of disease.

CERVICAL CARCINOMA IN PREGNANCY

This is not a common problem, although the incidence of cervical neoplasia in pregnancy varies markedly according to the overall incidence of the disease in the population under study. A review of 14 reports gave the incidence of carcinoma in situ in pregnancy as 1:770 pregnancies and for invasive carcinoma as 1:2205 pregnancies.[318] A complete pelvic examination and routine Papanicolaou smear in the prenatal period will avoid delay in diagnosis. All pregnant patients with abnormal smears should have colposcopy and directed biopsies. For lesions less than microinvasion (Fig. 19), close observation and follow-up with vaginal delivery and definitive treatment after delivery are appropriate. Suspected microinvasion usually requires cold knife conization to exclude frank invasion and allow planning of further therapy. Frankly invasive disease is treated according to the stage of the disease, the duration of the pregnancy, and the mother's desire for a child. Vaginal delivery itself does not appear to worsen the prognosis for cervical cancer,[318] but vaginal delivery through an invasive tumor is likely to produce severe hemorrhage and may disseminate tumor cells.

Cervical Intraepithelial Neoplasia (CIN 1, 2, and 3)
The patient is followed closely with colposcopy and allowed vaginal delivery. Reevaluation is carried out 6 to 8 weeks postpartum and appropriate therapy

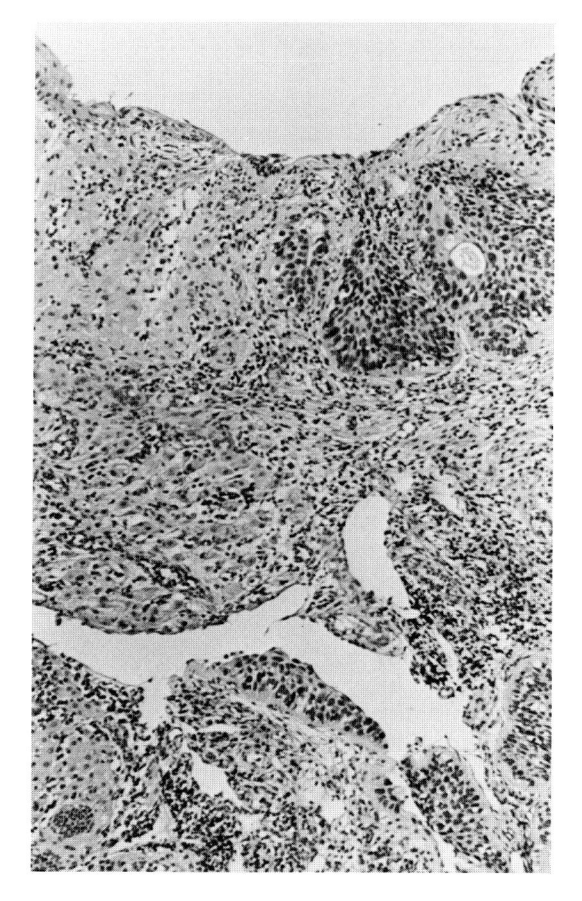

Figure 19. Carcinoma in situ of the cervix in pregnancy. The upper left field exhibits decidual change within the stroma of the cervix. Endocervical glands are involved, but there is no stromal invasion.

is planned. In a patient having a cesarean section for obstetric reasons, cesarean hysterectomy is a logical approach if the patient does not desire further children.

Microinvasion
If cone biopsy indicates the lesion is less than 3 mm in depth, without confluence or lymph-vascular permeation, the patient is followed carefully, allowed vaginal delivery, and treated definitively postpartum. If cesarean section is indicated, a cesarean hysterectomy may be performed.

Stages I B and II A
If the diagnosis is made before the twenty-fourth week of pregnancy, we advise radical hysterectomy and pelvic lymphadenectomy. Between the twenty-fourth and twenty-eighth weeks of pregnancy, treatment may be delayed until the fetus has a better chance of survival, provided the patient understands the risks involved. Specialists in maternal-fetal medicine and neonatology should be consulted. Once the fetus is sufficiently mature a radical cesarean hysterectomy and lymphadenectomy are performed. If the patient is a poor surgical candidate radiation is the treatment of choice.

Stages II B, III, and IV
Radiotherapy is the treatment of choice. In general 4000 to 5000 rads of teletherapy is given. In early pregnancy this will cause an abortion. In later pregnancy hysterotomy or cesarean section should be performed first, with neonatologists present to care for the baby. Radium or cesium applications complete the treatment after the uterus is evacuated.

FOLLOW-UP AFTER TREATMENT FOR CERVICAL CANCER

The majority of recurrences occur in the first 2 years after treatment. In a recent study 58 percent of recurrences were detected in the first year after primary therapy, 76 percent within 2 years, and only 5 percent after 5 years.[208] These figures are in broad agreement with those in earlier reports.[319-321] The most common site of recurrence is the pelvis,[319-321] although with better local control through improved techniques of radiotherapy and surgery it is likely that this pattern may change.

Patients should be seen every 1 to 2 months for the first year, every 2 to 4 months for the second year, and about every 4 to 6 months subsequently. The patient must understand the importance of follow-up. As most recurrences occur in the pelvis, and these are the type most amenable to treatment, it is essential that cytology be performed at least every 3 to 4 months and that careful inspection of the cervix and vagina be performed at each visit, together with a thorough rectovaginal examination. In the absence of regular intercourse the vagina tends to contract after radiotherapy, and patients not having regular coitus should be encouraged to use dilators to maintain vaginal patency, thus facilitating follow-up examination. Chest x-rays and intravenous pyelograms should be performed annually, or more often, when there is the suspicion of a recurrence.

In van Nagell's[208] series, only 10 percent of patients were asymptomatic at the time recurrence was diagnosed. This is in contrast with the findings of Munnell and Bonney[320] and of Halpin and colleagues[321] where the majority of recurrences were asymptomatic. The triad of weight loss, leg edema, and pelvic or sciatic pain is a particularly ominous set of symptoms. Although ureteric obstruction may result from radiation-induced fibrosis, this is extremely rare and a recurrent tumor is a more likely cause. If any form of curative procedure is to be performed it is essential that recurrences are detected early, and preferably well before there is sufficient tumor bulk to produce symptoms. The key to this is constant vigilance and the free use of biopsies when there is any suspicion of recurrence.

Documenting a suspected recurrence is often difficult. Shepherd and associates[322] showed that Papanicolaou smears accurately predicted recurrent cervical carcinoma in about 66 percent of cases and punch biopsies in about 80 percent. These errors can be explained by a variety of mechanisms, but in particular by the fact that recurrences may not be on the vaginal epithelium, or if they are, may be covered by a layer of necrotic tissue which prevent the correct diagnosis from being made. Because of this, Shepherd and colleagues[322] advised examination under anesthesia and needle biopsy of suspicious areas, and especially the deeper tissues of the cervix and parametrium using prostatic biopsy needles. This technique proved accurate in diagnosing recurrence in 96 percent of cases. On occasion the suspicion of recurrence may be so strong that even in the absence of demonstrable tumor a laparotomy may be advisable in an attempt to both document the lesion, and if it is present and resectable, to treat it.

While it is readily apparent that the cure of recurrent cervical cancer is dependent on early diagnosis, it is often difficult to accurately assess the amount of tumor present by clinical examination, as the combination of radiation and surgery will often produce dense fibrosis within the pelvis. In such cases laparotomy will often be the final arbiter of resectability, provided that the patient is a suitable candidate for pelvic exenteration.

REFERENCES

1. Jackson AR, quoted in Speert H: Obstetrics and Gynecology in America: A History. Chicago: Am Coll Obstet Gynecol, 1980, p 57
2. Munde P, quoted in Speert H: Obstetrics and Gynecology in America: A History. Chicago: Am Coll Obstet Gynecol, 1980, p 58
3. Ewing J: The prevention of cancer. In Cancer Control. Report of an International Symposium held under the auspices of the American Society for the Control of Cancer, Lake Mohonk, New York, 1926, p 169

4. Maclean JS: The life of Hans Hinselmann. Obstet Gynecol Survey 34:788, 1979
5. Schiller W: Looking back: Med J Aust, August 3, 1929, and Throsby T: A new clinical test for carcinoma of the cervix. Med J Aust 1:149, 1983
6. Schiller W: Early diagnosis of carcinoma of the cervix. Surg Gynecol Obstet 56:210, 1933
7. Babes A: Diagnosis of cancer of the uterine cervix by smears. La Presse Medicale 36:451, 1928 (Reprinted in translation in Acta Cytologica 11:217, 1967)
8. Papanicolaou GN: New cancer diagnosis. In Proceedings of the Third Race Betterment Conference, Battle Creek, Michigan. Race Betterment Foundation, 1928, p 528
9. Viana O: The early diagnosis of uterine cancer by smears. La Clinica Obstetrica 30:781, 1928 (Reprinted in translation in Acta Cytologica 14:544, 1970)
10. Papanicolaou GN, Traut HF: The diagnostic value of vaginal smears in carcinoma of the uterus. Am J Obstet Gynecol 42:193, 1943
11. Meigs JV, Graham RM, Fremont-Smith M, et al: The value of the vaginal smear in the diagnosis of uterine cancer. Surg Gynecol Obstet 77:449, 1943
12. Hinsey JC: George Nicholas Papanicolaou. Acta Cytol 6:483, 1962
13. Williams, quoted by Hertig AT: Early concepts of dysplasia and carcinoma in situ (a backward glance at a forward process): A brief historical review. Obstet Gynecol Survey 34:795, 1979
14. Schauenstein W: Histologishe untersuching uber atypisches plattenepithels an der portio und an der innenflache der cervix uteri. Arch Gynak 85:576, 1908
15. Rubin IC: The pathological diagnosis of incipient carcinoma of the uterus. Am J Obstet 62:668, 1910
16. Coppleson M: Cervical intraepithelial neoplasia: Clinical features and management. In Coppleson M (ed): Gynecologic Oncology: Fundamental Principles and Clinical Practice. New York: Churchill Livingstone, 1981, p 408
17. Richart RM: Colpomicroscopic studies of cervical intraepithelial neoplasia. Cancer 19:395, 1966
18. Richart RM: Cervical intraepithelial neoplasia. In Sommers SC (ed): Pathology Annual: 1973. New York: Appleton-Century-Crofts, 1973
19. Clark JG: More radical method of performing hysterectomy for cancer of the uterus. Johns Hopkins Hosp Bull 6:120, 1895
20. Wertheim E: Discussion on the diagnosis and treatment of cancer of the uterus. Br Med J 2:689, 1905
21. Schauta F: Die erweiterte vaginale total extirpation des uterus bei kollumkarzinom. Wien-Liepzig: Safar, 1908
22. Abbe, quoted by Kjellgren O: Clinical invasive carcinoma of cervix: Place of radiotherapy as primary treatment. In Coppleson M (ed): Gynecologic Oncology: Fundamental Principles and Clinical Practice. New York: Churchill Livingstone, 1981, p 482
23. Meigs JV: Carcinoma of the cervix. The Wertheim operation. Surg Gynecol Obstet 78:195, 1944
24. Meigs JV: The Wertheim operation for carcinoma of the cervix. Am J Obstet Gynecol 49:542, 1945
25. Devesa SS, Silverman DT: Cancer incidence and mortality trends in the United States: 1935–74. J Natl Cancer Inst 60:545, 1978
26. Lee HP, Cuello C, Singh K: Review of the epidemiology of cervical cancer in the Pacific basin. Natl Cancer Inst Monogr 62:197, 1982

27. Kim K, Rigal RD, Patrick JR, et al: The changing trends of uterine cancer and cytology. A study of morbidity and mortality trends over a 20 year period. Cancer 42:2439, 1978
28. Peters RK, Mack TM, Bernstein L: Parallels in the epidemiology of selected anogenital carcinomas. J Natl Cancer Inst 72:609, 1984
29. American Cancer Society: Cancer Facts and Figures, 1984. New York: American Cancer Society, 1984
30. Christopherson WM, Lundin FE, Mendel WM, Parker JE: Cervical cancer control. A study of mortality rates over a 20 year period. Cancer 38:1357, 1976
31. MacGregor JE, Teper S: Mortality from carcinoma of the cervix uteri in Britain. Lancet 2:774, 1978
32. Armstrong B, Holman D: Increasing mortality from cancer of the cervix in young Australian women. Med J Aust 1:460, 1981
33. Bourne RG, Grove WD: Invasive carcinoma of the cervix in Queensland. Change in incidence and mortality, 1959–1980. Med J Aust 1:156, 1983
34. Green GH: Rising cervical cancer mortality in young New Zealand women. N Z Med J 89:89, 1979
35. Anello C, Lao C: U.S. trends in mortality from cancer of the cervix. Lancet 1:1038, 1979
36. Stout AP: Observations on biopsy diagnosis of tumors. Cancer 10:912, 1957
37. Richart RM: CIN or not CIN? Dr. Richart replies. Acta Cytol 27:546, 1983
38. Koss LG: Dysplasia. Real concept or misnomer? Obstet Gynecol 51:374, 1978
39. Buckley CH, Butler EB, Fox H: Cervical intraepithelial neoplasia. J Clin Path 35:1, 1982
40. Stern E, Neely PM: Carcinoma and dysplasia of the cervix. A comparison of rates for new and returning populations. Acta Cytol 7:357, 1973
41. Fox CH: Biologic behavior of dysplasia and carcinoma in situ. Am J Obstet Gynecol 99:960, 1967
42. Barron BA, Richart RM: A statistical model of the natural history of cervical carcinoma based on a prospective study of 557 cases. J Natl Cancer Inst 41:1343, 1968
43. Richart RM, Barron BA: A follow-up study of patients with cervical dysplasia. Am J Obstet Gynecol 105:386, 1969
44. Nasiell K, Nasiell M, Vaclavinkova V: Behavior of moderate cervical dysplasia during long-term follow-up. Obstet Gynecol 61:609, 1983
45. Petersen O: Precancerous changes in the cervical epithelium in relation to manifest cervical carcinoma. Acta Radiologica (supp) 127, 1955
46. Lange P: Clinical and histological studies on cervical carcinoma. Precancerosis, Early Metastasis and Tubular Structures in the Lymph Nodes. Copenhagen: Munksgaard, 1960, p 27
47. Gad C: The management and natural history of severe dysplasia and carcinoma in situ of the uterine cervix. Br J Obstet Gynaecol 83:554, 1976
48. Barron BA, Cahill MC, Richart RM: A statistical model of the natural history of cervical neoplastic disease: The duration of carcinoma in situ. Gynecol Oncol 6:196, 1978
49. Coppleson LW, Brown B: Observations on a model of the biology of carcinoma of the cervix: A poor fit between observation and theory. Am J Obstet Gynecol 122:127, 1975
50. Bamford PN, Beilby JOW, Steele SJ, Vlies R: The natural history of cervical

intraepithelial neoplasia as determined by cytology and colposcopic biopsy. Acta Cytol 27:482, 1983
51. Beilby JOW, Bourne R, Guillebrand J, Steele SJ: Paired cervical smears: A method of reducing the false negative rate in population screening. Obstet Gynecol 60:46, 1982
52. Cramer DW, Cutler SJ: Incidence and histopathology of malignancies of the female genital organs in the United States. Am J Obstet Gynecol 118:443, 1974
53. Walton RJ, Blanchet M, Boyes DA, et al: Cervical cancer screening programs. 1. Epidemiology and natural history of carcinoma of the cervix. Can Med Assoc J 114:1003, 1976
54. Stern E: Epidemiology of dysplasia. Obstet Gynecol Survey 24:711, 1969
55. Feldman MJ, Kent DR, Pennington RL: Intraepithelial neoplasia of the uterine cervix in the teenager. Cancer 41:1405, 1978
56. Christopherson WM, Parker JE: A study of the relative frequency of carcinoma of the cervix in the negro. Cancer 13:711, 1960
57. Barron BA, Richart RM: An epidemiologic study of cervical neoplastic disease. Cancer 27:978, 1971
58. Rotkin ID: A comparison review of key epidemiologic studies in cervical cancer related to current searches for transmissible agents. Cancer Res 33:1353, 1973
59. Briggs RM: Dysplasia and early neoplasia of the uterine cervix. Obstet Gynecol Survey 34:70, 1979
60. Koss LG, Philips A: Summary and recommendations of the workshop on uterine cervical cancer. Cancer 33:1573, 1974
61. Harris RWC, Brinton LA, Cowdell RH, et al: Characteristics of women with dysplasia or carcinoma in situ of the cervix uteri. Br J Cancer 42:359, 1980
62. Handley WS: The prevention of cancer. Lancet 1:987, 1936
63. Terris M, Wilson F, Nelson JH: Relation of circumcision to cancer of the cervix. Am J Obstet Gynecol 117:1056, 1973
64. Cervical Cancer Screening Programs: Summary of the 1982 Canadian Task Force report. Can Med Assoc J 127:581, 1982
65. Gagnon F: Contribution to the study of etiology and prevention of cancer of the cervix and of the uterus. Am J Obstet Gynecol 60:516, 1950
66. Wynder EL: Epidemiology of carcinoma in situ of the cervix. Obstet Gynecol Survey 24:697, 1969
67. Nahmias AJ, Sawanabori S: The genital herpes-cervical cancer hypothesis. Ten years later. Prog Exp Tumor Res 21:117, 1978
68. Kessler II: Human cervical cancer as a venereal disease. Cancer Res 36:783, 1976
69. Melnick JL, Adam E: Epidemiological approaches to determining whether herpesvirus is the etiological agent of cervical cancer. Prog Exp Tumor Res 21:49, 1978
70. Royston I, Aurelian L: Immunofluorescent detection of herpes virus antigens in exfoliated cells from human cervical carcinoma. Proc Natl Acad Sci 67:204, 1970
71. Cabral GA, Fry D, Marciano-Cabral F, et al: A herpesvirus antigen in human premalignant and malignant cervical biopsies and explants. Am J Obstet Gynecol 145:79, 1983
72. Jariwalla RJ, Aurelian L, Tso PDP: Neoplastic transformation of Syrian hamster embryo cells by DNA of herpes simplex virus type 2. J Virol 30:404, 1979
73. Nahmias AJ, Roizman R: Infections with herpes simplex viruses 1 and 2. N Engl J Med 289:667, 1973

74. Franklin E, Jenkins R: Prospective studies of the association of genital herpes simplex infection and cervical anaplasia. Cancer Res 33:1491, 1973
75. Reid R: Genital warts and cervical cancer. II. Is human papillomavirus infection the trigger to cervical carcinogenesis? Gynecol Oncol 15:239, 1983
76. Crum CP, Egawa K, Barron B, et al: Human papillomavirus infection (condyloma) of the cervix and cervical intraepithelial neoplasia: A histologic and statistical analysis. Gynecol Oncol 15:88, 1983
77. Meisels A, Morin C: Human papillomavirus and cancer of the uterine cervix. Gynecol Oncol 12:S111, 1981
78. Syrjanen KJ: Human papillomavirus lesions in association with cervical dysplasias and neoplasias. Obstet Gynecol 62:617, 1983
79. Fujii T, Crum CP, Winkler B, et al: Human papillomavirus infection and cervical intraepithelial neoplasia: Histopathology and DNA content. Obstet Gynecol 63:99, 1984
80. Coppleson M: The origin and nature of premalignant lesions of the cervix uteri. Int J Gynecol Obstet 8:539, 1970
81. Singer A, Reid BL, Coppleson M: A hypothesis: The role of a high risk male in the etiology of cervical carcinoma. A correlation of epidemiology and molecular biology. Am J Obstet Gynecol 126:110, 1976
82. Reid BL, French PW, Singer A, et al: Sperm basic proteins in cervical carcinogenesis: Correlation with socioeconomic class. Lancet 2:60, 1978
83. Fish EN, Tobin SM, Cooter NBE, Papsin FR: Update on the relation of herpesvirus hominus type II to carcinoma of the cervix. Obstet Gynecol 59:220, 1982
84. Stafl A, Friedrich EG, Mattingly RF: Detection of cervical neoplasia. Reducing the risk of error. Clin Obstet Gynecol 16:238, 1973
85. Blaustein RL: Cytology of the female genital tract. In Blaustein A (ed): Pathology of the Female Genital Tract, 2nd ed. New York: Springer–Verlag, 1982, p 838
86. Johansen P, Arffmann E, Pallesen G: Evaluation of smears obtained by cervical scraping and an endocervical swab in the diagnosis of neoplastic diseases of the uterine cervix. Acta Obstet Gynecol Scand 58:265, 1979
87. Richart RM, Vaillant HW: Influence of cell collection technic upon cytologic diagnosis. Cancer 18:1474, 1965
88. Rubio CA, Stormby N, Kock Y, Thomassen P: Studies on the distribution of abnormal cells in cytological preparations. VI. Pressure exerted by the gynecologist during smearing. Gynecol Oncol 15:391, 1983
89. Morell ND, Taylor JR, Snyder RN, et al: False-negative cytology rates in patients in whom invasive cervical cancer subsequently developed. Obstet Gynecol 60:41, 1982
90. Stafl A, Mattingly RF: Colposcopic diagnosis of cervical neoplasia. Obstet Gynecol 41:168, 1973
91. Drescher CW, Peters WA, Roberts JA: Contribution of endocervical curettage in evaluating abnormal cervical cytology. Obstet Gynecol 62:343, 1983
92. Hollyock VE, Chanen W: The use of the colposcope in the selection of patients for cervical cone biopsy. Am J Obstet Gynecol 114:185, 1972
93. Donohue LR, Meriwether W: Colposcopy as a diagnostic tool in the investigation of cervical neoplasias. Am J Obstet Gynecol 113:107, 1972
94. Praphat H, Taylor H, Mehra H, et al: Comparison of colposcopic directed biopsy and cold conization in 100 patients with abnormal cytology. Surg Gynecol Obstet 142:333, 1976

95. Creasman WT, Rutledge FN: Carcinoma in situ of the cervix uteri. Obstet Gynecol 39:373, 1972
96. Hall JE, Boyce JG, Nelson JH: Carcinoma in situ of the cervix uteri. Obstet Gynecol 34:221, 1969
97. Way S, Hennigan M, Wright VC: Some experiences with preinvasive and microinvasive carcinoma of the cervix. J Obstet Gynaecol Br Commonw 75:593, 1968
98. American College of Obstetricians and Gynecologists: Technical Bulletin No. 24. Gynecologic Cancer. August, 1973
99. Boyes DA, Worth JA, Fidler HK: The results of treatment of 4389 cases of preclinical cervical squamous carcinoma. J Obstet Gynaecol Br Commonw 77:769, 1970
100. Brudenell M, Cox BS, Taylor CW: The management of dysplasia, carcinoma in situ and microcarcinoma of the cervix. J Obstet Gynaecol Br Commonw 80:673, 1973
101. Kolstad P, Klem V: Long-term follow-up of 1121 cases of carcinoma in situ. Obstet Gynecol 48:175, 1976
102. Burghardt E, Holzer E: Treatment of carcinoma in situ: Evaluation of 1609 cases. Obstet Gynecol 55:539, 1980
103. Bjerre B, Eliason G, Linell F, et al: Conization as only treatment of carcinoma in situ of the uterine cervix. Am J Obstet Gynecol 125:143, 1976
104. Jones HW, Buller RE: The treatment of cervical intraepithelial neoplasia by cone biopsy. Am J Obstet Gynecol 125:143, 1976
105. Ahlgren M, Ingermarsson I, Linberg LG, Nordqvist SR: Conization as treatment of carcinoma in situ of the uterine cervix. Obstet Gynecol 46:135, 1975
106. Schulman H, Cavanagh D: Intraepithelial carcinoma of the cervix. The predictability of residual carcinoma in the uterus from microscopic study of the margins of the cone biopsy specimen. Cancer 14:795, 1961
107. Devereux WP, Edwards CL: Carcinoma in situ of the cervix. Applicability of diagnostic and treatment methods in 632 cases. Am J Obstet Gynecol 98:497, 1967
108. Ostergard DR: Prediction of clearance of cervical intraepithelial neoplasia by conization. Obstet Gynecol 56:77, 1980
109. Hester LL, Read RA: An evaluation of cervical conization. Am J Obstet Gynecol 80:715, 1960
110. Weber T, Obel EB: Pregnancy complications following conization of the uterine cervix. Acta Obstet Gynecol Scand 58:347, 1979
111. Groonroos M, Liukko P, Kilkku P, Punnonen R: Pregnancy and delivery after conization of the cervix. Acta Obstet Gynecol Scand 58:477, 1979
112. Larsson G, Grundsell H, Gullberg B, Svennerud S: Outcome of pregnancy after conization. Acta Obstet Gynecol Scand 61:461, 1982
113. Jones JM, Sweetnam P, Hibbard BM: The outcome of pregnancy after cone biopsy of the cervix: A case control study. Br J Obstet Gynaecol 86:913, 1979
114. Leiman G, Harrison NA, Rubin A: Pregnancy following conization of the cervix. Complications related to cone size. Am J Obstet Gynecol 136:14, 1980
115. Jordan JA: The diagnosis and management of premalignant lesions of the cervix. Clin Obstet Gynaecol 3:295, 1976
116. Dorsey JH, Diggs ES: Microsurgical conization of the cervix by carbon dioxide laser. Obstet Gynecol 54:565, 1979

117. Larsson G, Gullberg B, Grundsell H: A comparison of complications of laser and cold knife conization. Obstet Gynecol 62:213, 1983
118. Crisp WE, Asadourian L, Romberger W: Application of cryosurgery to gynecologic malignancy. Obstet Gynecol 30:668, 1967
119. Charles EH, Savage EW: Cryosurgical treatment of cervical intraepithelial neoplasia. Obstet Gynecol Survey 35:539, 1980
120. Ostergard DR: Cryosurgical treatment of cervical intraepithelial neoplasia. Obstet Gynecol 56:231, 1980
121. Richart RM, Townsend DE, Crisp W, et al: An analysis of "long-term" follow-up results in patients with cervical intraepithelial neoplasia treated by cryotherapy. Am J Obstet Gynecol 137:823, 1980
122. Benedet JL, Nickerson KG, Anderson GH: Cryotherapy in the treatment of cervical intraepithelial neoplasia. Obstet Gynecol 58:725, 1981
123. Charles EH, Savage EW, Hacker N, Jones NC: Cryosurgical treatment of cervical intraepithelial neoplasia. Gynecol Oncol 12:83, 1981
124. Hatch KD, Shingleton HM, Austin JM, et al: Cryosurgery of cervical intraepithelial neoplasia. Obstet Gynecol 57:692, 1981
125. Javaheri G, Balin M, Meltzer RM: Role of cryosurgery in the treatment of intraepithelial neoplasia of the uterine cervix. Obstet Gynecol 58:83, 1981
126. Monaghan JM, Davis JA, Eddington PT: Treatment of cervical intraepithelial neoplasia by colposcopically directed cryosurgery and subsequent pregnancy experience. Br J Obstet Gynaecol 89:387, 1982
127. Peckham BM, Sonek MG, Carr WF: Outpatient therapy: success and failure with dysplasia and carcinoma in situ. Am J Obstet Gynecol 142:323, 1982
128. Stuart GC, Anderson RJ, Corlett BM, Maruncic MA: Assessment of failures of cryosurgical treatment in cervical intraepithelial neoplasia. Am J Obstet Gynecol 142:658, 1982
129. Coney P, Walton LA, Edelman DA, Fowler WC: Cryosurgical treatment of early cervical intraepithelial neoplasia. Obstet Gynecol 62:463, 1983
130. Van Lent M, Trimbos JB, Heintz AP, Van Hall EV: Cryosurgical treatment of cervical intraepithelial neoplasia (CIN III) in 102 patients. Gynecol Oncol 16:240, 1983
131. Creasman WT, Hinshaw WM, Clarke-Pearson DL: Cryosurgery in the management of cervical intraepithelial neoplasia. Obstet Gynecol 63:145, 1984
132. Figge DC, Creasman WT: Cryotherapy in the treatment of cervical intraepithelial neoplasia. Obstet Gynecol 62:353, 1983
133. Charles EH, Savage EW: Cryosurgical treatment of cervical intraepithelial neoplasia. Analysis of failures. Gynecol Oncol 9:361, 1980
134. Townsend DE, Richart RM, Marks E, Nielsen J: Invasive cancer following outpatient evaluation and therapy for cervical disease. Obstet Gynecol 57:145, 1981
135. Kaufman RH, Irwin JF: The cryosurgical therapy of cervical intraepithelial neoplasia. III. Continuing follow-up. Am J Obstet Gynecol 131:381, 1978
136. Sevin BU, Ford JH, Girtanner RD, et al: Invasive cancer of the cervix after cryosurgery. Pitfalls of conservative management. Obstet Gynecol 53:465, 1979
137. Singer A, Walker P: What is the optimal treatment of cervical premalignancy? Br J Obstet Gynaecol 89:335, 1982
138. Younge PA, Hertig AT, Armstrong D: A study of 135 cases of carcinoma in situ of the cervix at the Free Hospital for Women. Am J Obstet Gynecol 58:867, 1949

139. Richart RM, Sciarra JJ: Treatment of cervical dysplasia by outpatient electrocauterization. Am J Obstet Gynecol 101:200, 1968
140. Hollyock VE, Chanen W: Electrocoagulation diathermy for the treatment of cervical dysplasia and carcinoma in situ. Obstet Gynecol 47:196, 1976
141. Chanen W, Rome RM: Electrocoagulation diathermy for cervical dysplasia and carcinoma in situ. A 15 year survey. Obstet Gynecol 61:673, 1983
142. Hollyock VE, Chanen W, Wein R: Cervical function following treatment of intraepithelial neoplasia by electrocoagulation diathermy. Obstet Gynecol 61:79, 1983
143. Jako GL: Laser surgery of the vocal cords. Laryngoscope 82:2204, 1972
144. Kaplan I, Goldman J, Ger R: The treatment of erosion of the uterine cervix by use of the CO_2 laser. Obstet Gynecol 41:795, 1973
145. Stafl A, Wilkinson EJ, Mattingly RS: Laser treatment of cervical and vaginal neoplasia. Am J Obstet Gynecol 128:125, 1977
146. Carter R, Krantz KE, Hara GS, et al: Treatment of cervical intraepithelial neoplasia with a carbon dioxide laser beam. A preliminary report. Am J Obstet Gynecol 131:831, 1978
147. Baggish MS: High power density carbon dioxide laser therapy for early cervical neoplasia. Am J Obstet Gynecol 136:117, 1980
148. Bellina JH, Seto YJ: Pathologic and physiologic investigations into the CO_2 laser-tissue interactions with specific emphasis on cervical intraepithelial neoplasia. Lasers Surg Med 1:47, 1980
149. Burke H, Lovell L, Antonioli D: Carbon dioxide laser therapy of cervical intraepithelial neoplasia. Factors determining success rate. Lasers Surg Med 1:113, 1980
150. Bellina JH, Wright VC, Voros JI, et al: Carbon dioxide laser management of cervical intraepithelial neoplasia. Am J Obstet Gynecol 141:828, 1981
151. Benedet JL, Nickerson KG, White GW: Laser therapy for cervical intraepithelial neoplasia. Obstet Gynecol 58:188, 1981
152. Wright VC, Davies EM: The conservative management of cervical intraepithelial neoplasia. The use of cryosurgery and the carbon dioxide laser. Br J Obstet Gynaecol 88:663, 1981
153. Anderson MC: Treatment of cervical intraepithelial neoplasia with the carbon dioxide laser. Report of 543 patients. Obstet Gynecol 59:720, 1982
154. Popkin DR: Treatment of cervical intraepithelial neoplasia with the carbon dioxide laser. Am J Obstet Gynecol 145:177, 1983
155. Townsend DE, Richart RM: Cryotherapy and carbon dioxide laser management of cervical intraepithelial neoplasia. A controlled comparison. Obstet Gynecol 61:75, 1983
156. Wright VC, Davies E, Riopelle MA: Laser surgery for cervical intraepithelial neoplasia. Principles and results. Am J Obstet Gynecol 145:181, 1983
157. Creasman WT, Clarke-Pearson DL, Weed JC: Results of outpatient therapy of cervical intraepithelial neoplasia. Gynecol Oncol 12:S306, 1981
158. Richardson AC, Lyon JB: The effect of condom use on squamous cell cervical intraepithelial neoplasia. Am J Obstet Gynecol 140:909, 1981
159. Kitay DZ, Wentz WB: Cervical cytology in folic acid deficiency of pregnancy. Am J Obstet Gynecol 104:931, 1969
160. Webb JL: Nutritional effects of oral contraceptive use. A review. J Reprod Med 25:150, 1980

161. Butterworth CE, Hatch KE, Gore H, et al: Improvement in cervical dysplasia associated with folic acid therapy in users of oral contraceptives. Am J Clin Nutr 35:73, 1982
162. Elias PM, Williams ML: Retinoids, cancer, and the skin. Arch Dermatol 117:160, 1981
163. Bollag W: Therapy of epithelial tumors with an aromatic retinoic acid analogue. Chemotherapy 21:236, 1975
164. Romney SL, Palan PB, Duttagupta C, et al: Retinoids and the prevention of cervical dysplasias. Am J Obstet Gynecol 141:890, 1981
165. Bernstein A, Harris B: The relationship of dietary and serum vitamin A to occurrence of cervical intraepithelial neoplasia in sexually active women. Am J Obstet Gynecol 148:309, 1984
166. Surwit EA, Graham V, Droegmueller W, et al: Evaluation of topically applied transretinoic acid in the treatment of cervical intraepithelial lesions. Am J Obstet Gynecol 143:821, 1982
167. Ikic D, Nola P, Maricic Z, et al: Application of human leucocyte interferon in patients with urinary bladdar papillomas, breast cancer, and melanoma. Lancet 1:1022, 1981
168. Ikic D, Padovan I, Brodarec I, et al: Application of human leucocyte interferon in patients with tumors of the head and neck. Lancet 1:1025, 1981
169. Ikic D, Krusic J, Kirhmajor V, et al: Application of human leucocyte interferon in patients with carcinoma of the uterine cervix. Lancet 1:1027, 1981
170. Moller BR, Johannesen P, Osther K, et al: Treatment of dysplasias of the cervical epithelium with an interferon gel. Obstet Gynecol 62:625, 1983
171. Mestwerdt C: Probexcision und kolposkopie in der fruhdiagnose des portiokarcinoms. Zentralbl Gynaekol 4:326, 1947
172. Friedell GH, Graham JB: Regional lymph node involvement in small carcinoma of the cervix. Surg Gynecol Obstet 108:513, 1959
173. Averette HE, Nelson JH, Ng AB, et al: Diagnosis and management of microinvasive (Stage IA) carcinoma of the uterine cervix. Cancer 38:414, 1976
174. Ruch RM: Microinvasive carcinoma of the cervix. A confusing dilemma. Southern Med J 63:1123, 1970
175. Nelson JH, Averette HE, Richart RM: Detection, diagnostic evaluation and treatment of dysplasia and early carcinoma of the cervix. CA: A Cancer Journal for Clinicians 25:134, 1975
176. Benson WL, Norris HJ: A critical review of the frequency of lymph node metastases and death from microinvasive carcinoma of the cervix. Obstet Gynecol 49:632, 1977
177. Sedlis A, Sall S, Tsukada Y, et al: Microinvasive carcinoma of the uterine cervix: A clinicopathologic study. Am J Obstet Gynecol 133:64, 1979
178. Van Nagell JR, Greenwell N, Powell DF, et al: Microinvasive carcinoma of the cervix. Am J Obstet Gynecol 145:981, 1983
179. Foushee SJ, Greiss FC, Lock FR: Stage IA squamous cell carcinoma of the uterine cervix. Am J Obstet Gynecol 105:46, 1969
180. Roche WD, Norris HJ: Microinvasive carcinoma of the cervix. The significance of lymphatic invasion and confluent patterns of stromal growth. Cancer 36:180, 1975
181. Leman MH, Benson WL, Kurman RJ, Park RC: Microinvasive carcinoma of the cervix. Obstet Gynecol 48:571, 1976

182. Seski JC, Abell MR, Morley GW: Microinvasive squamous of the cervix. Definition, histologic analysis, late results of treatment. Obstet Gynecol 50:410, 1977
183. Taki I, Sugimuri H, Matsuyama T, et al: Treatment of microinvasive carcinoma. Obstet Gynecol Survey 34:839, 1979
184. Yajima A, Noda K: The results of treatment of microinvasive carcinoma (Stage IA) of the uterine cervix by means of simple and extended hysterectomy. Am J Obstet Gynecol 135:685, 1979
185. Hasumi K, Sakamoto A, Sugano H: Microinvasive carcinoma of the uterine cervix. Cancer 45:928, 1980
186. Averette HE, Ford JH, Dudan RC, et al: Staging of cervical cancer. Clin Obstet Gynecol 18(3):215, 1975
187. Barber HR, Somers SC, Rotterdam H, Kwon T: Vascular invasion as a prognostic factor in Stage IB cancer of the cervix. Obstet Gynecol 52:343, 1978
188. Burghardt E, Holzer E: Diagnosis and treatment of microinvasive carcinoma of the cervix uteri. Obstet Gynecol 49:641, 1977
189. Coppleson M: Preclinical invasive carcinoma of cervix (microinvasive and occult invasive carcinoma): Clinical features and management. In Coppleson M (ed): Gynecologic Oncology. Fundamental Principles and Clinical Practice. New York: Churchill Livingstone, 1981, p 451
190. Averette HE: Discussion of paper by Van Nagell and associates.[178] Am J Obstet Gynecol 145:989, 1983
191. Iverson T, Abeler V, Kjorstad KE: Factors influencing the treatment of patients with stage IA carcinoma of the cervix. Br J Obstet Gynaecol 86:593, 1979
192. Larsson G, Alm P, Gullberg B, Grundsell H: Prognostic factors in early carcinoma of the uterine cervix. A clinical, histopathological and statistical analysis of 343 cases. Am J Obstet Gynecol 146:145, 1983
193. Fidler HK, Boyes DA: Patterns of early invasion from intraepithelial carcinoma of the cervix. Cancer 12:673, 1959
194. Lohe KJ: Early squamous cell carcinoma of the uterine cervix. I. Definition and Histology. Gynecol Oncol 6:10, 1978
195. Lohe KJ, Burghardt E, Hillemans HG, et al: Early squamous cell carcinoma of the uterine cervix. II. Clinical results of a cooperative study in the management of 419 patients with early stromal invasion and microcarcinoma. Gynecol Oncol 6:31, 1978
196. Fennell RH: Microinvasive carcinoma of the uterine cervix. Obstet Gynecol Survey 33:406, 1978
197. Creasman WT, Parker RJ: Microinvasive carcinoma of the cervix. Clin Obstet Gynecol 16(2):261, 1973
198. Ng AB, Reagan JW, Lindner EA: The cellular manifestations of microinvasive carcinoma of the uterine cervix. Acta Cytol 16:5, 1972
199. Johnston WW, Myers B, Creasman WT, Owens SM: Cytopathology and the management of early invasive cancer of the uterine cervix. Obstet Gynecol 60:350, 1982
200. Sugimeri H, Matsuyama T, Kasimura M, et al: Colposcopic findings in microinvasive carcinoma of the uterine cervix. Obstet Gynecol Survey 34:804, 1979
201. Boronow RC: Stage I cervix cancer and pelvic node metatstasis. Special reference to the implications of the new and the recently replaced FIGO classifications of Stage IA. Am J Obstet Gynecol 127:135, 1977

202. Wilkinson EJ, Komorowski RA: Borderline microinvasive carcinoma of the cervix. Obstet Gynecol 51:472, 1978
203. Lunt R: Worldwide early detection of cervical cancer. Obstet Gynecol 63:708, 1984
204. Devesa SS: Descriptive epidemiology of cancer of the uterine cervix. Obstet Gynecol 63:605, 1984
205. Reagan JW, Wentz WB: Genesis of carcinoma of the uterine cervix. Clin Obstet Gynecol 10:883, 1967
206. Wentz WB, Reagan JW: Survival in cervical cancer with respect to cell type. Cancer 12:384, 1959
207. Swan DS, Roddick JW: A clinical-pathological correlation of cell type classification for cervical cancer. Am J Obstet Gynecol 116:666, 1973
208. Van Nagell JR, Rayburn W, Donaldson ES, et al: Therapeutic implications of patterns of recurrence in cancer of the uterine cervix. Cancer 44:2354, 1979
209. Nahhas WA, Chung CK, Stryker JA, et al: Relationship between histologic grading and extrapelvic nodal metastases in cervical carcinoma. Gynecol Oncol 11:191, 1981
210. Beecham JB, Halvorsen T, Kolbenstvedt A: Histologic classification, lymph node metastases, and patient survival in Stage IB cervical carcinoma. An analysis of 245 uniformly treated cases. Gynecol Oncol 6:95, 1978
211. Prempree T, Patanaphan V, Sewchand W, Scott RM: The influence of the patient's age and tumor grade on the prognosis of carcinoma of the cervix. Cancer 51:1764, 1983
212. Reagan JW: Cellular pathology and uterine cancer. Am J Clin Pathol 62:150, 1974
213. Sedlacek TV, Mangan CE, Giuntoli RC, et al: Exploratory celiotomy for cervical carcinoma: The role of histological grading. Gynecol Oncol 6:138, 1978
214. Rotmensch J, Rosenshein NB, Woodruff JD: Cervical sarcoma: A review. Obstet Gynecol Survey 38:456, 1983
215. Praphat H, Ruffolo EH, Copeland WJ, et al: Carcinoma of the cervix: A diagnostic problem. Am J Obstet Gynecol 137:514, 1980
216. Hendriksen E: The lymphatic spread of carcinoma of the cervix and of the body of the uterus. Am J Obstet Gynecol 58:924, 1949
217. Plentyl AA, Friedman E: Lymphatic system of the female genitalia. In The Morphologic Basis of Oncologic Diagnosis and Therapy, vol 2. Philadelphia: Saunders, 1971
218. Piver MS, Chung WS: Prognostic significance of cervical lesion size and pelvic node metastasis in cervical carcinoma. Obstet Gynecol 46:507, 1975
219. Burghardt E, Pickel H: Local spread and lymph node involvement in cervical cancer. Obstet Gynecol 52:138, 1975
220. Bleker OP, Ketting BW, Van Wayjen-Eecen GJ, et al: The significance of microscopic involvement of the parametrium and/or pelvic lymph nodes in cervical cancer stages IB and IIA. Gynecol Oncol 16:56, 1983
221. Martinbeau PW, Kjorstadt KE, Iversen T: Stage IB carcinoma of the cervix, the Norwegian Radium Hospital. II. Results when pelvic nodes are involved. Obstet Gynecol 60:215, 1982
222. Van Nagell JR, Donaldson ES, Wood EG, Parker JC: The significance of vascular invasion and lymphocytic infiltration in invasive cervical cancer. Cancer 41:288, 1978

223. Ucmakli A, Bonney WA, Palladino A: The nonlymphatic metastasis of carcinoma of the uterine cervix. Cancer 41:1027, 1978
224. Classification and Staging of Malignant Tumors of the Female Pelvis. ACOG Technical Bulletin No. 47, June, 1977
225. Villasanta V, Whitley NO, Haney PJ, Brenner D: Computed tomography in invasive carcinoma of the cervix: An appraisal. Am J Obstet Gynecol 62:218, 1983
226. Piver MS, Barlow, JJ: Para-aortic lymphadenectomy aortic node biopsy, and aortic lymphangiography in staging patients with advanced cervical cancer. Cancer 32:367, 1973
227. Brown RC, Buchsbaum HJ, Tewfik HH, Platz CE: Accuracy of lymphangiography in the diagnosis of para-aortic lymph node metastases from carcinoma of the cervix. Obstet Gynecol 54:571, 1979
228. Nordqvist SR, Sevin BV, Nadji M, et al: Fine needle aspiration cytology in gynecologic oncology. I. Diagnostic accuracy. Obstet Gynecol 54:719, 1979
229. Disaia PJ, Morrow CP, Haverback BJ, Dyce BJ: Carcinoembryonic antigen in cervical and vulvar cancer patients. Serum levels and disease progress. Obstet Gynecol 47:95, 1976
230. Fritsche HA, Freedman RS, Liu F, et al: A survey of tumor markers in patients with squamous cell carcinoma of the uterine cervix. Gynecol Oncol 14:230, 1982
231. Stage AH, Thomson JM: The use of pelvic artiography in assessing carcinoma of the cervix. Obstet Gynecol 52:151, 1978
232. Zaritsky D, Blake D, Willard J, Resnick M: Transrectal ultrasonography in the evaluation of cervical carcinoma. Obstet Gynecol 53:105, 1979
233. Kato H, Morioka H, Aramaki S, et al: Prognostic significance of the tumor antigen TA-4 in squamous cell carcinoma of the uterine cervix. Am J Obstet Gynecol 145:350, 1983
234. Berman ML, Lagasse LD, Watring WG, et al: The operative evaluation of patients with cervical carcinoma by an extraperitoneal approach. Obstet Gynecol 50:658, 1977
235. Averette HA, Dudan RC, Ford JH: Exploratory celiotomy for surgical staging of cervical cancer. Am J Obstet Gynecol 113:1090, 1972
236. Buchsbaum HJ: Para-aortic lymph node involvement in cervical carcinoma. Am J Obstet Gynecol 113:942, 1972
237. Nelson JH, Boyce J, Macaset M, et al: Incidence, significance and follow-up of para-aortic lymph node metastases in late invasive carcinoma of the cervix. Am J Obstet Gynecol 128:336, 1977
238. Sudarsanam A, Komandri C, Belinson J, et al: Influence of exploratory celiotomy on the management of carcinoma of the cervix: A preliminary report. Cancer 41:1049, 1978
239. Lagasse LD, Creasman WT, Shingleton HM, et al: Results and complications of operative staging in cervical cancer. Experience of the Gynecologic Oncology group. Gynecol Oncol 9:90, 1980
240. Wharton JT, Jones HW, Day TG, et al: Preirradiation celiotomy and extended field irradiation for invasive carcinoma of the cervix. Obstet Gynecol 49:333, 1977
241. Piver MS, Barlow JJ: High dose irradiation to biopsy confirmed aortic node metastases from carcinoma of the uterine cervix. Cancer 39:1243, 1977
242. Goldson AL, Delgado G, Hill LT: Intraoperative radiation of para-aortic nodes in carcinoma of the uterine cervix. Obstet Gynecol 52:713, 1978

243. Delgado G, Goldson AL, Ashayeri E, et al: Intraoperative radiation in the treatment of advanced cervical cancer. Obstet Gynecol 62:246, 1984
244. Buchsbaum HJ: Extrapelvic lymph node metastasis in cervical carcinoma. Am J Obstet Gynecol 133:814, 1979
245. Brandt B, Lifschitz S: Scalene node biopsy in advanced carcinoma of the cervix uteri. Cancer 47:1920, 1981
246. Piver MS, Barlow JJ, Krishnamsetty R: Five year survival (with no evidence of disease) in patients with biopsy-confirmed aortic node metastasis from cervical carcinoma. Am J Obstet Gynecol 139:575, 1981
247. Hamberger AD, Fletcher GH, Wharton JT: Results of treatment of early Stage I carcinoma of the uterine cervix with intracavitary radium alone. Cancer 41:980, 1978
248. Fletcher GH: Textbook of Radiotherapy, 3rd ed., Philadelphia: Lea & Febiger, 1980, p 720
249. Hoskins WJ, Ford JH, Lutz MH, Averette HE: Radical hysterectomy and pelvic lymphadenectomy for the management of early invasive carcinoma of the cervix. Gynecol Oncol 4:278, 1976
250. Blaikley JB, Ledarman M, Pollard W: Carcinoma of the cervix at Chelsea Hospital for Women. Five and ten year results of treatment. J Obstet Gynaecol Br Commw 76:729, 1969
251. Dickson RJ: Late results of radium treatment of carcinoma of the cervix. Radiol 23:528, 1972
252. Fletcher GH: Cancer of the uterine cervix. Am J Roentgenol Radium Ther Nucl 111:225, 1971
253. Kline JC, Schultz AE, Vermund H, Peckham BM: High dose radiotherapy for carcinoma of the cervix. Method and results. Am J Obstet Gynecol 104:479, 1969
254. Kottmeier, HL: Complications following radiation therapy in carcinoma of the cervix and their treatment. Am J Obstet Gynecol 88:854, 1964
255. Muirhead W, Green LS: Carcinoma of the cervix. Five year results and sequelae of treatment. Am J Obstet Gynecol 101:744, 1968
256. Wall JA, Collins VP, Hudgins PT, et al: Carcinoma of the cervix. Review of clinical experience during a 20-year period. Am J Obstet Gynecol 96:57, 1966
257. Kottmeier HL (ed): Annual Report of the Results of Treatment of Carcinoma of the Uterus, Vagina and Ovary, Vol 16. International Federation of Gynecologists and Obstetricians, Stockholm: 1976
258. Boronow RC, Rutledge F: Vesicovaginal fistula, radiation and gynecologic cancer. Am J Obstet Gynecol 111:85, 1971
259. Mickal A, Torres, JE, Schlosser JV: Complications of therapy for carcinoma of the cervix. Am J Obstet Gynecol 112:556, 1972
260. Peckham BM, Kline JC, Schultz HA, et al: Radiation dosage and complications in cervical cancer therapy. Am J Obstet Gynecol 104:485, 1969
261. Strockbine MF, Hancock JE, Fletcher GH: Complications in 831 patients with squamous cell carcinoma of the intact cervix treated with 3000 rads or more whole pelvis irradiation. Am J Roentgenol 108:293, 1970
262. Villasanta U: Complications of radiotherapy for carcinoma of the uterine cervix. Am J Obstet Gynecol 114:717, 1972
263. Piver MS, Barlow JJ, Vongtama V, Webster J: Hydroxyurea and radiation therapy in advanced cervical cancer. Am J Obstet Gynecol 120:969, 1974
264. Piver MS, Barlow JJ, Vongtama V, Blumenson L: Hydroxyurea: A radiation

potentiator in carcinoma of the uterine cervix. Am J Obstet Gynecol 147:803, 1983
265. Webb GA: The role of ovarian conservation in the treatment of carcinoma of the cervix with radical surgery. Am J Obstet Gynecol 122:476, 1975
266. Ellsworth LR, Allen HH, Nisker JA: Ovarian function after radical hysterectomy for stage I carcinoma of the cervix. Am J Obstet Gynecol 145:185, 1983
267. Brunschwig A, Barber HR: Surgical treatment of carcinoma of the cervix. Obstet Gynecol 27:21, 1966
268. Christenson A, Lange P, Neilson E: Surgery and radiotherapy for invasive cancer of the cervix. Surgical treatment. Acta Obstet Gynecol Scand 43:59, 1964
269. Ketcham AS, Hoye RC, Taylor PT, Decker PJ: Radical hysterectomy and lymphadenectomy for carcinoma of the uterine cervix. Cancer 28:1272, 1971
270. Liu W, Meigs JV: Radical hysterectomy and pelvic lymphadenectomy: A review of 473 cases including 244 for primary invasive carcinoma of the cervix. Am J Obstet Gynecol 69:1, 1955
271. Masterson JG: The role of surgery in the treatment of early carcinoma of the cervix. Clin Obstet Gynecol 10:922, 1967
272. Park RC, Patow WE, Rogers RR, Zimmerman EA: Treatment of Stage I carcinoma of the cervix. Obstet Gynecol 41:117, 1973
273. Webb MJ, Symmonds RE: Wertheim hysterectomy: A reappraisal. Obstet Gynecol 54:140, 1979
274. Webb MJ, Symmonds RE: Radical hysterectomy: Influence of recent conization on morbidity and complications. Obstet Gynecol 53:290, 1979
275. De Cenzo JA, Malo T, Cavanagh D: Factors affecting cone hysterectomy-morbidity. Am J Obstet Gynecol 110:380, 1971
276. Morley GW, Seski GC: Radical pelvic surgery versus radiation for Stage I carcinoma of the cervix (exlusive of microinvasion). Am J Obstet Gynecol 126:785, 1976
277. Newton M: Radical hysterectomy or radiotherapy for Stage I cervical cancer. A prospective comparison with 5- and 10-year follow-up. Am J Obstet Gynecol 123:535, 1975
278. Surwit EA, Fowler WC, Montana GS: Radical hysterectomy with preoperative intracavitary therapy for Stage IB squamous cell carcinoma of the cervix. Int J Radiation Oncology Biol Phys 4:865, 1978
279. Stallworthy J: Clinical invasive carcinoma of cervix: Combined radiotherapy and radical hysterectomy as primary treatment. In Coppleson M (ed): Gynecologic Oncology: Fundamental Principles and Clinical Practice. New York: Churchill Livingstone, 1981, p 508
280. Bonar L: Results of radical surgical procedures after radiation for treatment of invasive carcinoma of the uterine cervix in a private practice. Am J Obstet Gynecol 136:1006, 1980
281. Hansen MK: Surgical and combination therapy of cancer of the cervix uteri stages IB and IIA. Gynecol Oncol 11:275, 1981
282. Marziale P, Atlante G, Le Pera V, et al: Combined radiation and surgical treatment of stages IB and IIA carcinoma of the cervix. Gynecol Oncol 11:175, 1981
283. De Graaf J: The Mitra-Schauta operation in combination with preoperative irradiation as treatment for carcinoma of the cervix. Gynecol Oncol 10:267, 1980
284. Quigley MM, Knab DR, McMahon EB: Carcinoma of the cervix. A third treatment. Obstet Gynecol 45:650, 1975

285. Jampolis S, Andras EJ, Fletcher GH: Analysis of sites and causes of failures or irradiation in invasive squamous cell carcinoma of the intact uterine cervix. Radiology 115:681, 1975
286. Fletcher GH, Rutledge FN, Chau PM: Policies of treatment in cancer of cervix uteri. Am J Roentgenol Ther Radium Nucl Med 87:6, 1962
287. Nelson AJ, Fletcher GH, Wharton JT: Indications for adjunctive conservative extrafascial hysterectomy in selected cases of carcinoma of the uterine cervix. Am J Roentgenol 123:91, 1975
288. Truelson F: Cancer of the Uterine Cervix. A Report of 2918 Cases. London: Lewis and Co, 1949
289. Douglas RG, Sweeney WJ: Exenteration operations in the treatment of advanced pelvic cancer. Am J Obstet Gynecol 73:1169, 1957
290. Parsons L, Friedell GH: Radical surgical treatment of cancer of the cervix. Proc Nat Cancer Conf 5:241, 1964
291. Brunschwig A: What are the indications and results of pelvic exenteration? JAMA 194:274, 1965
292. Kiselow M, Butcher HR, Bricker EM: Results of the radical surgical treatment of advanced pelvic cancer. A 15-year study. Ann Surg 166:425, 1967
293. Krieger JS, Embree HK: Pelvic exenteration. Cleveland Clinic Quart 36:1, 1969
294. Ketcham AS, Deckers TJ, Sugarbaker EV, et al: Pelvic exenteration for carcinoma of the uterine cervix. Cancer 26:513, 1970
295. Symmonds RE, Pratt JH, Webb MJ: Exenterative operations. Experience with 198 patients. Am J Obstet Gynecol 121:907, 1975
296. Rutledge FN, Smith JP, Wharton JT, O'Quinn AG: Pelvic exenteration. Analysis of 296 patients. Am J Obstet Gynecol 129:881, 1977
297. Morley GW, Lindenaur SM: Pelvic exenteration therapy for gynecologic malignancy. An analysis of 70 cases. Cancer 38:581, 1976
298. Symmonds RE: Morbidity and complications of radical hysterectomy with pelvic lymph node dissection. Am J Obstet Gynecol 94:663, 1966
299. Williams GA: Congenital absence of the vagina. A simple operation for its relief. J Obstet Gynaecol Br Comm 71:511, 1964
300. Watring WG, Lagasse LD, Smith ML, et al: Vaginal reconstruction for treatment for pelvic cancer. Am J Obstet Gynecol 125:809, 1976
301. Cavanagh D, Martin DS, Hernandez-Roman P: Closed pelvic perfusion. A new approach to the problem of advanced gynecologic malignancy. Am J Obstet Gynecol 92:996, 1965
302. Cavanagh D, Hovadhanakul P, Comas MR: Regional chemotherapy: A comparison of pelvic perfusion and intraarterial infusion in patients with advanced gynecologic cancer. Am J Obstet Gynecol 123:435, 1975
303. Lifshitz S, Railsback LD, Buchsbaum HJ: Intraarterial pelvic perfusion chemotherapy in advanced gynecologic. Obstet Gynecol 52:373 1978
304. Llorens AS: Chemotherapy of squamous cell carcinoma of the cervix. Obstet Gynecol 55:373, 1980
305. Trope C, Johnsson JE, Grundson H, Mattsson W: Adriamycin-methotrexate combination chemotherapy of advanced carcinoma of the cervix: A third look. Obstet Gynecol 55:488, 1980
306. Daghestani AN, Hakes TB, Lynch G, Lewis JL: Cervix carcinoma. Treatment with combination cisplatin and bleomycin. Gynecol Oncol 16:334, 1983
307. Friedlander M, Kaye SB, Sullivan A, et al: Cervical carcinoma. A drug respon-

sive tumor. Experience with combined cisplatin, vinblastine and bleomycin therapy. Obstet Gynecol 16:275, 1983
308. Lele SB, Piver MS, Barlow JJ: Cyclophosphamide, adriamycin and platinum chemotherapy in treatment of advanced and recurrent cervical carcinoma. Gynecol Oncol 16:15, 1983
309. Sorbe B, Frankendal B: Bleomycin-adriamycin-cisplatin combination chemotherapy in the treatment of primary advanced and recurrent cervical carcinoma. Obstet Gynecol 63:167, 1984
310. Rutledge FN, Galatatos AE, Wharton JT, Smith JP: Adenocarcinoma of the uterine cervix. Am J Obstet Gynecol 122:236, 1975
311. Korhonen MO: Epidemiological differences between adenocarcinoma and squamous cell carcinoma of the uterine cervix. Gynecol Oncol 10:312, 1980
312. Tamimi HK, Figge DC: Adenocarcinoma of the uterine cervix. Gynecol Oncol 13:335, 1982
313. Shingleton HM, Gore H, Bradely DH, Soong SJ: Adenocarcinoma of the cervix. I. Clinical evaluation and pathologic features. Am J Obstet Gynecol 139:799, 1981
314. Cuccia CA, Bloedorn FG, Onal M: Treatment of primary adenocarcinoma of the cervix. Am J Roentgenol 99:371, 1967
315. Abad RS, Kurohara SS, Graham JB: Clinical significance of adenocarcinoma of the cervix. Am J Obstet Gynecol 104:517, 1969
316. Rutledge FN, Gutteirez AG, Fletcher GH: Management of stage I and II adenocarcinoma of the cervix in an intact uterus. Am J Roentgenol 102:161, 1965
317. Kagan RA, Nussbaum H, Chan PY, Ziel HK: Adenocarcinoma of the uterine cervix. Am J Obstet Gynecol 117:464, 1973
318. Hacker NF, Berek JS, Lagasse LD, et al: Carcinoma of the cervix associated with pregnancy. Obstet Gynecol 59:735, 1982
319. Barber HRK, O'Neil WH: Recurrent cervical cancer after treatment by a primary surgical program. Obstet Gynecol 37:165, 1971
320. Munnell EW, Bonney WA: Critical points of failure in the therapy of cancer of the cervix. A study of 250 recurrences. Am J Obstet Gynecol 81:521, 1961
321. Halpin, JF, Frick HC, Munnell EW: Critical points of failure in the therapy of cancer of the cervix: A reappraisal. Am J Obstet Gynecol 114:755, 1972
322. Shepherd JH, Cavanagh D, Ruffolo EH, Praphat, H: The value of needle biopsy in the diagnosis of gynecologic cancer. Gynecol Oncol 11:309, 1981

CHAPTER 4
Carcinoma of the Endometrium

Endometrial carcinoma is the most frequently diagnosed invasive malignancy of the female genital tract in the United States. It is estimated that almost 40,000 new cases were diagnosed in 1984, and that about 3000 women died from the disease.[1] In 1956, Peel[2] commented that as a resident in the 1930s he had been taught that endometrial cancer was "a benign form of neoplasm with a very good prognosis from not very radical surgery" but that attitudes to the disease had subsequently "undergone a slow but radical change." There is little evidence of any radical change in the attitudes of the majority of gynecologists to endometrial cancer, and many who readily refer patients with other gynecologic tumors to specialist centers feel competent to manage this malignancy themselves.[3,4]

Stallworthy,[5] in 1973, "expressed concern about the generally optimistic view of endometrial cancer, the actual reported survival figures, and about the poor approach of the occasional surgeon." That his concern was justified was clearly demonstrated by Jones[6] who reported in 1975 that worldwide 5-year survival figures for endometrial cancer averaged only 68 percent. In 1976, Boronow[4] discussed "four prevalent myths" relating to endometrial cancer. The first, that endometrial cancer is relatively benign, he refuted by showing that, stage for stage, the prognosis of endometrial cancer was the same as for cervical cancer, and that despite a preponderance of early stage lesions the overall 5-year survival rates in the United States were less than 70 percent. The other "myths" that he exposed were that the best therapy and the prognostic factors had been defined and that the lymph nodes were of little importance in endometrial cancer.

There is no more cause for complacency today. Overall 5-year survival figures for four large series from North America published since 1978 average only 75 percent (Table 1).[7-10] Furthermore, the fact that the majority of cases are diagnosed at an early stage means that the majority of deaths occur in patients with Stage I disease (Table 2). Both increasing incidence rates for endometrial cancer and the high cure rates may in part be due to overdiagnosis, an error that appears to be particularly common in regions with a high incidence of postmenopausal estrogen usage. In one study, three pathologists independently reviewing histologic specimens from a group of women who had undergone hysterectomy for endometrial cancer, could only agree among themselves on the diagnosis in 74 percent of cases.[11] In another study, it was concluded that 18 percent of women diagnosed as having endometrial cancer actually had benign or premalignant lesions.[12] A recent pathologic review of specimens from women who underwent hysterectomy for endometrial cancer in a major university medical center showed that 27 percent actually had endometrial hyperplasia rather than frank carcinoma.[13]

A major cause for concern is the fact that although endometrial cancer is far less common among blacks, their survival rates by stage, and within Stage I, by tumor grade, is markedly worse than for whites.[10] This observation may be related to the fact that black women are significantly older at diagnosis. For women of all races the prognosis is markedly worse with advancing age, an important observation as this is a disease of older women, and the aging population is increasing significantly. Older women do tend to have more advanced and less well-differentiated tumors, but this does not fully explain the findings, and it may be that aging immunodefense mechanisms play a part.

In considering the management of endometrial cancer, one must bear in mind that among Stage I tumors, those with deep myometrial involvement or

TABLE 1. OVERALL 5-YEAR SURVIVAL RATES FOR ENDOMETRIAL CARCINOMA IN 4 NORTH AMERICAN SERIES PUBLISHED SINCE 1978

Author	Institution	Number of Cases	Overall 5-year Survival (%)
Malkasian (1978)[7]	Mayo Clinic	523	73.8
Beck (1979)[8]	University of Alberta	509	75.4
McCabe and Sagerman (1979)[9]	Upstate Medical Center, New York	379	74
Connelly et al. (1982)[10]	Louisville, Kentucky	811	77.1
Total		2222	75.4

TABLE 2. PROPORTION OF PATIENTS IN 4 SERIES WHO HAD STAGE I ENDOMETRIAL CARCINOMA, AND THE PROPORTION OF THE DEATHS IN EACH SERIES DUE TO PATIENTS WITH STAGE I DISEASE

Author	Proportion of Patients in Series Stage I (%)	Proportion of All Deaths Occurring in Series in Stage I Patients (%)
Malkasian (1978)[7]	78	53
Beck (1979)[8]	86	58
McCabe and Sagerman (1979)[9]	81	57
Connelly et al. (1982)[10]	91	81

anaplastic tumors have para-aortic node involvement in 45.5 and 37.5 percent of cases, respectively.[14] Furthermore, peritoneal cytology is positive in over 15 percent of women with Stage I disease.[15] There is increasing emphasis on subtypes of tumors such as papillary adenocarcinoma, clear cell adenocarcinoma, and adenosquamous carcinoma, all of which carry a much poorer prognosis than does adenocarcinoma.[16-18] Adenosquamous carcinoma appears to be increasing in incidence.[19]

EPIDEMIOLOGY

Racial and Geographic Factors

The white population of the United States has the highest age standardized incidence of endometrial cancer in the world, India and Japan have the lowest, and the European countries occupy intermediate positions.[20] Black women in the United States have incidence rates roughly one-half those of whites. Data from various cancer registries in the Pacific basin provide striking evidence of the geographic and racial variations in incidence (Table 3).[21]

Compared with white women in the United States, women of Spanish descent in Colombia, Cuba, and Puerto Rico have relative risks of developing endometrial carcinoma of 0.16, 0.26, and 0.20 respectively.[22] In Los Angeles County, immigrant and indigenous women of Spanish descent have relative risks of 0.36 and 0.69, respectively, compared with whites.

The incidence of endometrial cancer among Chinese, Japanese, and Spanish-American women who migrate from countries of low incidence appears to increase in proportion to their time in the United States.[22]

In Israel, Jewish women born in Europe or America have an incidence of endometrial cancer almost six times higher than Jewish women of Asian or African origin, who in turn have a slightly higher incidence of the disease than Israeli-born Jews or non-Jews.[23]

TABLE 3. ANNUAL AGE STANDARDIZED INCIDENCE RATES FOR CORPUS CARCINOMA IN THE PACIFIC BASIN

Registry	Japanese	Chinese	Spanish-American	Black	White
Osaka, Japan	7.7	—	—	—	—
Hong Kong	—	4.0	—	—	—
Singapore	—	4.9	—	—	—
New Zealand	—	—	—	—	10.4
Recife, Brazil	—	—	2.2	—	—
Cali, Colombia	—	—	5.1	—	—
Hawaii, U.S.A.	15.6	19.7	—	—	28.8
El Paso, U.S.A.	—	—	9.5	—	—
San Francisco, U.S.A.	—	16.1	—	13.3	29.9
Los Angeles, U.S.A.	19.9	7.9	17.6	15.0	35.5

Age

Between 75 and 80 percent of women diagnosed with endometrial carcinoma are postmenopausal, and the mean age at diagnosis is about 60 years.[7,10] The greatest number of cases are diagnosed in the 55 to 60-year age group, while the peak incidence per 100,000 women in the population is in the 65 to 70-year age group.[24] Less than 5 percent of endometrial carcinomas occur in women under 40 years of age.[25] Figure 1 shows the proportion of cases diagnosed in each age group, based on the findings of the Third National Cancer Survey.[26]

There are racial variations in age-specific incidence rates within the United States. Among white women, the peak incidence of 87.2/100,000 occurs in the 65 to 69-year age group, while for black women, the peak incidence rate is 78.9/100,000 in the 75 to 79-year age group.[26]

Socioeconomic Factors

Consideration must be given to the possibility that racial and geographic factors are explained by the difference in socioeconomic status in various

Figure 1. Proportion of cases of endometrial carcinoma diagnosed in various age groups in the third National Cancer Survey. (*From Cutler SJ, Young JL: Nat Cancer Inst Monogr 41, 1975, with permission.*)[26]

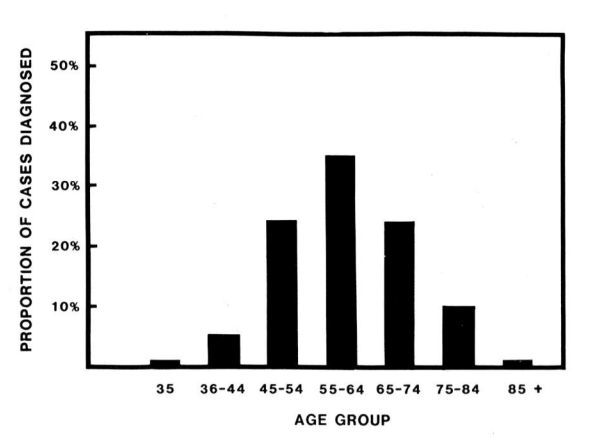

countries. This may be indirectly related, but European countries, Australia, and New Zealand, which have incidence rates only half those of the United States are not significantly less affluent. Japan, with one of the lowest incidence rates in the world, is certainly more affluent than many countries with far higher rates. Studies in Great Britain failed to show different incidence rates between the social classes,[27] but among white women in Los Angeles County incidence rates rose from the lowest to the highest social classes.[28]

The "Corpus Cancer Syndrome"

Yahia and colleagues[29] coined this term in 1963 to encompass obesity, hypertension, diabetes mellitus, and prolonged or unopposed estrogen stimulation as predisposing factors for endometrial cancer.

Undoubtedly, a significant proportion of women with endometrial carcinoma are obese. Wynder and colleagues[30] found obesity to be the single most important factor associated with endometrial cancer. They estimated that women 21 to 50 pounds overweight had 3 times the risk, and those 51 or more pounds overweight 9 times the risk of developing endometrial cancer compared with women of average or less than average weight. On the other hand, controlled studies by Fox and Sen[31] and Brown[32] failed to support a relationship. Many women with endometrial carcinoma are obese, but screening the heaviest one-third of the population would not detect more than one-half of patients with the disease even if the highest association rates are correct.[33]

Hypertension is also frequently present in women with endometrial cancer. A recent Finnish study showed that 27 percent of patients had diastolic blood pressures of 100 mm Hg or more[34] and a large study from the United States found 45 percent of patients to have blood pressures greater than 140/90 mm Hg.[10] Such figures may simply reflect the effects of age and possibly obesity. A Mayo Clinic study found comparable rates of hypertension among patients with endometrial carcinoma and women of similar age in the general population.[35]

The association between diabetes and endometrial carcinoma was first described by Crossen and Hobbs[36] in 1935, and is generally accepted. Nevertheless, Peel[2] found a very low incidence of endometrial carcinoma among maturity-onset diabetics, and Kessler[37] found the age-specific mortality rate for endometrial carcinoma among over 100,000 women to be lower than for the general population. Way[38] found frank diabetes to be present in 30 percent of endometrial cancer patients, and "prediabetic" glucose tolerance curves in a further 43 percent. It has been suggested that diabetics have almost three times the risk of developing endometrial cancer,[33] whereas some controlled studies show no preponderance of diabetics.[31] Part of the confusion may relate to equating abnormal glucose tolerance curves with diabetes. In a controlled study, Brown[39] showed that frank diabetes was not unduly frequent in patients with endometrial cancer, but that abnormal glucose tolerance was very common. Reviewing the data, Elwood and associates[40] conclude that diabetes per se is not a risk factor, but that the diagnosis of abnormal glucose tolerance is frequently made concurrently or subsequent to the diagnosis of endometrial cancer. It seems likely that the impaired glucose tolerance is often due to obesity.

The final feature of the "corpus cancer syndrome" is prolonged, unopposed estrogen stimulation. This subject will be dealt with next under a separate heading.

Unopposed Estrogen Action

Estrogens undoubtedly play an important role in the etiology of endometrial carcinoma. A number of epidemiologic studies illustrate the point.

Functioning Ovarian Tumors. Functioning ovarian tumors provide a "natural experiment" with markedly raised endogenous estrogen levels. Schroder,[41] in 1922, reported the coexistence of endometrial carcinoma and a functioning ovarian tumor, and since then, reports have indicated that up to 27 percent of women with estrogen-producing tumors have endometrial carcinoma. Among granulosa-theca cell tumors referred to the Emil Novak Ovarian Tumor Registry, 23 percent were associated with endometrial carcinoma and 65 percent with endometrial hyperplasia, but this may reflect a bias in referral of "interesting cases."[42] A more realistic assessment of the risk may be that of Larson,[43] who concluded from a review of the world literature that 4.8 percent of all women with feminizing tumors developed endometrial carcinoma, although this was rare in premenarchial girls and younger women, with the figure reaching 10 percent for postmenopausal women. Later studies have confirmed the risk to be of this magnitude,[44,45] but although it is lower than suggested by some authors, there is still a very significant risk.

Polycystic Ovarian Disease. The Stein-Leventhal syndrome is characterized by infertility, menstrual dysfunction, hirsutism, and often obesity. The anovulatory ovaries contribute to the significantly increased pool of circulating androgens, which are metabolized by peripheral nonglandular conversion to estrogens, principally estrone. Thus, the endometrium is stimulated by consistently elevated estrone levels, and in the absence of ovulation there is no cyclic progesterone secretion to counter this stimulus. Dockerty and colleagues,[46] wrote that there had been insufficient emphasis on the possibility of endometrial carcinoma complicating polycystic ovarian disease. Between 19 and 25 percent of women who develop endometrial carcinoma before the age of 40 have been said to have evidence of polycystic ovarian disease.[47] The proportion of women with polycystic disease who develop endometrial cancer is not certain: one study of 43 patients found 38 percent to have developed endometrial carcinoma.[48] Subsequent reviews have suggested that these figures are excessive, and that the risk, though increased, is of far lesser magnitude.[49]

Ovarian Dysgenesis. Ovarian dysgenesis (Turner's syndrome) is frequently managed with estrogen replacement therapy. In the absence of such therapy, endometrial carcinoma is rare in women with this condition, but 14 patients with ovarian dysgenesis treated with estrogen replacement therapy have been reported to have developed endometrial carcinoma.[47] Ostor and colleagues[25] have reported four women, two with pure XO genotype, and two with XO mosaicism, who in the absence of replacement estrogens, developed endometrial carcinoma, but such occurrences are rare.

Sequential Oral Contraceptives. Sequential oral contraceptives were introduced in the United States in 1963, with the promise of a more "natural" effect on the endometrium. They were withdrawn from the market in 1976 after it was noted that although this type of medication accounted for only 10 percent of oral contraceptives marketed in the United States, 20 of the first 30 patients in a registry of young women developing endometrial carcinoma following oral contraceptive use had taken sequential agents. Among women taking oral contraceptives at the time of diagnosis, 17 were using sequential and 2 combined formulations.[50] Whether this was due to the stimulation of neoplasia by sequential agents, or a protective effect of combined agents, is not clear.[51] The most commonly used sequential agent did, however, have a relatively high estrogenic potency, 100 μg of ethinyl estradiol, with only 5 days of a relatively weak gestagen, 25 mg of dimethesterone.

Estrogen Replacement Therapy. Although animal experiments had shown the association of estrogens with endometrial hyperplasia and carcinoma, and case reports of endometrial carcinoma in women using estrogen replacement therapy had been published previously, the first controlled study showing increased estrogen usage among women with endometrial carcinoma was not published until 1954. Jensen and Østergaard[52] demonstrated that 33 percent of 105 endometrial cancer patients had used estrogens compared to 21 percent of controls. In 1961, Gusberg and Hall[53] published observations on 23 long-term estrogen users, all but 2 of them receiving hormones for menopausal symptoms, who developed endometrial carcinoma, and concluded that a relationship between prolonged, continuous, and unopposed estrogen action and a proportion of endometrial cancers was highly likely. Subsequent studies by Wynder and colleagues[30] in 1966 and Dunn and Bradbury[54] in 1967 failed to substantiate a significant relationship. However, in 1975, the first case-control studies linking estrogen replacement therapy and endometrial carcinoma appeared, and these have been followed by a series of papers substantiating the association (Table 4).[55-70] The initial reports generated considerable con-

range of descriptive terminology, diagnostic labels, and treatment plans that have "conspired to confuse both the pathologist (in the formulation of meaningful diagnoses) and the gynecologist (in therapeutic decision-making)."[82]

In 1974, Vellios[83] commented that the so-called "hyperplasias" of the endometrium would be more appropriately termed "dysplasias," in a manner analogous to lesions of the cervix. This led us to review the work of Richart[84] on the classification of the precursors of cervical carcinoma. He developed the unifying concept of cervical intraepithelial neoplasia (CIN) to replace the profusion of terms describing the precursors of invasive cervical cancer, such as atypical hyperplasia, basal cell hyperactivity, anaplasia, and mild, moderate, or severe dysplasia. Noting the arbitrary nature of the division between severe dysplasia and carcinoma in situ, in terms of both diagnosis and prognosis, he included both in the category CIN 3. This classification has been widely accepted and has at once simplified and clarified the diagnostic and therapeutic aspects of premalignant cervical lesions.

The present authors believe that a similar concept is eminently suitable for classifying premalignant endometrial lesions. The changes are confined to the glandular epithelium, without invasive carcinoma. Architectural and cytologic changes are both involved in a continuum ranging from mild aberrations to those often considered as carcinoma in situ. We have proposed a classification of endometrial hyperplasias analogous to CIN of the cervix, termed "glandular intraepithelial neoplasia" (GIN).[85] Such a concept seems likely to be acceptable to both gynecologists and pathologists in view of the general acceptance of the concept of cervical intraepithelial neoplasia by both groups.

We propose a simple classification of GIN 1, 2, and 3. Table 5 shows the correlation between this classification and existing terminologies, and Figures 2 through 4 illustrate the lesions.

GIN 1 (Fig. 2) includes cystic hyperplasia and adenomatous hyperplasia without atypia.

GIN 2 (Fig. 3) refers to adenomatous hyperplasias of moderate degree and to atypical hyperplasia. The cellular atypia falls short of what has previously been designated "borderline" lesions, such as the severe atypical hyperplasias and carcinoma in situ.

GIN 3 (Fig. 4) would include lesions termed by Gusberg and Kaplan[88] as "marked adenomatous hyperplasia," by Vellios[87] as "severe atypical hyperplasia," and by Hertig and Sommers[80] as "carcinoma in situ." It is of paramount importance to separate this group from invasive carcinoma. Kurman and Norris[92] have designated this lesion "AH-CIS" and defined precise criteria for its diagnosis on the basis of endometrial curettings. The four criteria of stromal invasion in endometrial curettings were:

1. Irregular infiltration of glands associated with an altered fibroblastic stroma or desmoplastic response.
2. A pattern of confluent glands where individual glands are not inter-

gested that these figures are excessive, and that the risk, though increased, is of far lesser magnitude.[49]

Ovarian Dysgenesis. Ovarian dysgenesis (Turner's syndrome) is frequently managed with estrogen replacement therapy. In the absence of such therapy, endometrial carcinoma is rare in women with this condition, but 14 patients with ovarian dysgenesis treated with estrogen replacement therapy have been reported to have developed endometrial carcinoma.[47] Ostor and colleagues[25] have reported four women, two with pure XO genotype, and two with XO mosaicism, who in the absence of replacement estrogens, developed endometrial carcinoma, but such occurrences are rare.

Sequential Oral Contraceptives. Sequential oral contraceptives were introduced in the United States in 1963, with the promise of a more "natural" effect on the endometrium. They were withdrawn from the market in 1976 after it was noted that although this type of medication accounted for only 10 percent of oral contraceptives marketed in the United States, 20 of the first 30 patients in a registry of young women developing endometrial carcinoma following oral contraceptive use had taken sequential agents. Among women taking oral contraceptives at the time of diagnosis, 17 were using sequential and 2 combined formulations.[50] Whether this was due to the stimulation of neoplasia by sequential agents, or a protective effect of combined agents, is not clear.[51] The most commonly used sequential agent did, however, have a relatively high estrogenic potency, 100 µg of ethinyl estradiol, with only 5 days of a relatively weak gestagen, 25 mg of dimethesterone.

Estrogen Replacement Therapy. Although animal experiments had shown the association of estrogens with endometrial hyperplasia and carcinoma, and case reports of endometrial carcinoma in women using estrogen replacement therapy had been published previously, the first controlled study showing increased estrogen usage among women with endometrial carcinoma was not published until 1954. Jensen and Østergaard[52] demonstrated that 33 percent of 105 endometrial cancer patients had used estrogens compared to 21 percent of controls. In 1961, Gusberg and Hall[53] published observations on 23 long-term estrogen users, all but 2 of them receiving hormones for menopausal symptoms, who developed endometrial carcinoma, and concluded that a relationship between prolonged, continuous, and unopposed estrogen action and a proportion of endometrial cancers was highly likely. Subsequent studies by Wynder and colleagues[30] in 1966 and Dunn and Bradbury[54] in 1967 failed to substantiate a significant relationship. However, in 1975, the first case-control studies linking estrogen replacement therapy and endometrial carcinoma appeared, and these have been followed by a series of papers substantiating the association (Table 4).[55-70] The initial reports generated considerable con-

TABLE 4. RELATIVE RISKS FOR DEVELOPMENT OF ENDOMETRIAL CARCINOMA IN 16 PUBLISHED SERIES

Author	Institution/Study Population	No. of Patients	Overall Relative Risk	Notes
Smith et al. (1975)[55]	University of Washington	317	4.5	Highest risks in women without predisposing constitutional factors.
Ziel and Finkle (1975)[56]	Kaiser Permanente Hospital, Los Angeles	94	7.6	Relative risk related to length of exposure—5.6 for 1 to 5 years, and 13.9 for 7 or more years' exposure.
Mack et al. (1976)[57]	Retirement Community, Los Angeles	63	8.0	Dose-response effect demonstrated relative risk 5.0 for 0.3 mg conjugated estrogen and 9.4 for 1.25 mg.
McDonald et al. (1977)[58]	Mayo Clinic	145	4.9	Dose- and time-related risk. For 3 or more years use relative risk 7.9.
Gray et al. (1977)[59]	Private Practice, Louisville, Ky.	205	3.1	Dose-related risk. No increase for less than 5 years' exposure. For 10 or more years, relative risk 11.5.
Hoogerland et al. (1978)[60]	Wisconsin Clinical Cancer Center	587	2.2	Risk only increased in women *without* predisposing constitutional factors.
Horwitz et al. (1978)[61]	Yale-New Haven Medical Center	119	1.7–11.9	Rate dependent on control group used. See text.
Wigle et al. (1978)[62]	Province of Alberta, Canada	202	2.2	For current users relative risk 2.7, past users 2.0, for 1–4 years use relative risk 1.8, for 5 or more years 5.2.
Antunes et al. (1979)[63]	Greater Baltimore Area, Maryland	451	6	For over 5 years use relative risk 15.

Study	Location	N	Relative Risk	Comments
Jick et al. (1979)[64]	Group Health Cooperative, Seattle, Washington	67	10	For current users relative risk 20.
Jelovsek et al. (1980)[65]	Duke University Medical Center, Durham, N.C.	431	2.38	Relative risk 4.8 for 5–10 years of use. Greatest risk group is white women with over 5 years use.
Hulka et al. (1980)[66]	North Carolina Memorial Hospital	256	3.6	Relative risk 5 to 8 among non-obese, normotensive whites with over 3½ years' use. Latency period of 3–6 years after first exposure. After 2 years of estrogens, risk reduced to normal level.
Shapiro et al. (1980)[67]	Multiple Areas of U.S.A. and Canada	149	3.9	Relative risk for 1–4 years' use was 2.6 and for 5 or more years, 6.0 relative risk decline after 1 year off estrogens.
Stravraky et al. (1981)[68]	Victoria Hospital, London, Canada	206	Between 1.5 and 4.8	Relative risk 105 when patients with gynecologic disease controls, and 4.8 of controls are patients with nongynecologic disease.
Spengler et al. (1981)[69]	Metropolitan Toronto, Canada	134	2.9	For 5 or more years, use relative risk 8.6.
Obrink et al. (1981)[70]	Radiumhemmet, Stockholm, Sweden	622	5	Relative risk of 5 is calculated for 3–6 year use only.

troversy and a degree of hysteria. Although this has largely settled now, there are valid criticisms of all these studies. The chief problem relates to choice of control groups, and Horwitz and Feinstein were able to demonstrate a relative risk of almost 12 when cases were matched with controls with other gynecologic cancer, but only 1.7 when matched with controls who had been screened for endometrial cancer.[61] They argued that estrogen merely induced bleeding in patients with occult cancer, thereby increasing detection rates. To support the concept of a large pool of undetected endometrial carcinoma in the community, they later reported that data from two necropsy series suggested that occult endometrial carcinoma was present four to five times more often than it was clinically detected.[71] It was subsequently demonstrated that this study compared lifetime risk with annual rate, and that using the same data the pool of occult cancer was about one-fifth as large as they had calculated.[72] While it is clear that control groups are difficult to select, better types of study are unlikely to be performed and one must accept that estrogen replacement therapy does carry an increased risk of endometrial carcinoma. It should be noted, however, that the preparation most commonly used has been conjugated estrogen, and it may be that other estrogen preparations are less likely to produce such problems.

There were criticisms, too, that the studies relating to estrogen use were misdiagnosing endometrial hyperplasias as carcinoma. While demonstrating that this did occur, Gordon and colleagues,[11] after reviewing the specimens from the original Ziel and Finkle study,[56] found that even with the reclassification, the original risk estimate was appropriate. Likewise, a review of the pathologic specimens in the original study of Smith and associates[55] and exclusion of several cases substantiated their original risk estimates.[73]

Following the publication of the early studies, sales of conjugated estrogens have fallen markedly in many areas of the United States and subsequently there has been a decline in incidence of endometrial carcinoma.[64,74,75]

Other Epidemiologic Observations

Among both married and single women there is a markedly increased risk of endometrial carcinoma associated with *nulliparity*. Up to one-third of women with endometrial carcinoma are nulliparous. More significantly, the risks of endometrial carcinoma appear to decline in proportion to the parity.[40] A Boston study concluded that nulliparous women had twice the risk of women with one child, and over three times the risk of women with five or more children.[33]

Although it must be carefully distinguished from abnormal bleeding in the perimenopausal period, *late menopause* appears to be related to development of endometrial carcinoma.[40] One study suggested that a menopause occurring at age 52 or later conferred a 2.4 times increased risk, compared with women whose menopause occurred at age 49 or less.[33]

Endometrial carcinoma and *leiomyomas* of the uterus are frequently associated, but no etiologic relationship has been established.

PRECURSORS OF ENDOMETRIAL CARCINOMA

A range of hyperplastic lesions of the endometrium has long been recognized, often in association with frank malignancy, or in women considered at high risk for endometrial carcinoma. In 1900, Cullen[76] suggested an etiologic relationship between the endometrial hyperplasias and cancer, and reviews by Taylor[77] and Novak and Yui[78] supported this view. In 1947, Gusberg[79] labeled the entire spectrum of hyperplastic lesions "adenomatous hyperplasia," drew attention to their production by both endogenous and exogenous estrogenic stimulation, and emphasized their role as precursors of frank carcinoma. The first complete classification of endometrial hyperplasia was that of Hertig and Sommers,[80] published in 1949. From among 389 cases of endometrial carcinoma, they were able to review endometrial curettings performed between 1 and 23 years prior to the diagnosis in 32 cases. In all cases where the biopsy was taken less than 15 years before the diagnosis of cancer, some form of hyperplasia was noted. Their classification included cystic hyperplasia, adenomatous hyperplasia, anaplasia, and carcinoma in situ. Cystic hyperplasia was present in earlier biopsies of 17 of the 32 patients who subsequently developed endometrial carcinoma, but they commented that its incidence declined steadily from 10 or more years before cancer to "a year or two before," and therefore was a "remote rather than immediate forerunner of carcinoma." Adenomatous hyperplasia was the most frequently encountered lesion, and its frequency increased as the time of diagnosis of cancer approached. Where cystic hyperplasia was characterized by spherically dilated glands containing secretion and lined by columnar epithelium, adenomatous hyperplasia had glands that showed outpouchings like fingers of a glove into the stroma which when pinched off formed small back-to-back glands. Neither lesion showed atypical cellular changes. Their next grouping was "anaplasia," characterized by variations in size, shape, polarity, and staining characteristics of the cellular lining of the hyperplastic endometrium. Such anaplasia was noted more frequently as the time of diagnosis of endometrial carcinoma approached. Their final group of hyperplastic endometria was termed carcinoma in situ. This was characterized by glands with large, eosinophilic cells containing abundant cytoplasm. Nuclei were irregular, with folded or scalloped membranes, and were pale with fine granular chromatin. They considered this lesion, in contrast to others, to be irreversible. Of the six patients in their original study who had this lesion, all developed invasive carcinoma in 1 to 11 years. This lesion was further defined in a subsequent study to include cell disorientation, varying cell size, and stratification. Crowded, but not back-to-back, glands were said to be present, with reduplication of the lumina.[81] When the effects of progestins had been more clearly defined, the authors conceded that some cases of carcinoma in situ might be reversible if these agents were used.

Subsequent to these early studies, numerous authors have attempted to classify endometrial hyperplasias, but unfortunately the results have been a range of descriptive terminology, diagnostic labels, and treatment plans that have "conspired to confuse both the pathologist (in the formulation of meaningful diagnoses) and the gynecologist (in therapeutic decision-making)."[82]

In 1974, Vellios[83] commented that the so-called "hyperplasias" of the endometrium would be more appropriately termed "dysplasias," in a manner analogous to lesions of the cervix. This led us to review the work of Richart[84] on the classification of the precursors of cervical carcinoma. He developed the unifying concept of cervical intraepithelial neoplasia (CIN) to replace the profusion of terms describing the precursors of invasive cervical cancer, such as atypical hyperplasia, basal cell hyperactivity, anaplasia, and mild, moderate, or severe dysplasia. Noting the arbitrary nature of the division between severe dysplasia and carcinoma in situ, in terms of both diagnosis and prognosis, he included both in the category CIN 3. This classification has been widely accepted and has at once simplified and clarified the diagnostic and therapeutic aspects of premalignant cervical lesions.

The present authors believe that a similar concept is eminently suitable for classifying premalignant endometrial lesions. The changes are confined to the glandular epithelium, without invasive carcinoma. Architectural and cytologic changes are both involved in a continuum ranging from mild aberrations to those often considered as carcinoma in situ. We have proposed a classification of endometrial hyperplasias analogous to CIN of the cervix, termed "glandular intraepithelial neoplasia" (GIN).[85] Such a concept seems likely to be acceptable to both gynecologists and pathologists in view of the general acceptance of the concept of cervical intraepithelial neoplasia by both groups.

We propose a simple classification of GIN 1, 2, and 3. Table 5 shows the correlation between this classification and existing terminologies, and Figures 2 through 4 illustrate the lesions.

GIN 1 (Fig. 2) includes cystic hyperplasia and adenomatous hyperplasia without atypia.

GIN 2 (Fig. 3) refers to adenomatous hyperplasias of moderate degree and to atypical hyperplasia. The cellular atypia falls short of what has previously been designated "borderline" lesions, such as the severe atypical hyperplasias and carcinoma in situ.

GIN 3 (Fig. 4) would include lesions termed by Gusberg and Kaplan[88] as "marked adenomatous hyperplasia," by Vellios[87] as "severe atypical hyperplasia," and by Hertig and Sommers[80] as "carcinoma in situ." It is of paramount importance to separate this group from invasive carcinoma. Kurman and Norris[92] have designated this lesion "AH-CIS" and defined precise criteria for its diagnosis on the basis of endometrial curettings. The four criteria of stromal invasion in endometrial curettings were:

1. Irregular infiltration of glands associated with an altered fibroblastic stroma or desmoplastic response.
2. A pattern of confluent glands where individual glands are not inter-

TABLE 5. CLASSIFICATIONS OF HYPERPLASIAS OF ENDOMETRIUM

Proposed	GIN 1	GIN 2	GIN 3
WHO (1975)[86]	Cystic hyperplasia and adenomatous hyperplasia	Adenomatous hyperplasia	Atypical hyperplasia
Vellios (1972)[87]	Cystic hyperplasia and adenomatous hyperplasia	Atypical hyperplasia	Carcinoma in situ
Gore and Hertig (1966)[81]	Cystic hyperplasia and adenomatous hyperplasia	Anaplasia	Carcinoma in situ
Gusberg and Kaplan (1963)[88]	Mild adenomatous hyperplasia	Moderate adenomatous hyperplasia	Marked adenomatous hyperplasia
Campbell and Barter (1961)[89]	Benign hyperplasia Atypical hyperplasia	Atypical hyperplasia Type II Type I	Atypical hyperplasia Type III
Beutler, et al. (1963)[90]	Cystic proliferation and glandular hyperplasia		Glandular hyperplasia with atypical epithelial proliferation

(Modified from Tavassoli F, Kraus FT: N Engl J Med 70:770, 1978, with permission.)[91]

    rupted by stroma, merging to form a cribiform pattern of stromal replacement.
  3. An extensive papillary pattern.
  4. Replacement of stroma by masses of squamous epithelium.

To allow the diagnosis of invasion to be made, the second, third, and fourth criteria must be present in at least one-half of a low-power field. Use of the criteria proved extremely reliable in predicting the presence or absence of invasive disease in the uteri of 204 women.[92]

Cystic hyperplasia, which would be classified as GIN 1 in our proposed classification, must be carefully distinguished from postmenopausal cystic atrophy, where the glandular epithelium is flattened and atrophic and the stroma is reduced in quantity and often fibrous. The malignant potential of true cystic hyperplasia is uncertain. McBride[93] followed 544 postmenopausal women with this diagnosis for up to 24 years, and found that cancer developed in only 0.4 percent. Nevertheless, the true cystic hyperplasia, correctly diagnosed, is evidence of estrogenic stimulation and patients with this diag-

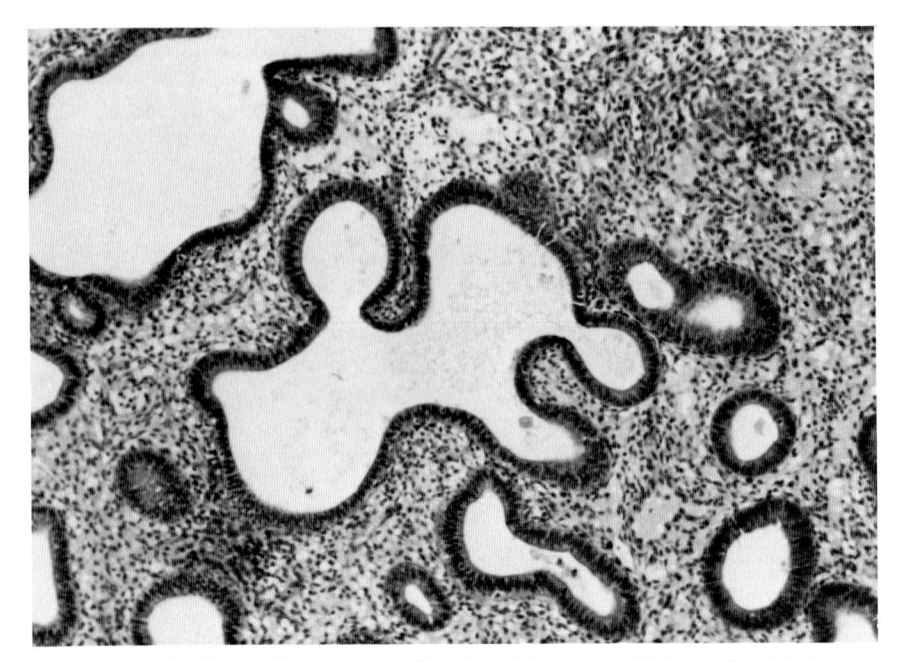

Figure 2A. GIN 1—There is cystic dilatation of the glands with branching, "pinching off" to form additional small glands. Original magnification. X80.

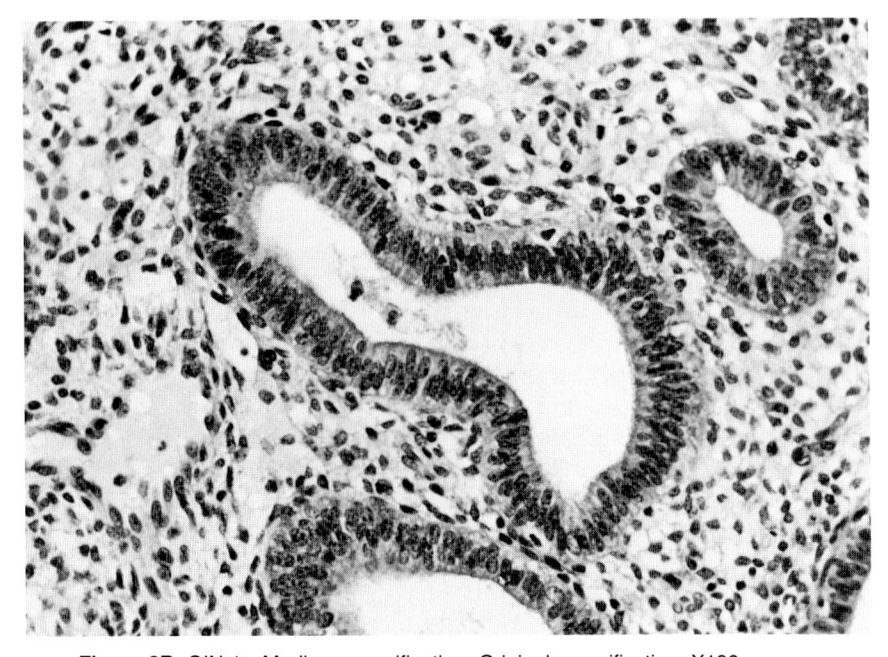

Figure 2B. GIN 1—Medium magnification. Original magnification. X190.

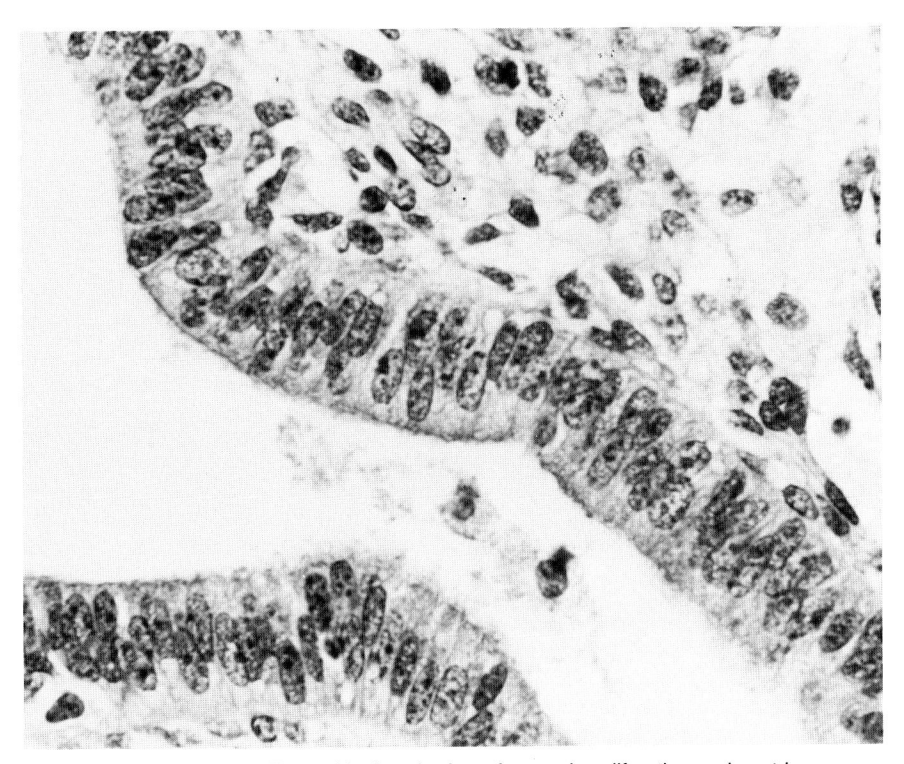

Figure 2C. GIN 1—The epithelium is that of normal proliferative endometrium. The cells are pseudostratified with oval nuclei, mutually polarized to a vertical or perpendicular orientation to the lumen. The nuclear membranes are delicate and the chromatin rather evenly distributed without definite nucleoli. These changes have been referred to as cystic and mild adenomatous hyperplasia. Original magnification. X500.

nosis should be followed carefully. McBride excluded postmenopausal women with cystic hyperplasia from his study.

The likelihood of progression of the various grades of GIN can be estimated from various reports. Wentz[94] studied 115 patients with 2 curettage specimens at least 8 weeks apart showing what we would term GIN. In follow-up of 2 to 8 years without therapy, he found that 27 percent of those with what we would call GIN 1, 82 percent with GIN 2, and 100 percent with GIN 3 developed invasive cancer. Sherman[95] studied 204 patients and concluded that patients with what we would classify as GIN 1 have a 20 percent chance of developing invasive cancer 2 to 10 years later, while for those with GIN 2 and GIN 3, the figure was the same, 57 percent. The number of patients with GIN 3 was very small, which may have affected the results, as may the exclusion from the study of patients within 2 years of curettage.[95]

We agree entirely with Kurman and Norris,[92] who state:

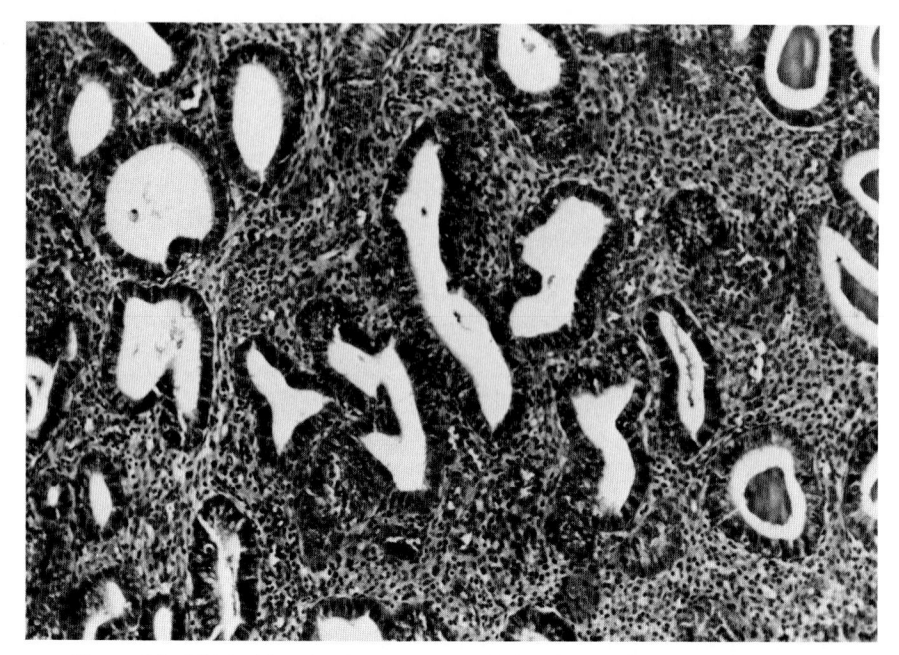

Figure 3A. GIN 2—The glands appear crowded and are rather large with persistent branching. Normal stroma separates the glands. The glandular epithelium appears crowded. Original magnification. X80.

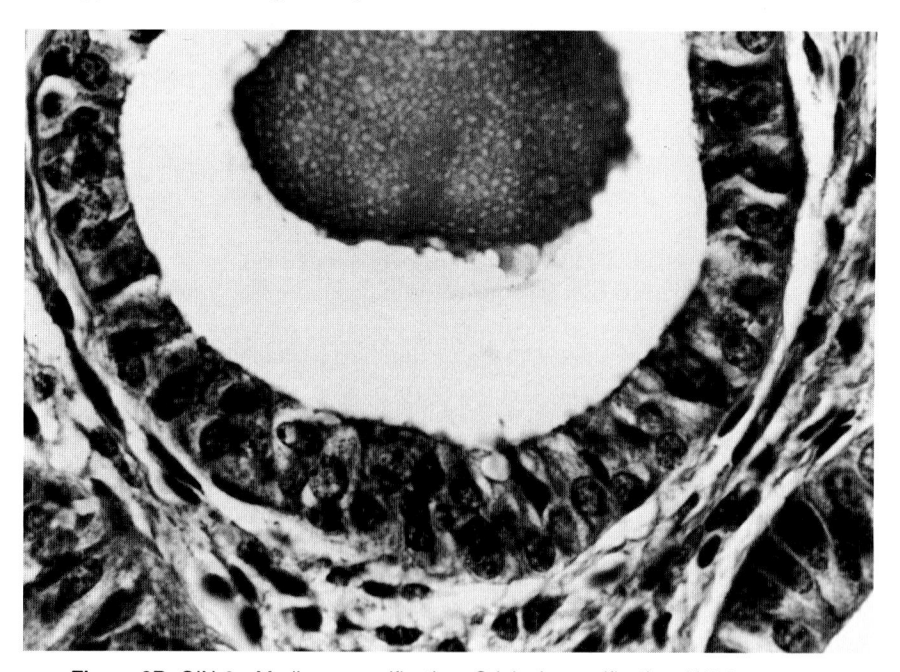

Figure 3B. GIN 2—Medium magnification. Original magnification. X190.

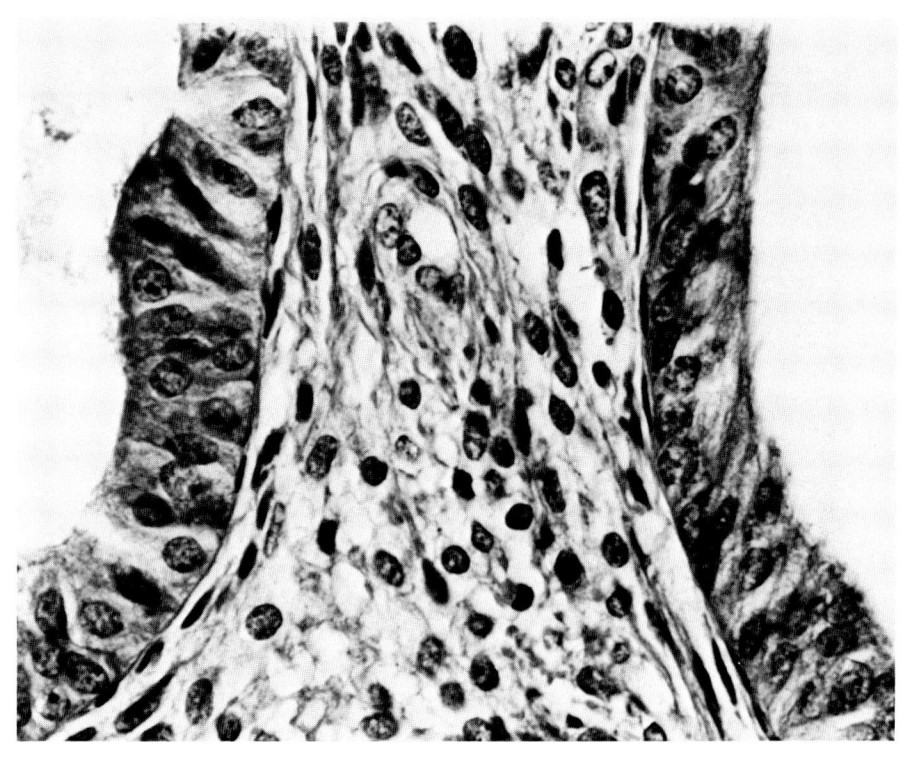

Figure 3C. GIN 2—True stratification is seen in the lower left. The nuclei have partially lost their oval shape and appear rounder. There is beginning loss of nuclear polarity to one another as well as to the glandular lumen. There is little variation in size. The chromatin pattern remains grainy without distinct nucleoli. The nuclear membranes appear regular. Cytoplasm is similar in density and staining characteristic to GIN 1. These changes have been referred to atypical hyperplasia or moderate adenomatous hyperplasia. Original magnification. X500.

Advances in the histologic diagnosis and understanding of endometrial neoplasia have been impeded by nomenclatures that subdivide lesions that merge imperceptibly . . . these subdivisions have little clinical merit, and the implication that they exist as discrete entities only perpetuates the existing confusion.

It is our belief that the concept of glandular intraepithelial neoplasia will form a practical alternative to previous classifications, and form a practical basis for the diagnosis and management of the precursors of endometrial carcinoma.

THE DIAGNOSIS OF ENDOMETRIAL CARCINOMA
Mode of Presentation
Most women diagnosed with endometrial carcinoma seek medical advice because of abnormal genital bleeding. In three recent studies 90 percent of

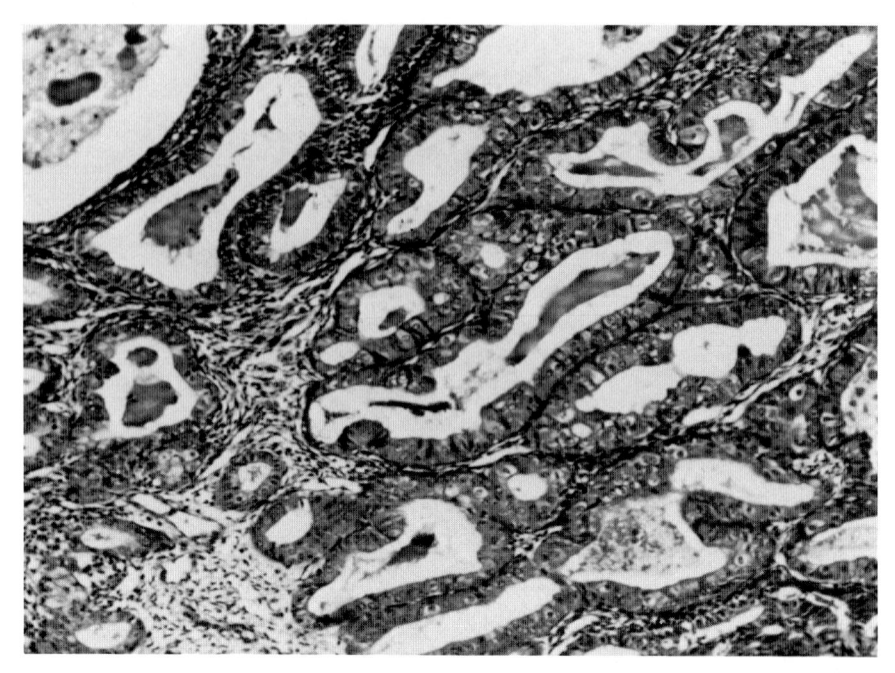

Figure 4A. GIN 3—The glands appear crowded, some being "back-to-back," but separated by delicate fibers of endometrial stroma. Even at this magnification the glandular epithelium has a disorganized appearance. Original magnification. X80.

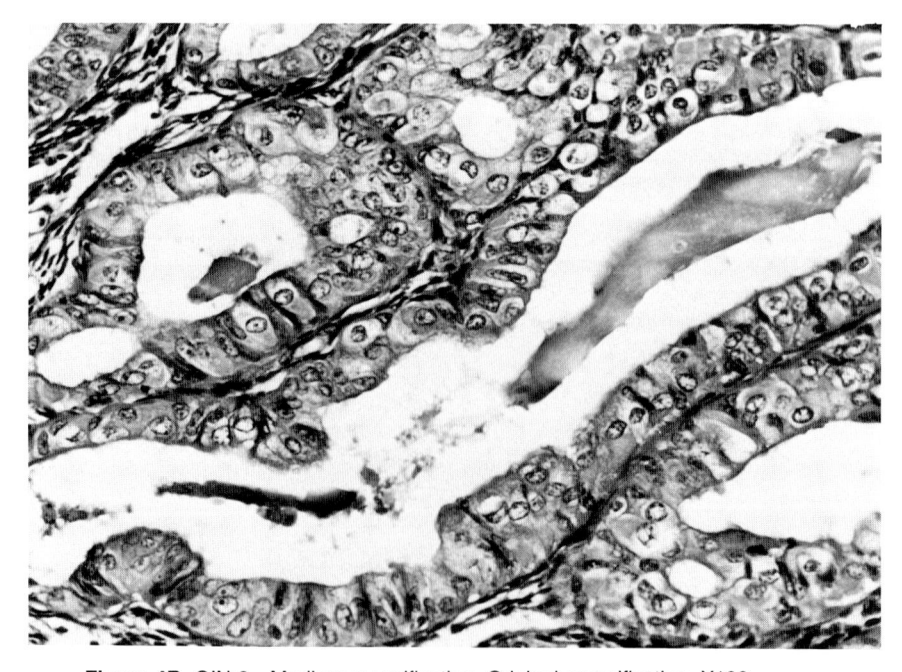

Figure 4B. GIN 3—Medium magnification. Original magnification. X190.

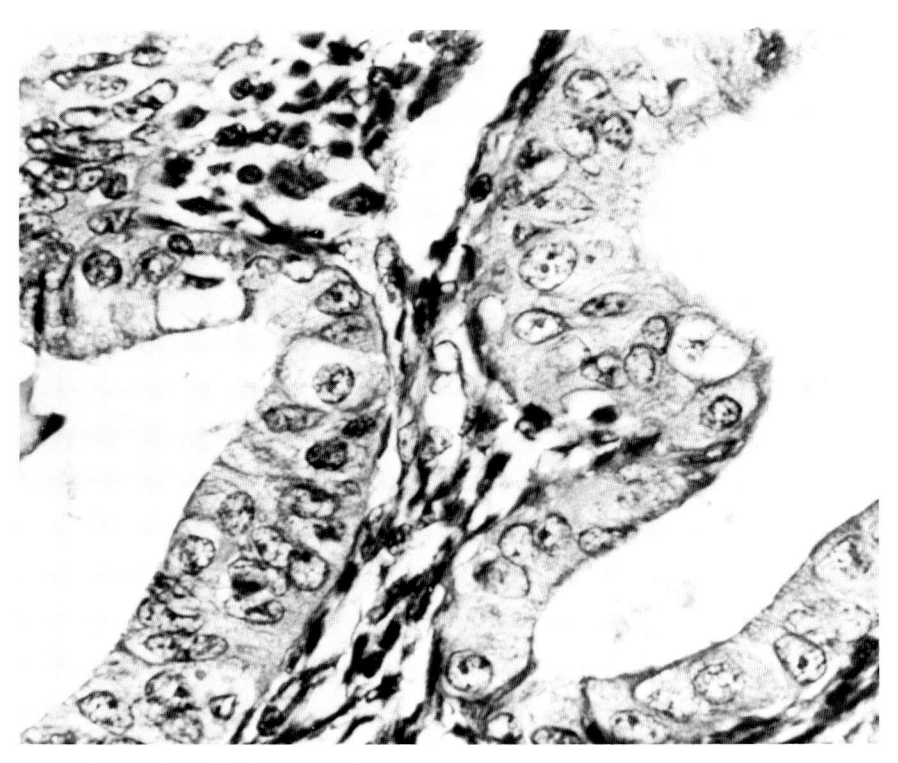

Figure 4C. GIN 3—The endometrial glands are separated by normal stroma, lacking desmoplasia. The cellular cytoplasm is abundant and pale. True stratification of cells is present. The nuclei are mostly round, differ in size, and exhibit loss of polarity to one another as well as the glandular lumen. The nuclear membranes are irregular. There is chromatin clearing, lending a vesicular appearance to the nuclei. Eosinophilic nucleoli are present. These changes have been referred to as severe atypical hyperplasia or carcinoma in situ. Original magnification. X500.

patients had been investigated for this complaint,[10,96,97] and this is typical of other studies. As the majority of patients with endometrial carcinoma are in the perimenopausal or postmenopausal age group, abnormal bleeding at that time is especially important. Nevertheless, it is important to remember that any abnormal uterine bleeding can be related to endometrial cancer, and should be properly investigated. Particular care should be taken in investigating the obese woman with a long history of "dysfunctional bleeding" or other menstrual abormalities, infertility, or stigmata of polycystic ovarian disease. Various techniques of endometrial sampling will be discussed later. One should emphasize that the definitive test is a formal dilation and thorough fractional curettage. This will ensure that carcinoma is detected if present, and if it is not, the procedure may be therapeutic.

Perimenopausal women with abnormal bleeding may believe that their bleeding is the result of "the change of life." Any women in this age group with more frequent or heavier periods, or intermenstrual bleeding, should be investigated until either proved to have uterine cancer or until it is excluded by a formal dilation and curettage. Similarly, one should be most cautious with women having "regular periods" after age 52.

The chance of detecting genital carcinoma during the investigation of postmenopausal bleeding is generally of the order of 20 percent,[98] although higher rates have been quoted. Among earlier papers, cervical cancer was found more frequently than endometrial, but the proportion of endometrial tumors may well be increasing. One must be particularly aware of the fact that the presence of one lesion, which could explain bleeding, such as atrophic vaginitis, does not rule out malignancy. All patients with postmenopausal bleeding must be investigated until endometrial carcinoma is excluded. The proportion of patients with postmenopausal bleeding who have malignancy increases with age and duration of menopause.[98] Although the duration and amount of bleeding is variable, even small amounts of bleeding must be investigated. In general, any amount of frank bleeding, and more than minimal amounts of bloody discharge, merit investigation. The recent use of estrogen should not be allowed to delay investigation on the assumption that the cause is "withdrawal bleeding."

A small proportion of women with endometrial carcinoma will present because of pyometra. The signs and symptoms are purulent, often bloody, vaginal discharge, and lower abdominal pain. The cervix will often appear small and atrophic, and on bimanual examination it may be difficult to assess uterine size. In such cases, passage of a uterine sound is important. This is a procedure that is potentially dangerous. In general, if a uterine sound cannot be passed easily in the office, it is wisest to perform the procedure under anesthesia to avoid perforation of the uterus, which is potentially fatal. Generally, once drainage is established, curettage is postponed for several weeks to avoid systemic infection and uterine perforation.

It is disquieting that between 10 and 20 percent of patients in two recent studies had symptoms present for over 1 year before the diagnosis was made.[35,97] The causes of delay may be the reluctance of elderly women to seek advice about genital problems, their ignorance of the significance of postmenopausal bleeding, or the failure of health care personnel to assess adequately patients with such complaints. Education is the solution to all these problems.

In most series, the number of asymptomatic patients found to have endometrial cancer is very low. This may mean that virtually all tumors produce symptoms early, or that there is a pool of occult carcinoma present. If this is the case, then there is clearly a need for effective screening procedures.

Evaluation of Symptomatic Patients

We wish to reiterate our warning that patients with symptoms suggestive of endometrial cancer must be investigated until the diagnosis of endometrial carcinoma has been made, or until it has been excluded by cervical dilation and thorough curettage. The availability of numerous endometrial sampling devices for office use should not be allowed to change this dictum. It may be reasonable to attempt office biopsy or sampling in an effort to hasten the diagnosis, but a negative result demands a thorough curettage. Endometrial sampling or biopsy can be difficult, painful, and possibly dangerous in this age group. The main danger is uterine perforation, at the isthmus or the fundus.

Screening Asymptomatic Patients

Two groups must be distinguished here: those with no apparent predilection for endometrial carcinoma, and those with either constitutional risk factors or those who are using estrogens. Screening the entire obese population would detect only about half of the cases of endometrial carcinoma, and although exogenous estrogens appear to increase markedly the incidence of endometrial carcinoma, the great majority of patients are not using estrogens. Hence, if a screening program is to affect the incidence of endometrial carcinoma, it would need to cover the entire postmenopausal population. Of course, even in the absence of such a program, routine screening of all women using estrogens postmenopausally is justified to minimize the danger of the therapeutic agent.

Papanicolaou smears are relatively poor for detecting endometrial carcinoma, even in symptomatic patients. An extensive review of the literature indicates that samples from the posterior fornix and ectocervix, and from the endocervix by aspiration will detect about 70 percent of endometrial carcinomas, while the standard vaginal/ectocervical/endocervical smear on a single slide detects only about 40 percent of tumors.[99] Both doctors and patients must be aware that a routine Papanicolaou smear is a poor way of excluding endometrial cancer (Fig. 5).

Endometrial sampling techniques may involve obtaining specimens for histologic or cytologic examination. Before considering the relative merits of each technique, a note of caution must be sounded. Most reports of the efficacy of the techniques are based on the examination of symptomatic patients, a totally different situation from examining asymptomatic women. The detection rates obtained may therefore be rather better than can be obtained by routine use.

Vuopala[99] has collated the results reported in the literature for a variety of screening techniques, and these are presented in Table 6.

A large number of ingenious techniques have been designed to sample the endometrium. All produce specimens for either cytologic or histologic evaluation. Koss and associates[100] provide an overview of the various techniques and point out that, manufacturers' claims to the contrary, cytologic smears of the endometrium are very difficult to interpret. The problems of diagnosing hyperplasia on cytologic smears are even greater. Gusberg and Milano[101] favor the histologic examination of specimens obtained by vacuum aspiration of the endometrium, claiming ease of interpretation, a 90 percent successful sampling rate, and over 97 percent accuracy in detecting carcinoma. Further, the state that the technique accurately diagnoses hyperpla-

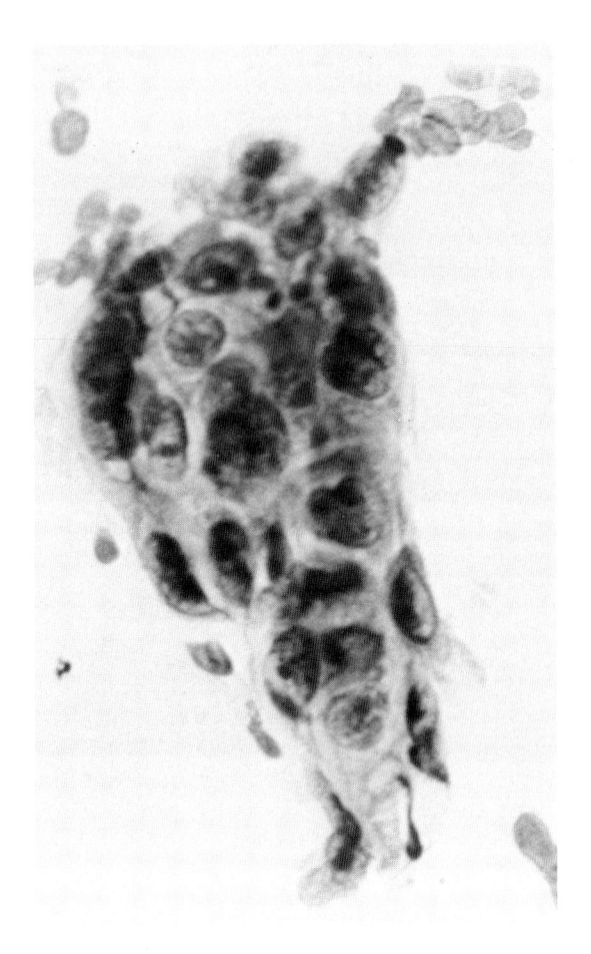

Figure 5. A Papanicolaou smear showing malignant endometrial cells, apparently forming a tight epithelial structure. Individual cells differ in size, shape, and chromatin structure. (Pap smears are positive in about 50 percent of cases of endometrial carcinoma).

TABLE 6. POOLED RESULTS IN DIAGNOSIS OF ENDOMETRIAL CANCER FROM A NUMBER OF PUBLISHED SERIES UTILIZING VARIOUS CYTOLOGIC AND HISTOLOGIC TECHNIQUES OF ENDOMETRIAL SAMPLING

Technique	No. of Patients in Study	No. with Endometrial Cancer	Accuracy in Diagnosing Cancer (%)
Aspiration	12,480	331	88.5
Lavage	2805	206	81.6
Endometrial brush	1354	278	87.4
Jet wash			
Direct smear	2258	90	86.7
Millipore filter	1234	64	75.0
Cell block	4701	184	87.5
Endometrial biopsy	1679	445	87.4
Aspiration curettage	1135	40	97.5

(Modified from Vuopala S: Acta Obstet Gynecol Scand [Suppl] 70:8, 1977, with permission.)[99]

sias in almost 92 percent and that 90 percent of women are willing to accept the procedure again. Perforation occurred in only 7 out of 4500 patients in their series.

Koss and colleagues[100] evaluated the feasibility of screening for endometrial neoplasia on a routine basis on ambulatory, asymptomatic patients. They employed a technique utilizing both cytologic and histologic examination of specimens, claiming that the two are complementary. They reported on 2007 women screened, 80 percent of whom were postmenopausal. The success rate of obtaining satisfactory samples on the first attempt was 86 percent: in 7 percent of patients the sampling instrument could not be passed through the cervical canal because of pain or stenosis. Sampling was successful in 95 percent of women under 60 years of age, but only in 83 percent of women over 70. In 7 percent of patients, samples were obtained but were inadequate for interpretation. Ten cases of endometrial carcinoma occurred in this asymptomatic population. Eight were detected by the endometrial sampling procedure and one by examination of a vaginal pool Papanicolaou smear, and one became symptomatic 6 months after a negative sampling. The authors concluded that it was too early to assess whether such screening procedures would lower morbidity and mortality from endometrial cancer.

STAGING ENDOMETRIAL CARCINOMA

The generally accepted staging system for endometrial carcinoma is that adopted by the International Federation of Gynecology and Obstetrics (FIGO) in 1971 (Table 7).[102] The system is based on clinical findings obtained prior to definitive therapy. The findings at examination, preferably under anesthesia, which include inspection, palpation, and fractional curettage are essential. Findings on hysteroscopy, cystoscopy, and protoscopy are acceptable for staging purposes, as are chest x-rays, skeletal x-rays, and intravenous pyelograms.

Fractional Curettage. This procedure allows the uterine size to be assessed and the diagnosis to be confirmed with adequate curettings. It also allows recognition of endocervical involvement (Stage II). The technique is critical. The procedure is best performed under anesthesia. After sounding of the uterine cavity but *before* dilation of the cervix, *thorough* curettage of the endocervical canal is performed and the specimen put in a labeled container. Then the cervix is dilated and the uterine corpus curetted in a systematic and thorough manner, with the endometrial curettings placed in a separate labeled container. The endocervical and endometrial curettings are evaluated separately by the pathologist.

The incidence of endocervical involvement in endometrial carcinoma has varied widely in different reports. Rutledge[103] found that in 17 studies published between 1961 and 1973, involving over 7000 cases, Stage II disease was diagnosed in from 3 to 24 percent, with a mean of 12 percent. One reason for the variation may be a failure to perform endocervical curettage, although

TABLE 7. THE FIGO CLINICAL STAGING FOR INVASIVE ENDOMETRIAL CARCINOMA

Stage I	The carcinoma is confined to the corpus
Stage I A	The length of the uterine cavity is 8 cm or less
Stage I B	The length of the uterine cavity is more than 8 cm
	It is desirable that the Stage I cases be subgrouped with regard to the histologic type of the adenocarcinoma as follows:
G 1	Highly differentiated adenomatous carcinoma
G 2	Moderately differentiated adenomatous carcinoma with partly solid areas
G 3	Predominantly solid or entirely undifferentiated carcinoma
Stage II	The carcinoma has involved the corpus and the cervix but has not extended outside the uterus
Stage III	The carcinoma has extended outside the uterus but not outside the true pelvis
Stage IV	The carcinoma has extended outside the true pelvis or has obviously involved the mucosa of the bladder or rectum. A bullous edema as such does not permit a case to be allotted to stage IV
Stage IV A	Spread of the growth to adjacent organs
Stage IV B	Spread to distant organs

(From The American Joint Committee for Cancer Staging and End-results Reporting: Manual for Staging of Cancer, Chicago, American Joint Committee, 1978, with permission.)[102]

Kneale[104] found that where subsequent histology showed a 20 percent incidence of endocervical involvement, fractional curettage had detected only 10 percent.

Homesley and colleagues[105] found that of 538 patients treated for Stage I disease, 90 (17 percent) had endocervical involvement on retrospective examination of the hysterectomy specimen. They concluded that both grossly apparent cervical involvement and microscopic involvement carried a high risk of extrauterine spread, and an equally poor prognosis. This argues strongly for careful fractional curettage in all cases.

Several histologic variants of apparent endocervical involvement are possible. Tumor from the corpus may inadvertently be picked up by the endocervical curette, appearing separate from endocervical tissue. Tumor may spread by contiguous growth over the surface of the endocervical canal, may involve the stroma, or may completely replace endocervical tissue. Kadar and associates[106] demonstrated that any form of true endocervical involvement carried the same prognostic connotations, but suggested that tissue space or lymphatic spread was more common than contiguous spread. Early spread of this type could not be detected by anything but the most thorough curettage.

Hysteroscopy. Marsden and Correy[107] have shown that this is a technique that can be quickly mastered by any gynecologist, using either special hysteroscopes, or pediatric or adult cystoscopes, although considerable experience is required for reliable examinations. It is particularly useful in patients with postmenopausal bleeding to confirm the presence of a normal endometrial cavity when no curettings are obtained. It should also be useful in detecting Stage II lesions. Kneale[104] found this to be the case, as did Anderson.[108] Hysteroscopy is not widely practiced in the United States at the present time.

Hysterography. Hysterography has been advocated by some authors,[108,109] but we are not yet convinced of its value. However, fears that hysterography may lead to spread of tumor and subsequent poorer prognosis seem to be unfounded.[109]

Cystoscopy. Cystoscopy may be used for staging, but caution is essential. Misdiagnosis of bladder involvement by inexperienced observers is an ever-present risk, and biopsy can be hazardous if direct extension of the tumor has occurred. Vesicouterine or vesicocervical and vesicovaginal fistulas are most unpleasant complications, and difficult to explain to the patient.

Prognostic Significance of FIGO Staging

There is a broad correlation between FIGO stage of disease and outcome, as shown in Table 8. Substages I A and I B appear to have little significance, but as will be discussed later, the tumor differentiation is of great importance in Stage I disease.

While the FIGO staging is useful for correlation of worldwide results, and in particular to help set standards to be achieved in developing countries, we believe it should be supplanted, or supplemented, by a surgical staging system. The reasons for this will become apparent when we discuss the pathology of endometrial carcinoma and the other prognostic factors.

HISTOPATHOLOGY OF ENDOMETRIAL CARCINOMA

Tumor Subtypes

Carcinoma of the endometrium occurs in a number of subtypes, each varying in its propensity for myometrial invasion and metastasis. The relative frequen-

TABLE 8. ENDOMETRIAL CARCINOMA: SURVIVALS BY STAGE REPORTED IN RECENT PAPERS

Author	Percentage 5-Year Survival			
	Stage I	Stage II	Stage III	Stage IV
Malkasian (1978)[7] (523 cases)	82	75	59	13
Beck (1979)[8] (509 cases)	89	31	33	9
McCabe and Sagerman (1979)[9] (379 cases)	82	60	17	0
Connelly et al. (1982)[10] (811 cases)	81	41	42	9
Kauppila et al. (1982)[34] (1113 cases)	78	61	29	5

cies of the various types of endometrial carcinoma have varied with time, and from one institution to another. Table 9 shows the proportion of tumors of each subtype in two recently published studies from the United States.

Adenocarcinoma. Adenocarcinoma is the most common variety of subtype and is seen in almost two-thirds of cases. Histologically it is characterized by the proliferation of abnormal glands in an abnormal relationship to one another. Little or no stroma separates the glands. The lining epithelium may be infolded or papillary. Cells are enlarged and often pseudostratified, with variable numbers of mitotic figures. In accordance with the FIGO staging systems, it is usual to classify the tumor as grade 1, well differentiated; grade 2, moderately differentiated with partly solid areas; and grade 3, predominantly solid, or entirely undifferentiated. Examples of adenocarcinoma of the endometrium and each grade of differentiation are shown in Figures 6 through 9.

Adenoacanthoma. Adenoacanthoma is an adenocarcinoma with areas of benign squamous epithelium, usually scattered throughout the tumor but occasionally localized (Fig. 6). Ng and colleagues[19] demonstrated a slight increase in the frequency of this tumor over a 30-year period. Areas of squamous epithelium are said to be detectable by thorough searching in most endometrial adenocarcinomas and have been recognized for at least 95 years, occasionally being attributed to estrogens.[110]

Adenosquamous Carcinoma. Adenosquamous carcinoma is characterized by the presence of both malignant glandular and squamous elements (Fig. 7). The squamous component may be interspersed among the malignant glands or superimposed. Glandular malignancy is the dominant component in 60 percent and squamous in 40 percent of cases. The glandular component tends to be well differentiated much less frequently than in pure adenocarcinoma.[111] The incidence of adenosquamous malignancies rose dramatically in the

TABLE 9. FREQUENCY OF HISTOLOGIC SUBTYPES AMONG 989 CASES OF PRIMARY ENDOMETRIAL CARCINOMA IN TWO RECENT STUDIES

Tumor Type	Christopherson et al. (1982)[16] (%)	Reagan and Fu (1981)[110] (%)
Adenocarcinoma	59.6	65
Adenoacanthoma	21.7	19
Adenosquamous carcinoma	6.9	14
Clear cell carcinoma	5.7	1
Papillary adeno-carcinoma	4.7	—
Secretory carcinoma	1.5	1

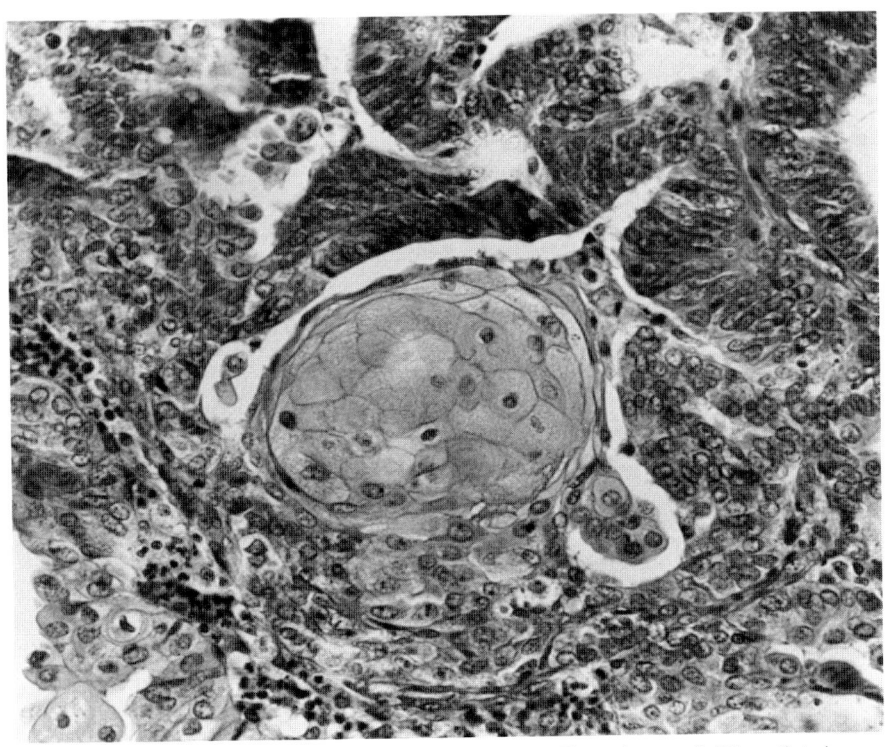

Figure 6. Adenoacanthoma of the endometrium. There is a well-differentiated adenocarcinoma with foci of benign squamous metaplasia. It is important to differentiate between this tumor and adenosquamous carcinoma (Fig. 7), which has a much poorer prognosis.

30-year period studied by Ng and colleagues,[19] but Alberhasky and colleagues[18] found no such increase. They did, however, find a dramatic increase in the incidence of adenoacanthomas.

Clear Cell Adenocarcinoma. Clear cell adenocarcinoma (Fig. 8) consists of polygonal, hobnail-shaped or flattened cells arranged in solid masses, or papillary, tubular or cystic patterns. Psammoma bodies may be present. The cells are PAS-positive.

Papillary Carcinoma. Papillary carcinoma (Fig. 9) is distinguished from the papillary clear cell carcinoma by the absence of a significant clear cell component. The cells have sparse, basophilic or amphophilic cytoplasm and are PAS-negative.

Secretory Adenocarcinoma. Secretory adenocarcinoma is characterized by a basically glandular pattern with cells showing uniform, subnuclear vacuolization, similar to that seen in the luteal phase of the menstrual cycle.

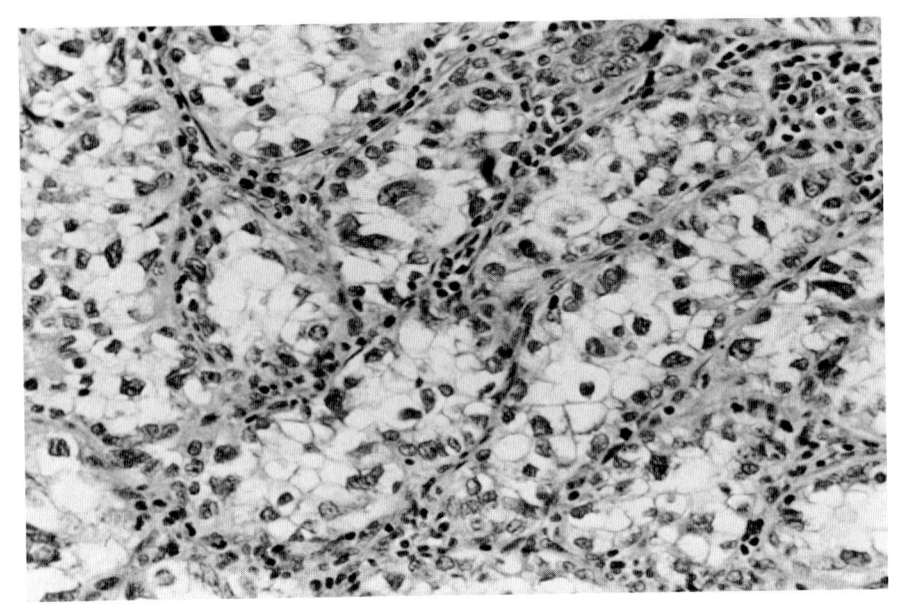

Figure 8. Clear cell adenocarcinoma of the endometrium. Tumor cells form solid sheets, and tubular, papillary, or cystic structures. Prominent nuclei create a hobnail appearance. The histologic appearance of this tumor is identical regardless of where it arises in the Müllerian system, i.e., endometrium, ovary, or cervix.

incidence of lymph node involvement. Table 10 shows the relationship between tumor grade and depth of myometrial invasion, as reported by Cheon.[112] The prognostic relationship of various combinations of these variables is presented in Table 11.

Lymph Node Involvement

One of the "myths" exposed by Boronow[4] is that "traditional" teaching tends to minimize the importance of lymph node involvement in endometrial carcinoma. It is becoming increasingly evident that lymph node involvement is far more common than was once thought, and that it is essential to search it out as a routine part of the surgical assessment of all patients, regardless of the stage of disease. Only recently has the importance of lymph node spread been recognized, and thus reliable data on its incidence are difficult to obtain. Moreover, if only "suspicious" nodes are sampled, then a proportion of metastases will be missed. It is our belief that undetected extrauterine spread that is present at the time of surgery is the most common cause of treatment failure in early stage lesions.

In an attempt to clarify the situation, Creasman and colleagues[114] performed "selective" pelvic lymphadenectomies on 140 women with Stage I endometrial carcinoma, and para-aortic lymphadenectomy in 102 of these patients. Pelvic node metastases were found in 11.4 percent and para-aortic node metastases in 5.7 percent. Of particular importance was the fact that in

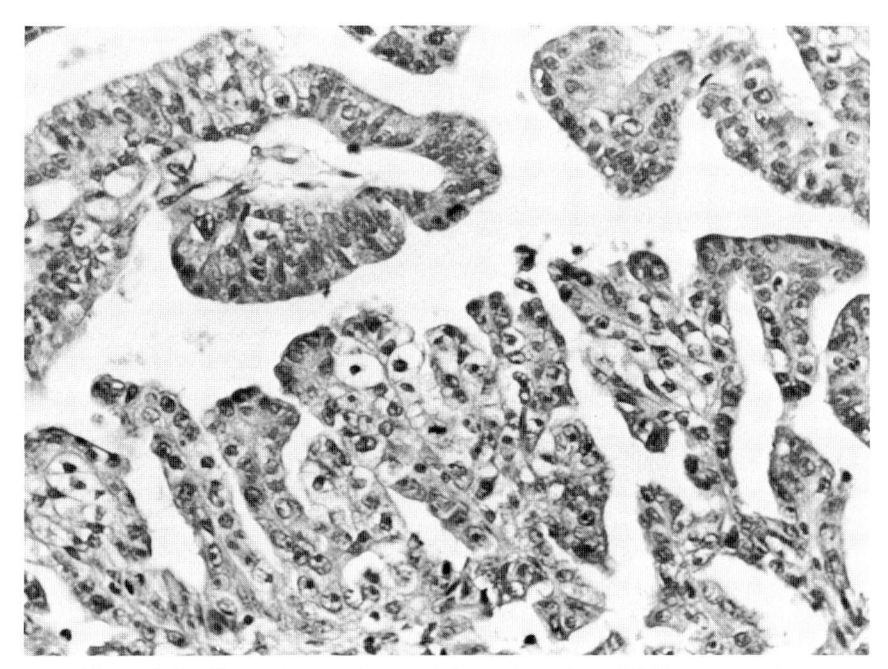

Figure 9. Papillary adenocarcinoma of the endometrium. (**A**) The tumor cells are supported on thin fibrovascular cores forming delicate papillary fronds.

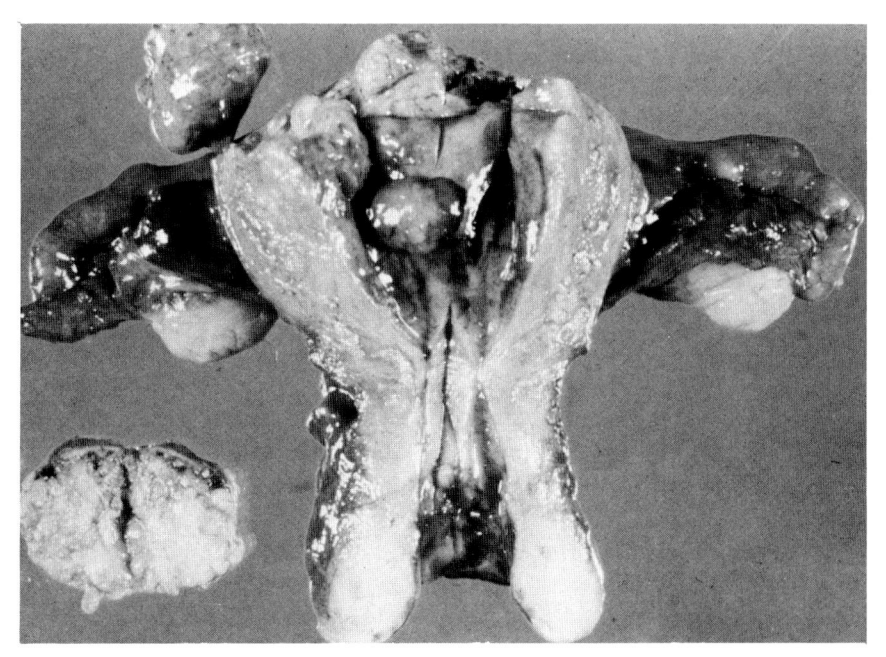

Figure 9B. This 60 gram uterus contains a papillary adenocarcinoma of the endometrium, which invades to the middle third and extends to the endocervix. An enlarged right internal iliac lymph node contained metastatic tumor.

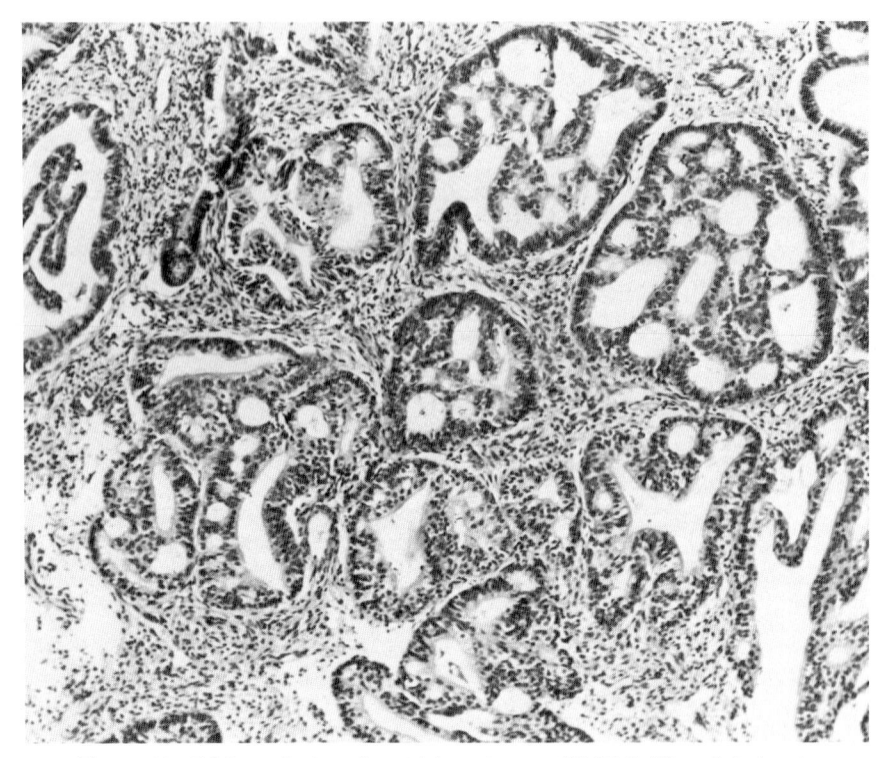

Figure 10. FIGO grade 1 endometrial carcinoma. **(A)** Well-differentiated endometrial cells form glandular structures, which in this case are cribriform. There are no solid masses of tumor cells.

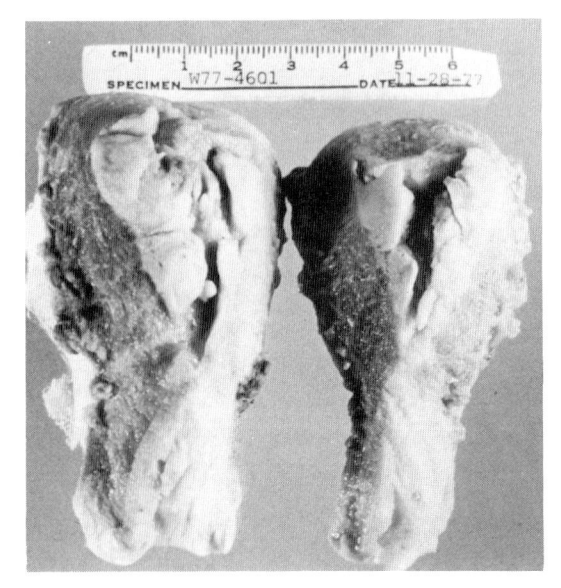

Figure 10B. This 80 gram uterus contains a diffuse FIGO grade 1 endometrial carcinoma, with no myometrial invasion. There is a sharp line of demarcation apparent between the tumor and the myometrium.

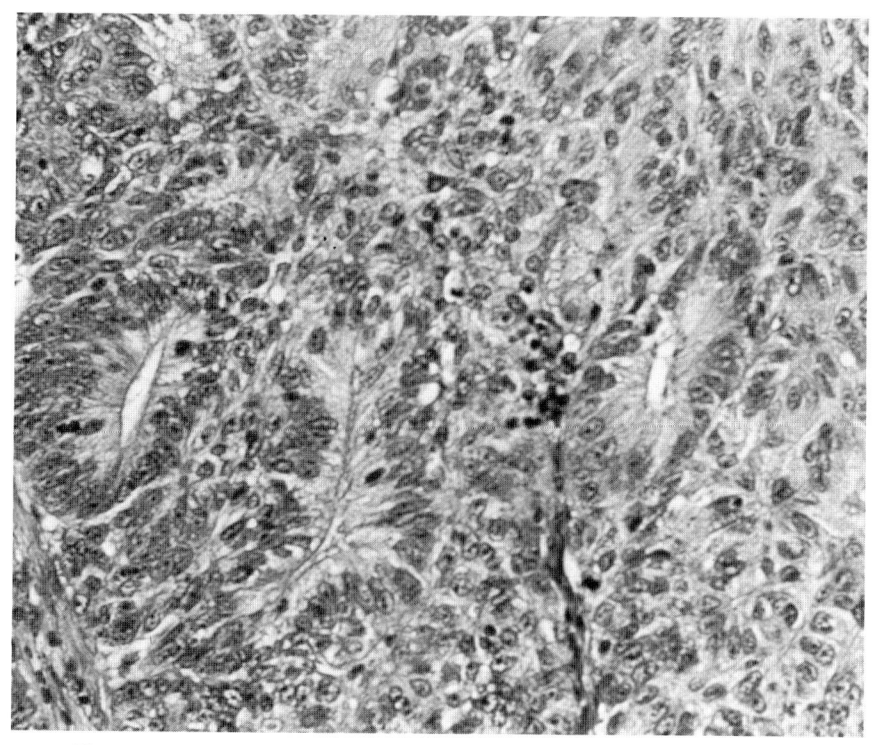

Figure 11A. FIGO grade 2 endometrial adenocarcinoma. The tumor consists of moderately well-differentiated malignant cells. There are areas of solid tumor interspersed with glandular tumor elements.

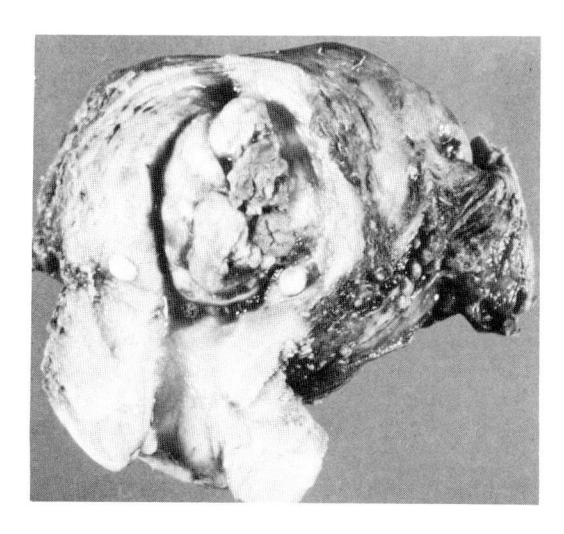

Figure 11B. A 250 gram uterus containing a FIGO grade 2 endometrial carcinoma, which appears as a polypoid mass macroscopically invading to the middle third of the myometrium.

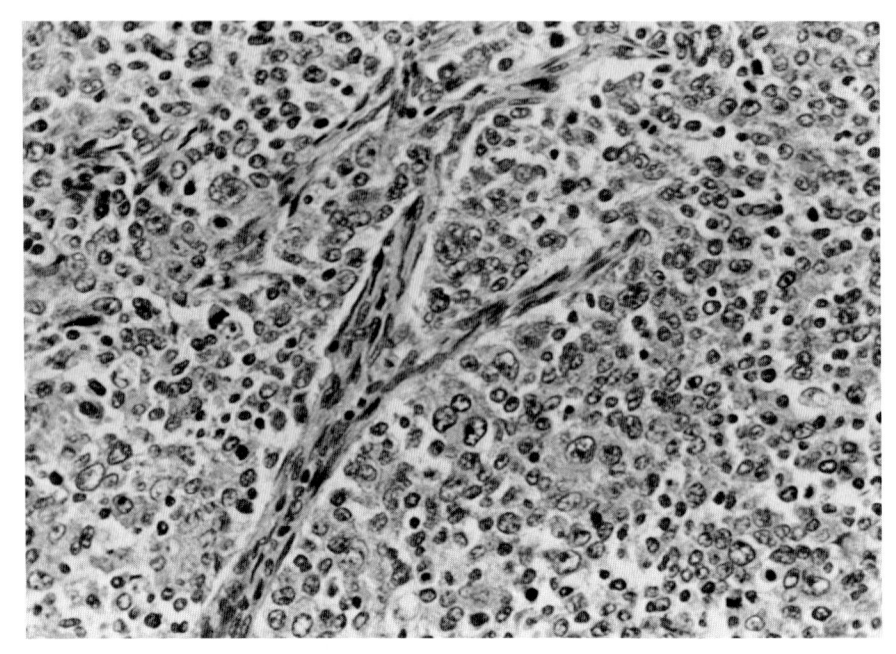

Figure 12A. FIGO grade 3 adenocarcinoma of the endometrium. The tumor consists of solid sheets of malignant cells, with no attempt to form glandular structures.

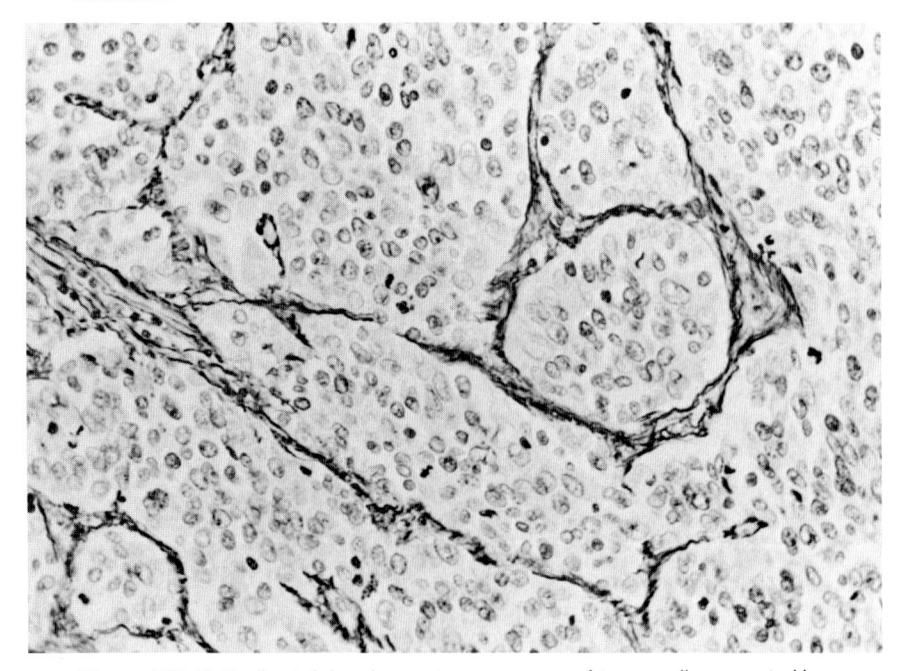

Figure 12B. Reticulin staining demonstrates masses of tumor cells separated by strands of connective tissue. Endometrial stromal sarcoma, and lymphomas show intercellular reticulin fibers, facilitating the differential diagnosis.

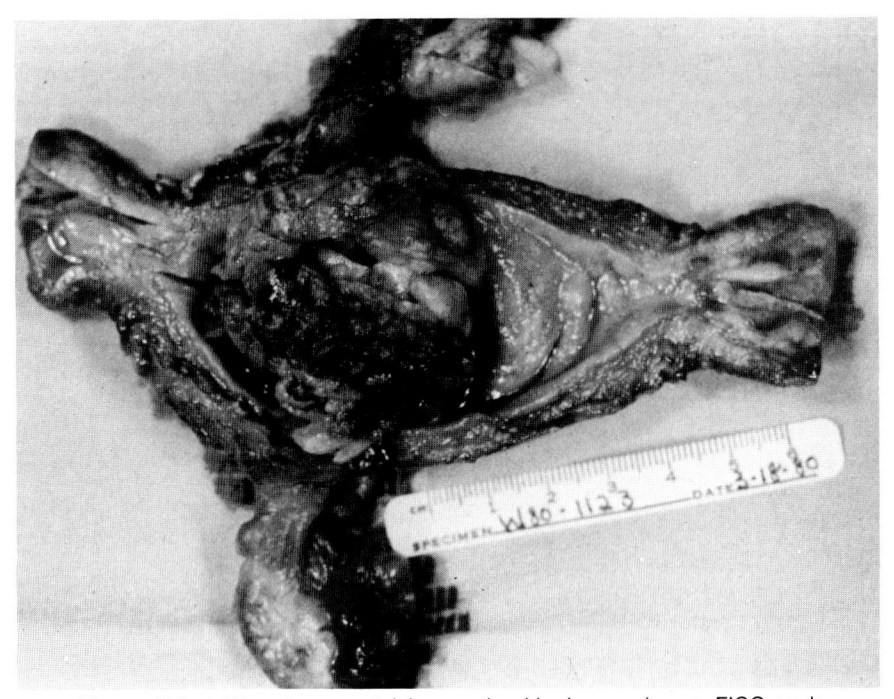

Figure 12C. A 72-g uterus containing a polypoid adenocarcinoma, FIGO grade 3, which invades to half way through the myometrium and which microscopically showed lymph vascular permeation.

only one-fourth of the patients with positive para-aortic nodes were they clinically suspicious for metastases. Table 12 shows the relationship of stage, grade, and myometrial invasion to the incidence of lymph node metastasis. In Stage I B, grade 3 lesions, 36 percent of patients had positive pelvic nodes, and 28 percent positive para-aortic nodes. Kneale[104] reported the results of nonselected lymphadenectomies on 206 consecutive patients with endometrial carcinoma, and found that overall 8.4 percent had positive pelvic nodes: among patients with Stage I disease, 7.4 percent had positive pelvic nodes.

Piver and colleagues[14] performed para-aortic lymphadenectomy on 41 women with Stage I endometrial carcinoma, and found positive nodes in 14.6 percent of cases. There were no positive para-aortic nodes among women with grade 1 lesions, but there were 14 percent with grade 2 and 38 percent with grade 3 lesions. When tumor was confined to the endometrium, no para-aortic nodes were positive, but with superficially invasive or deeply invasive lesions the rates were 5 and 46 percent, respectively.

Peritoneal Cytology

Creasman and Rutledge[115] drew attention to the importance of peritoneal cytology in gynecologic malignancy in 1971, but most gynecologists have not

TABLE 10. THE INTERRELATIONSHIP OF MYOMETRIAL INVASION AND TUMOR GRADE

FIGO Grade	Depth of Myometrial Invasion		
	None (%)	Superficial (%)	Deep (%)
Grade 1	58	30	12
Grade 2	51	28	20
Grade 3	38	16	46

(From Cheon HK: Obstet Gynecol 34:680, 1963, with permission.)[112]

accepted their warning, and few perform the examination routinely. In a recent paper, Creasman and colleagues[15] reported the findings on peritoneal cytology in 167 patients with Stage I endometrial carcinoma (Table 13). Recurrences occurred in 34 percent of patients with positive cytology and in only 10 percent of those with negative cytology.

PRETREATMENT WORK-UP

Endometrial cancer patients are often old, and may be obese or suffer from such medical conditions as diabetes, hypertension, and cardiopulmonary disease. Careful but sensible pretreatment assessment is essential to maximize the effectiveness and minimize the danger of therapy.

History and physical examination should be systematic and thorough, with particular emphasis on preexisting medical conditions and their treatment. Cardiopulmonary status should be especially carefully assessed, and one should not hesitate to seek specialist consultation for concurrent medical conditions.

It should be remembered that the age and constitution of patients with endometrial carcinoma make them more likely than the average to have concomitant or subsequent tumors, especially of the breast and bowel. A total of 92 other malignancies were found prior to, concomitant with, or subsequent to the endometrial tumor among 577 Stage I patients at the Mayo Clinic,[35]

TABLE 11. THE 5-YEAR SURVIVAL RATES OF PATIENTS WITH ENDOMETRIAL CARCINOMA WITH VARYING COMBINATIONS OF TUMOR DIFFERENTIATION AND MYOMETRIAL INVASION

FIGO Grade	Depth of Myometrial Invasion		
	None (%)	Superficial (%)	Deep (%)
Grade 1	95	92	33
Grade 2	93	72	50
Grade 3	63	50	18

(Data from Ng AB, Reagan JW: Obstet Gynecol 35:437, 1970, with permission.)[113]

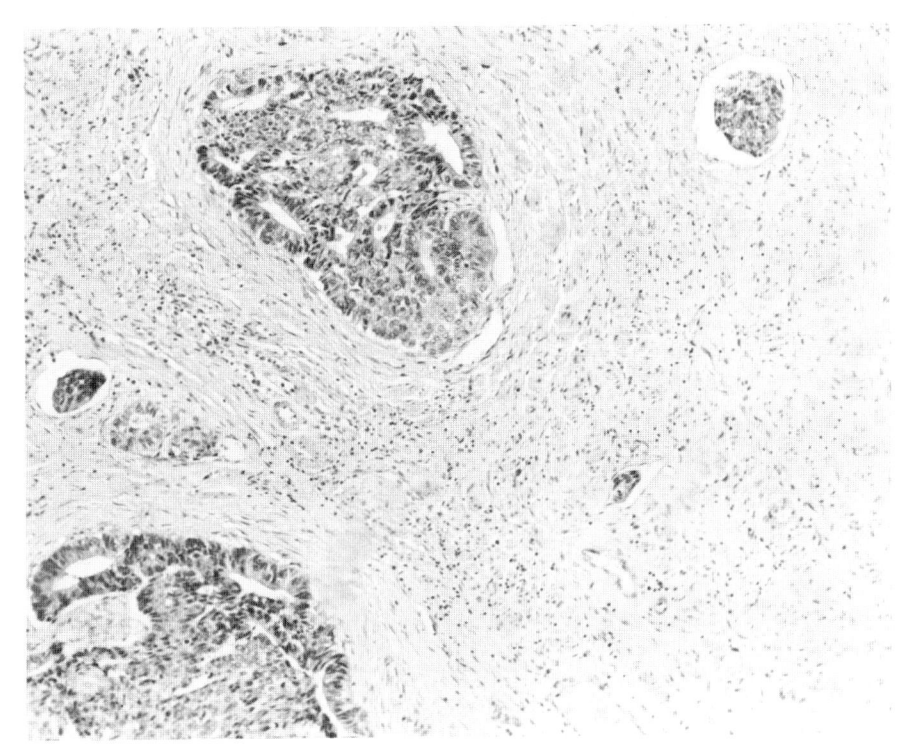

Figure 13. Well-differentiated tumors may on occasion show myometrial invasion. This FIGO grade 1 tumor shows deep myometrial invasion and emboli in lymphatic or vascular spaces.

TABLE 12. STAGE I ENDOMETRIAL CARCINOMA: RELATIONSHIP BETWEEN TUMOR STAGE, GRADE, AND MYOMETRIAL INVASION AND THE INCIDENCE OF LYMPH NODE INVOLVEMENT

	Pelvic Nodes Positive (%)	Para-aortic Nodes Positive (%)
Stage I A	6	4
Stage I B	18	12
Grade 1	3	2
Grade 2	10	4
Grade 3	36	28
Myometrial invasion		
Endometrium only	4	2
Superficial	12	10
Intermediate	10	0
Deep	43	21

(Data from Creasman WT, et al: Gynecol Oncol 4:239, 1976, with permission.)[114]

TABLE 13. STAGE I ENDOMETRIAL CARCINOMA. INCIDENCE OF POSITIVE PERITONEAL CYTOLOGY

Stage I A	17%
Stage I B	13%
Grade 1	9%
Grade 2	22%
Grade 3	16%
Myometrial invasion	
Endometrium only	8%
Superficial	15%
Intermediate	30%
Deep	32%

(Data from Creasman WT, et al: Am J Obstet Gynecol 110:773, 1971, with permission.)[115]

and in approximately 7 percent of over 1000 patients in the series of Kauppila and associates.[34]

Breast examination should be carefully performed. Emphasis should be put on careful pelvic examination with emphasis on examination of the entire vagina and cervix for metastases or concomitant tumor. Biopsies of suspicious areas are essential. Bimanual and rectovaginal examination, although often difficult, must be done with great thoroughness.

Blood work should include full blood counts, SMA complete, and blood grouping. Where diabetes is present or suspected, fasting and postprandial glucose levels may be obtained.

Radiologic investigation must include a chest x-ray and intravenous pyelogram. We include a barium enema, on the grounds that colorectal carcinoma is relatively common in this age group. Mammography is included in our protocol because of the relative frequency of breast cancer, and similarities in epidemiology and hormonal profiles for women with endometrial or breast cancer.

CT scanning of the abdomen has been most disappointing as a routine screening test in our hospital, and among patients referred from other institutions, and we recommend it only in exceptional cases. Bone scanning and liver-spleen scanning should only be used where indicated by specific signs or symptoms.

We consider lymphography to be of little value in these cases.

Electrocardiograms should be done on all patients.

Consultation with specialists in cardiopulmonary medicine or endocrinology is frequently required. It is advisable to consult the anesthesiologist several days in advance should surgery be planned in the obese or medically compromised patient.

Special testing of cardiopulmonary status should be performed as indicated. The insertion of a Swan-Ganz catheter is occasionally necessary preoperatively.

Respiratory and physical therapy may profitably begin *before* surgery in patients at high risk. For patients to know their therapists and understand the exercises and equipment that will be used after surgery can greatly facilitate the postoperative course.

Radiotherapy consultation should be obtained prior to the examination under anesthesia in all cases where radiation is being considered as a possible part of management. This allows the gynecologic and the radiation oncologist the opportunity to discuss the problem, examine the patient, and decide on the best course of management.

TREATMENT

Stages I and II

The true extent of endometrial carcinoma can only be ascertained after exploratory laparotomy, and so we believe that the primary approach to almost all patients with Stages I and II disease should be surgical. For many years it was standard practice to give preoperative radiotherapy by either external beam or the intracavitary route. This was aimed at reducing tumor bulk, "sealing" lymphatics, and "sterilizing" the tumor to prevent intraoperative spread and central recurrence. The incidence of vaginal vault recurrence was said to fall from 10 percent to less than 5 percent in different series, but survival did not appear to change significantly.[6] Surgery was customarily delayed for 4 to 6 weeks after radiation to allow radiation-damaged tissues to recover. Unfortunately, by that time radiation effects had "destroyed the evidence" in terms of the factors now known to be prognostically important, such as myometrial invasion and cervical involvement. Some have advocated intracavitary radiation followed by immediate surgery (within 48 hours) to circumvent this problem.[116] It has, however, been demonstrated that preoperative and postoperative radiation are equally effective in preventing pelvic recurrences.[6] Currently, we believe that all patients fit for surgery should have the operation first, and that only those with the presence of anaplastic or adenosquamous tumors, unsuspected cervical involvement, deep myometrial penetration, or extrauterine extension should be considered for radiotherapy.

Surgery is performed through a generous vertical incision. Peritoneal washings are obtained immediately on entering the abdominal cavity. The upper abdomen is carefully explored for metastatic disease. Thereafter, paraaortic lymphadenectomy is performed. The bowel is then packed away and the pelvis explored. We perform bilateral pelvic lymphadenectomies in all cases: the procedure is rather less fastidious than in the radical operation for cervical carcinoma, involving removal of all enlarged or suspicious nodes, and generous samples of apparently normal nodes from each major group. We then perform an extrafascial hysterectomy and bilateral salpingo-ophorectomy in patients with Stage I disease. Fit patients with Stage II disease receive a radical hysterectomy. Following completion of the surgery, the vault is drained with a T-tube, and the pelvic lymphadenectomy sites with suction drains brought out through the abdominal wall.

We close the abdominal incision with a continuous "bulk-closure" technique utilizing No. 2 Vicryl or Dexon sutures through peritoneum, muscle and fascia. The subcutaneous tissues are then approximated with a few No. 000 sutures, and the skin is closed with staples.

We believe that nursing with the foot of the bed elevated 30 degrees, and early postoperative mobilization are the most important steps in preventing thromboembolism, and doctors, nurses, and physical therapists are all actively involved in achieving this.

When the pathologist confirms that the disease is totally confined to the uterus, with little or no myometrial invasion and a well-differentiated Stage I tumor, we do not employ radiotherapy. Patients with Stage I or Stage II disease and poorly differentiated or deeply invasive tumors, or those with evidence of pelvic lymphatic involvement, or involvement of other pelvic organs, receive a full course of radiotherapy to the pelvis, utilizing a linear accelerator. Radiotherapy starts 2 to 4 weeks after surgery. It is our practice to start these patients on megestrol acetate (Megace) in doses of 80 to 160 mg per day on discharge from hospital.

Although we favor radical hysterectomy as the treatment of choice for Stage II disease, in many institutions Stage II disease is treated with radiotherapy as for a carcinoma of the cerivx, together with an extrafascial hysterectomy and bilateral salpingo-oophorectomy.

At laparotomy, a small proportion of patients with clinical Stage I or Stage II disease will be found to have extrauterine spread, and the management of these patients presents a difficult problem. Where the only evidence of extrauterine spread was positive peritoneal cytology, Creasman and associates[15] found that the instillation of radioactive chromium phosphate appeared to reduce the incidence of tumor recurrence. The radiocolloid was administered through a peritoneal dialysis catheter about 2 weeks after surgery. The actual significance of positive peritoneal cytology in patients with early stage endometrial carcinoma remains to be clarified. Yazigi and colleagues[117] performed peritoneal cytology on 93 patients with Stage I endometrial cancer, and followed the patients for a minimum of 10 years, or until death if it came sooner. Neither the recurrence rate nor the actuarial survival rates differed significantly between the 83 patients with negative cytology and the 10 with positive cytology.

For patients with positive para-aortic nodes, but no other evidence of extrauterine spread, we advise pelvic radiotherapy in an attempt to reduce the chance of central recurrence, and provided that a supraclavicular node biopsy is negative, we would consider radiotherapy to the para-aortic nodal region. Gestagens are given as mentioned above. Patients with macroscopic intraperitoneal metastases at the time of surgery generally have a very poor prognosis. Greer and Hamberger[118] reported on the use of whole abdominal radiation and a "pelvic boost" in the treatment of 31 patients with this type of disease. Their overall actuarial 5-year survival rates with this treatment were 63 percent. Where residual tumor masses were less than 2 cm in diameter the corrected survival rate was 80 percent, whereas if the residual tumor masses were over 2 cm in diameter no patient survived 5 years. These results appear impressive, but it should be remembered that whole abdominal radiotherapy is a far from benign form of therapy. The reason such treatments are even considered is the fact that no other truly effective therapy is known at present.

Stage III

Clinical Stage III disease is treated by whole pelvis radiotherapy and gestagens. Nevertheless, unless parametrial extension is clinically present, patients classified as Stage III on the basis of an adnexal mass should have a laparotomy, preferably before radiation. This allows assessment of peritoneal cytology and para-aortic nodes, as well as accurate assessment of the nature of the adnexal mass. If the parametrium is free but tumor has spread to the serosa of the uterus or to the ovaries, but not to such an extent as to prevent hysterectomy, we prefer to perform total hysterectomy and bilateral salpingo-oophorectomy unless it appears hazardous to the patient. Patients with such extensive disease do poorly, but removal of the tumor bulk and subsequent pelvic radiation may help prevent troublesome sequelae form a mass of necrotic tumor in the pelvis.

Vaginal metastases are usually managed by intravaginal applications of cesium. The distribution of sources and types of applicators depend upon whether the vault, midvagina, or suburethral area is most obviously involved.

Aalders and associates[119] drew attention to the difference in prognosis for patients with clinical Stage III disease, and those patients with clinical Stage I or II disease who at laparotomy are found to have extrauterine but intrapelvic spread of tumor (so-called "surgical Stage III"). The 5-year survival rates for the former group was only 16 percent, whereas for the latter group it was 40 percent. They attributed this difference to the fact that it was frequently impossible to surgically remove all of the tumor in patients with clinical Stage III disease, and that if this was possible the survival rates were comparable to those patients with subclinical extrauterine spread. Similarly, Bruckman and associates[120] showed that patients with extrauterine metastases confined to the tube or ovary had a better prognosis than those where other pelvic structures or the vagina were involved. Patients who were only discovered to have metastases to the tube or ovary at the time of surgery had an actuarial 5-year tumor-free survival of 80 percent, whereas for those with spread to other pelvic structures or to the vagina it was only 15 percent.

Stage IV

In a study of 83 patients with Stage IV endometrial carcinoma, the most common sites of metastases were the lung, seen in 36 percent of cases, the inguinal, supraclavicular or axillary lymph nodes, seen in 13 percent, and the bladder, also seen in 13 percent.[121] In 23 percent of patients metastases were present in multiple sites. The overall actuarial 5-year survival rate was 10 percent, although 28 percent of the patients who had a tumor in the pelvis obtained local control by pelvic radiation in combination with surgery or gestagens.

Treatment of patients with extrapelvic metastases generally involves the use of gestagens such as megesterol acetate (80 to 160 mg/day), the antiestrogen tamoxifen (20 to 40 mg/day), or a combination of these agents. Surgery is occasionally indicated to prevent or control hemorrhage or drain a pyometra. Whole pelvis radiotherapy may allow temporary control of local disease, improve patient comfort, or prevent or control bleeding. Occasionally, dramatic pain relief for symptomatic metastases, especially those in bone, can be achieved with "spot" radiotherapy to a dose of approximately 2000 rads.

Systemic chemotherapy will be discussed later in this chapter.

Recurrent Endometrial Cancer

Although early stage disease may recur several years after the completion of treatment, about 70 percent of recurrences appear within 2 years.[122] If radiotherapy has not been used, recurrences tend to be within the pelvis and are amenable to radiotherapy. Extrapelvic recurrences, or recurrences after failure of radiotherapy, generally require systemic chemotherapy or hormonal therapy. "Spot" radiotherapy may have palliative value in selected cases.

Exenteration is rarely indicated for recurrent endometrial carcinoma because it usually fails to control the disease. Our understanding of the frequency of lymphatic involvement in even early disease provides a ready explanation of this fact. Barber and Brunschwig[123] reported that only 5 of 36 patients with recurrent endometrial carcinoma survived 5 years after exenteration, with 26 percent of patients requiring a second operative procedure.

Hormonal Therapy and Chemotherapy

In 1961, Kelley and Baker[124] described significant regression in about one-third of patients with metastatic endometrial cancer treated with gestagens, and this mode of therapy has been used widely since. Response rates are highest for well-differentiated tumors and late recurrences. We use megestrol acetate 80 to 160 mg/day orally. The treatment appears most effective for nonpelvic recurrences. In 1979, Martin and colleagues[125] drew attention to the fact that gestagens can only be expected to produce a clinical response if progesterone receptors are present in the tumor cells. Benraad and associates[126] were able to predict the clinical response of metastatic endometrial carcinoma to gestagens by assaying estrogen and progesterone receptors in specimens obtained at the time of initial diagnosis. Levy and colleagues[127] proposed that a dynamic test be used to determine potential tumor responsiveness to gestagens. They proposed that after the initial biopsy diagnosis of endometrial carcinoma, the patient should be given tamoxifen 20 mg b.i.d. for 7 days, and then a further biopsy performed. Patients whose progesterone receptor levels rose would be considered most likely to respond to gestagen therapy. Ehrlich and associates[128] demonstrated a highly significant relationship between the progesterone receptor status and response to gestagens. Further studies of receptor status and response to hormonal therapy are clearly warranted.

The nonsteroidal "antiestrogen" tamoxifen, in a dose of 10 to 20 mg twice daily, has been used to treat advanced or recurrent endometrial carcinoma, including treatment failures after gestagens. Response rates are encouraging, but may take 6 weeks or more to develop.[129] Using a dosage of 40 to 60 mg per day, Bonte and associates[130] achieved a 50 percent objective response rate. This agent may be a significant tool in the management of these vexing problems.

Swenerton[131] reported favorable results with tamoxifen, and suggested that it might have an important role in combination with gestagens. As tamoxifen can induce the production of progesterone receptors in malignant endometrial cells, it was proposed that patients should be treated by alternating courses of tamoxifen, to induce progesterone receptor production, followed by gestagens. In the nude mouse model, Mortel and associates[132] demonstrated that the sequential administration of tamoxifen and gestagen was more effective than gestagen alone in the treatment of transplanted human endometrial carcinoma. Carlson and colleagues[133] used such a regimen on patients with recurrent endometrial carcinoma, and found the response rate was no better than for gestagen alone. Nevertheless, we believe that this approach merits further study.

A wide range of nonhormonal chemotherapeutic agents have been used in endometrial carcinoma, but results have generally been disappointing. With adriamycin, only about one-third of patients have responded, and the median survival of responders has been reported to be 14 months for complete responders, and 7 months for partial responders.[134] Other agents evaluated included 5-fluorouracil, cyclophosphamide, chlorambucil, 6-mercaptopurine and nitrogen mustard, and all gave equally poor responses.[134]

In 1982, three regimens of chemotherapy were evaluated by Horton and associates.[135] These included megestrol acetate, cyclophosphamide, and doxorubicin, or these three drugs combined with 5-fluorouracil, or an alternative regimen of megestrol, phenylalanine mustard, and 5-fluorouracil. The response rates for all regimens were of the order of 20 percent. Whether survival rates are increased is another question.

Our own results using cyclophosphamide, doxorubicin, and *cis*-platinum have been uniformly poor.

CONCLUSIONS

"Old habits die hard," and the attitude of most gynecologists to endometrial carcinoma supports this adage. Despite frequent warnings over many years, this tumor remains underrated and its management more casual than its virulence warrants. That it is, overall, the least aggressive of gynecologic malignancies, should not be permitted to obscure the fact that for many women this tumor is a cause of considerable morbidity. Indeed many who have what is generally assumed to be an easily curable, early stage lesion die from it.

The optimal treatment of early stage endometrial carcinoma will not be defined until all women with the disease are investigated and treated in a manner that allows the assessment of known prognostic factors. Other as yet unrecognized prognosticators must be aggressively sought by clinical and laboratory research. New methods of therapy for extensive, disseminated, or recurrent disease must be carefully evaluated.

For all women who suffer from this disease in the future, it is essential that consultation with a gynecologic oncologist be obtained as freely as for the other gynecologic malignancies.

REFERENCES

1. American Cancer Society: Cancer Facts and Figures, 1984. New York: American Cancer Society, 1984
2. Peel JH: Observations upon the etiology and treatment of carcinoma of the corpus uteri. Am J Obstet Gynecol 71:718, 1956
3. Berman ML, Ballon SC, Lagasse LD, et al: Prognosis and treatment of endometrial cancer. Am J Obstet Gynecol 136:679, 1980
4. Boronow RC: Endometrial cancer. Not a benign disease. Obstet Gynecol 47:630, 1976
5. Stallworthy J, quoted by Gusberg SB: Discussion: Treatment. Gynecol Oncol 2:429, 1974
6. Jones HW III: Treatment of adenocarcinoma of the endometrium. Obstet Gynecol Survey 30:146, 1975
7. Malkasian GD: Carcinoma of the endometrium: effect of stage and grade on survival. Cancer 41:996, 1978
8. Beck RP: Experience in treating two hundred and eighty-eight patients with endometrial carcinoma from 1968 to 1972. Am J Obstet Gynecol 133:260, 1979
9. McCabe JB, Sagerman RH: Treatment of endometrial cancer in a regional radiation therapy center. Analysis of 379 consecutive patients. Cancer 43:1052, 1979
10. Connelly PJ, Alberhasky RC, Christopherson WM: Carcinoma of the endometrium. III. Analysis of 865 cases of adenocarcinoma and adenoacanthoma. Obstet Gynecol 59:569, 1982
11. Gordon J, Reagan JW, Finkel WD, et al: Estrogens and endometrial carcinoma. An independent pathology review supporting original risk estimate. N Engl J Med 297:570, 1977
12. Szekely DR, Weiss NS, Schweid AI: Incidence of endometrial carcinoma in King County, Washington: A standardized histologic review. J Natl Cancer Inst 60:985, 1978
13. Hendrickson M, Ross J, Eifel PJ, et al: Andenocarcinoma of the endometrium: Analysis of 256 cases with carcinoma limited to the uterine corpus. Gynecol Oncol 13:373, 1982

14. Piver MS, Lele SB, Barlow JJ, et al: Paraaortic lymph node evaluation in Stage I endometrial carcinoma. Obstet Gynecol 59:97, 1982
15. Creasman WT, DiSaia PJ, Blessing J, et al: Prognostic significance of peritoneal cytology in patients with endometrial cancer and preliminary data concerning therapy with intraperitoneal radiopharmaceuticals. Am J Obstet Gynecol 141:921, 1981
16. Christopherson WM, Alberhasky RC, Connelly PJ: Carcinoma of the endometrium. II. Papillary carcinoma: A clinical pathological study of 46 cases. Am J Clin Pathol 77:534, 1982
17. Christopherson WM, Alberhasky RC, Connelly PJ: Carcinoma of the endometrium. I. A clinicopathologic study of clear-cell carcinoma and secretory carcinoma. Cancer 49:1511, 1982
18. Alberhasky RC, Connelly PJ, Christopherson WM: Carcinoma of the endometrium. IV. Mixed adenosquamous carcinoma. Am J Clin Path 77:655, 1982
19. Ng AB, Reagan JW, Storaasli JP, et al: Mixed adenosquamous carcinoma of the endometrium. Am J Clin Path 59:765, 1973
20. Waterhouse J, Muir C, Correa P, et al (eds): Cancer Incidence in Five Continents, vol III. IARC Sci Publ No. 15. Lyon: IARC, 1976
21. Menck HR, Henderson BE: Cancer incidence rates in the Pacific Basin. Natl Cancer Inst Monogr 53:115, 1979
22. Thomas DB: Epidemiologic studies of cancer in minority groups in the Western United States. Natl Cancer Inst Monogr 53:103, 1979
23. Schenker JG, Birkenfeld A, Schwartz S: Endometrial cancer in Israel, 1969–1975. Int J Gyneacol Obstet 20:455, 1982
24. Silverberg E: Gynecologic Cancer: Statistical and Epidemiologic Information. New York: American Cancer Society, 1975
25. Ostor AG, Adam R, Butteridge BH, et al: Endometrial carcinoma in young women. Aust NZ J Obstet Gynaecol 22:38, 1982
26. Cutler SJ, Young JL (eds): Third National Cancer Survey: Incidence data. Nat Cancer Inst Monogr 41, 1975
27. Registrar General's Decennial Supplement—England and Wales, 1961: Occupational mortality tables. London: Her Majesty's Stationary Office, 1971
28. Mack TM, Casagrande JT: Epidemiology of gynecologic cancer. II. Endometrium, ovary, vagina, vulva. Coppleson M (ed). Gynecologic Oncolocy, Fundamental Principles and Clinical Practice. Edinburgh: Churchill Livingstone, 1981, p 21
29. Yahia C, Benirschke K, Sturgis SH: Carcinoma of the endometrium. Meigs JV, Sturgis SH (eds). Progress in Gynecology, vol IV. New York: Grune and Stratton, 1963, p 410
30. Wynder EL, Escher GC, Mantel N: An epidemiological investigation of cancer of the endometrium. Cancer 19:489, 1966
31. Fox H, Sen DK: A controlled study of the constitutional stigmata of endometrial adenocarcinoma. Br J Cancer 24:30, 1970
32. Brown R: Clinical features associated with endometrial carcinoma. J Obstet Gynaecol Br Cwlth 81:933, 1974
33. MacMahon B: Risk factors for endometrial cancer. Gynecol Oncol 2:122, 1974
34. Kauppila A, Grönroos M, Nieminen U: Clinical outcome in endometrial cancer. Obstet Gynecol 60:473, 1982
35. Malkasian GD, Annegers JF, Fountain KS: Carcinoma of the endometrium, Stage I. Am J Obstet Gynecol 136:872, 1980

36. Crossen RJ, Hobbs JE: Relationship of late menstruation to carcinoma of the corpus uteri. J Missouri St Med Assoc 32:361, 1935
37. Kessler II: Cancer mortality among diabetics. J Natl Cancer Inst 44:673, 1970
38. Way S: The aetiology of carcinoma of the body of the uterus. J Obstet Gynaec Br Emp 61:46, 1954
39. Brown R: Carbohydrate metabolism in patients with endometrial carcinoma. J Obstet Gynaecol Br Cwlth 81:940, 1974
40. Elwood M, Cole P, Rothman KJ, et al: Epidemiology of endometrial cancer. J Natl Cancer Inst 59:1055, 1977
41. Schroder, quoted by Ingram JM, Novak E: Endometrial carcinoma associated with feminizing tumors. Am J Obstet Gynecol 61:774, 1951
42. Novak ER, Kutchmeshgi J, Mupas RS, et al: Feminizing gonadal stromal tumors. Analysis of the granulosa-theca cell tumors of the ovarian tumor registry. Obstet Gynecol 38:701, 1971
43. Larson JA: Estrogens and endometrial carcinoma. Obstet Gynecol 3:551, 1954
44. Koller O: Granulosa and theca cell tumors and genital cancer. Acta Obstet Gynecol Scand 45:114, 1966
45. Fox H, Agrawal K, Langley FA: A clinicopathological study of 92 cases of granulosa cell tumor of the ovary with special reference to the factors influencing prognosis. Cancer 35:231, 1975
46. Dockerty MB, Lovelady SB, Foust FT: Carcinoma of the corpus uteri in young women. Am J Obstet Gynecol 61:966, 1951
47. Ziel HK: Estrogen's role in endometrial cancer. Obstet Gynecol 60:509, 1982
48. Jackson RL, Dockerty MB: The Stein-Leventhal syndrome: Analysis of 43 cases with special reference to association with endometrial carcinoma. Am J Obstet Gynecol 73:161, 1957
49. Yen SSC: The polycystic ovary syndrome. Clin Endocr 12:177, 1980
50. Silverberg SG, Makowski EL, Roche WD: Endometrial carcinoma in women under 40 years of age. Cancer 39:592, 1977
51. Huggins GR, Giuntoli RL: Oral contraceptives and neoplasia. Fertil Steril 32:1, 1979
52. Jensen EI, Østergaard E: Clinical studies concerning the relationship of estrogens to the development of cancer of the corpus uteri. Am J Obstet Gynecol 67:1094, 1954
53. Gusberg SB, Hall RE: Precursors of corpus cancer. III. The appearance of cancer of the endometrium in estrogenically conditioned patients. Obstet Gynecol 17:397, 1961
54. Dunn LJ, Bradbury JT: Endocrine factors in endometrial carcinoma. A preliminary report. Am J Obstet Gynecol 97:465, 1967
55. Smith DC, Prentice R, Thompson DJ, et al: Association of exogenous estrogen and endometrial carcinoma. N Engl J Med 293:1164, 1975
56. Ziel HK, Finkle WD: Increased risk of endometrial carcinoma among users of conjugated estrogens. N Engl J Med 293:1167, 1975
57. Mack TM, Pike MC, Henderson BE, et al: Estrogens and endometrial cancer in a retirement community. N Engl J Med 294:1262, 1976
58. McDonald, TW, Annegers JF, O'Fallon WM, et al: Exogenous estrogen and endometrial carcinoma: Case-control and incidence study. Am J Obstet Gynecol 127:572, 1977
59. Gray LA, Christopherson WM, Hoover RN: Estrogens and endometrial carcinoma. Obstet Gynecol 49:385, 1977

60. Hoogerland DL, Buchler DA, Crowley JJ, et al: Estrogen use—risk of endometrial carcinoma. Gynecol Oncol 6:451, 1978
61. Horwitz RI, Feinstein AR: Alternative analytic methods for case control studies of estrogens and endometrial cancer. N Engl J Med 299:1089, 1978
62. Wigle DT, Grace M, Smith ES: Estrogen use and cancer of the uterine corpus in Alberta. Can Med Assoc J 118:1276, 1978
63. Antunes CM, Stolley PD, Rosenshein NB, et al: Endometrial cancer and estrogen use. Report of a large case controlled study. N Engl J Med 300:9, 1979
64. Jick H, Watkins RN, Hunter JR, et al: Replacement estrogens and endometrial cancer. N Engl J Med 300:218, 1979
65. Jelovsek FR, Hammond CB, Woodard BH: Risk of exogenous estrogen therapy and endometrial cancer. Am J Obstet Gynecol 137:85, 1980
66. Hulka BS, Fowler WC, Kaufman DG, et al: Estrogen and endometrial cancer. Cases and two control groups from North Carolina. Am J Obstet Gynecol 137:92, 1980
67. Shapiro S, Kaufman DW, Slone D, et al: Recent and past use of conjugated estrogens in relation to adenocarcinoma of the endometrium. N Engl J Med 303:485, 1980
68. Stravraky KM, Collins JA, Donner A, et al: A comparison of estrogen use of women with endometrial cancer, gynecologic disorders and other illnesses. Am J Obstet Gynecol 141:574, 1981
69. Spengler RF, Clarke EA, Woolever CA, et al: Exogenous estrogens and endometrial cancer: A case control study and assessment of potential biases. Am J Epidemiol 114:497, 1981
70. Obrink A, Bunne G, Collen J, et al: Estrogen regimen of women with endometrial carcinoma. Acta Obstet Gynecol Scand 60:191, 1981
71. Horwitz RI, Feinstein AR, Horwitz SM, et al: Necropsy diagnosis of endometrial cancer and detection bias in case control studies. Lancet 2:66, 1981
72. Hulka BS, Grimson RC, Greenberg BG: Endometrial cancer and detection bias. Lancet 2:817, 1981
73. Merletti F, Cole P: Detection bias and endometrial cancer. Lancet 2:579, 1981
74. Smith DC, Prentice RL, Bauerrmeister DE: Endometrial carcinoma: Histopathology, survival, and exogenous estrogens. Gynecol Obstet Invest 12:169, 1981
75. Austin DF, Roe KM: The decreasing incidence of endometrial cancer: Public Health Implications. Am J Public Health 72:65, 1982
76. Cullen TS: Cancer of the Uterus. New York: D. Appleton and Co., 1900
77. Taylor HC: Endometrial hyperplasia and carcinoma of the body of the uterus. Am J Obstet Gynecol 23:309, 1932
78. Novak E, Yui E: Relationship of endometrial hyperplasia to adenocarcinoma of the uterus. Am J Obstet Gynecol 32:674, 1936
79. Gusberg SB: Precursors of corpus carcinoma: Estrogens and adenomatous hyperplasia. Am J Obstet Gynecol 54:905, 1947
80. Hertig AT, Sommers SC: Genesis of endometrial carcinoma. I. Study of prior biopsies. Cancer 2:946, 1949
81. Gore H, Hetig AT: Carcinoma in situ of the endometrium. Am J Obstet Gynecol 94:134, 1966
82. Scully RE: Definition of endometrial carcinoma precursors. Clin Obstet Gynecol 25(1):39, 1982
83. Vellios L: Endometrial hyperplasia and carcinoma in situ. Gynecol Oncol 2:152, 1974

84. Richart, RM: Cervical intraepithelial neoplasia. Pathology Annual. New York: Appleton-Century-Crofts, 1973, p.301
85. Ruffolo EH, Cavanagh D, Marsden DE: Glandular intraepithelial neoplasia (GIN). A unifying concept of the precursors of endometrial carcinoma. Aust NZJ Obstet Gynaecol 23:220, 1983
86. Poulsen HE, Taylor CW: International classification of tumors. No. 13. Histological typing of female genital tract tumors. Geneva, WHO, 1975
87. Vellios L: Endometrial hyperplasias, precursors of endometrial carcinoma. Sommers SC (ed): Pathology Annual. New York: Appleton-Century-Crofts, 1972, p 201
88. Gusberg SB, Kaplan AL: Precursors of corpus cancer. IV. Adenomatous hyperplasia as stage O carcinoma of the endometrium. Am J Obstet Gynecol 87:662, 1963
89. Campbell PE, Barter RA: The significance of atypical endometrial hyperplasia. J Obstet Gynaecol Br Commow 68:668, 1961
90. Beutler HK, Dockerty MB, Randall LM: Precancerous lesions of the endometrium. Am J Obstet Gynecol 86:433, 1963
91. Tavassoli F, Kraus FT: Endometrial lesions in uteri resected for atypical endometrial hyperplasia. N Engl J Med 70:770, 1978
92. Kurman RJ, Norris HJ: Evaluation of criteria for distinguishing atypical endometrial hyperplasia from well-differentiated carcinoma. Cancer 49:2547, 1982
93. McBride JM: Premenopausal cystic hyperplasia and endometrial carcinoma. J Obstet Gynaecol Br Emp 66:288, 1959
94. Wentz WB: Progestin therapy for endometrial hyperplasia. Gynecol Oncol 2:362, 1964
95. Sherman AI: Precursors of endometrial cancer. Israel J Med Sc 14:370, 1978
96. Kennedy AW, Casey MJ, Gondos B, et al: Carcinoma of the endometrium: Review of experience at a community hospital, 1971–1977. Gynecol Oncol 14:164, 1982
97. De Palo G, Kenda R, Andreola S, et al: Endometrial carcinoma: Stage I. A retrospective analysis of 262 patients. Obstet Gynecol 60:225, 1982
98. Caspi E, Perpinial S, Reif A: Incidence of malignancy in Jewish women with postmenopausal bleeding. Israel J Med Sci 13:299, 1977
99. Vuopala S: Diagnostic accuracy and clinical applicability of cytological and histological methods for investigating endometrial carcinoma. Acta Obstet Gynecol Scand (supp) 70:8, 1977
100. Koss LG, Schreiber K, Moussouris H, et al: Endometrial carcinoma and its precursors: Detection and screening. Clin Obstet Gynecol 25(1):49, 1982
101. Gusberg SB, Milano C: Detection of endometrial cancer and its precursors. Cancer 47:1173, 1981
102. American Joint Committee for Cancer Staging and End-results Reporting: Manual for Staging of Cancer, 1978. Chicago: American Joint Committee, 1978, p 92
103. Rutledge FN: The role of radical hysterectomy in adenocarcinoma of the endometrium. Gynecol Oncol 2:331, 1974
104. Kneale BL: The current status of surgery for endometrial carcinoma: Facts and fantasy. Aust NZ J Surg 49:327, 1979
105. Homesley HD, Boronow RC, Lewis JL: Stage II endometrial adenocarcinoma: Memorial Hospital for cancer, 1949–1965. Obstet Gynecol 49:604, 1977
106. Kadar NR, Kohorn EI, LiVolsi VA, et al: Histologic variants of cervical involvement by endometrial carcinoma. Obstet Gynecol 59:85, 1982

107. Marsden DE, Correy JF: An evaluation of hysteroscopy in clinical gynaecologic practice. Asia-Oceana J Obstet Gynaecol 7:51, 1981
108. Anderson B: Diagnosis and staging of endometrial carcinoma. Clin Obstet Gynecol 25(1):75, 1982
109. Devore GR, Schwartz PE, Morris JM: Hysterography: A 5 year follow up in patients with endometrial carcinoma. Obstet Gynecol 60:369, 1982
110. Baggish MS, Woodruff JD: The occurrence of squamous epithelium in the endometrium. Obstet Gynecol Survey 22:69, 1967
111. Reagan JW, Fu YS: Pathology of endometrial carcinoma. Coppleson M (ed): Gynecologic Oncology: Fundamental Principles and Clinical Practice. New York: Churchill Livingstone, 1981, p 546
112. Cheon HK: Prognosis of endometrial carcinoma. Obstet Gynecol 34:680, 1963
113. Ng AB, Reagan JW: Incidence and prognosis of endometrial carcinoma by histologic grade and extent. Obstet Gynecol 35:437, 1970
114. Creasman WT, Boronow RC, Morrow CP, et al: Adenocarcinoma of the endometrium: its metastatic lymph node potential. A preliminary report. Gynecol Oncol 4:239, 1976
115. Creasman WT, Rutledge F: The prognostic value of peritoneal cytology in gynecologic malignant disease. Am J Obstet Gynecol 110:773, 1971
116. Boronow RC: Editorial comment: A fresh look at corpus cancer management. Obstet Gynecol 42:448, 1973
117. Yazigi R, Piver MS, Blumenson L: Malignant peritoneal cytology as prognostic indicator in Stage I endometrial cancer. Obstet Gynecol 62:359, 1983
118. Greer BE, Hamberger AD: Treatment of intraperitoneal metastatic adenocarcinoma of the endometrium by the whole-abdomen moving-strip technique and pelvic boost irradiation. Gynecol Oncol 16:365, 1983
119. Aalders JG, Abeler V, Kolstad P: Clinical (Stage III) as compared to subclinical intrapelvic extrauterine tumor spread in endometrial carcinoma: A clinical and histopathological study of 175 patients. Gynecol Oncol 17:64, 1984
120. Bruckman JE, Bloomer WD, Marck A, et al: Stage III endometrial carcinoma: Two prognostic groups. Gynecol Oncol 9:12, 1980
121. Aalders JG, Abeler V, Kolstad P: Stage IV endometrial carcinoma: A clinical and histopathological study of 83 patients. Gynecol Oncol 17:75, 1984
122. Salazar OM, Feldstein ML, De Papp EW, et al: Endometrial carcinoma. Analysis of failures with special emphasis on the use of initial preoperative external pelvic radiation. Int J Radiation Oncol Biol Phys 2:1011, 1977
123. Barber HRK, Brunschwig A: Treatment and results of recurrent cancer of corpus uteri in patients receiving anterior and total pelvic exenteration, 1947–1963. Cancer 22:949, 1968
124. Kelley RM, Baker WH: Progestational agents in the treatment of carcinoma of the endometrium. N Engl J Med 264:216, 1961
125. Martin PM, Rolland PH, Gammerre M, et al: Estradiol and progesterone receptors in normal and neoplastic endometrium: Correlations between receptors, histopathological examinations, and clinical responses under progestin therapy. Int J Cancer 23:321, 1979
126. Benraad TJ, Friberg LG, Koenders AJ, et al: Do estrogen and progesterone receptors (E2R and PR) in metastasizing endometrial cancers predict the response to gestagen therapy? Acta Obstet Gynecol Scand 59:155, 1980
127. Levy C, Robell P, Wolff JP, et al: Hormone receptors as indicators of the biologi-

cal properties of neoplastic tissues. In Fox BW (ed): Advances in Medical Oncology, Research and Education, vol 5. Oxford: Pergammon Press, 1979, p 213
128. Ehrlich CE, Young PC, Cleary RE: Cytoplasmic progesterone and estradiol receptors in normal, hyperplastic, and carcinomatous endometria: Therapeutic implications. Am J Obstet Gynecol 141:539, 1981
129. Swenerton KD, White GW, Boyes DA: Treatment of advanced endometrial carcinoma with tamoxifen. N Engl J Med 301:105, 1979
130. Bonte J, Ide P, Billiet G, et al: Tamoxifen as a possible chemotherapeutic agent in endometrial adenocarcinoma. Gynecol Oncol 11:140, 1981
131. Swenerton KD: Treatment of advanced endometrial adenocarcinoma with tamoxifen. Cancer Treat Rep 64:805, 1980
132. Mortel R, Zaino R, Satyaswaroop PG: Response of endometrial carcinoma to sequential treatment with tamoxifen and progestin in the nude mouse model. Abstract 5: Fifteenth Annual Meeting of the Society of Gynecologic Oncologists, Miami, 1984
133. Carlson JA, Allegra JC, Day TG, et al: Tamoxifen and endometrial carcinoma: Alterations in estrogen and progesterone receptors in untreated patients and combination hormonal therapy in advanced neoplasia. Abstract 1: Fifteenth Annual Meeting of the Society of Gynecologic Oncologists, Miami, 1984
134. Thigpen JT, Buchsbaum HJ, Mangan C, et al: Phase II trial of Adriamycin in the treatment of advanced or recurrent endometrial carcinoma: a Gynecologic Oncology group study. Cancer Treat Rep 63:21, 1979
135. Horton J, Elson P, Gordon P, et al: Combination chemotherapy for advanced endometrial cancer. An evaluation of three regimens. Cancer 49:2441, 1982

CHAPTER 5
Sarcomas of the Uterus

Sarcomas of the uterus are among the most lethal tumors encountered by the gynecologist. Their existence has been recognized since 1860 when the first case was presented to the Berlin Obstetrical Society by Meyer, the pathology being described by Virchow.[1]

Sarcomas account for approximately 3 percent of all malignant tumors of the uterine corpus. They tend to occur in the fifth and sixth decades of life and are more common in nulliparous women. They differ from the epithelial tumors because of their increased propensity to metastasize via the bloodstream so that hepatic, pulmonary, and cerebral metastases are more common. Thus, the clinical stage of the disease is generally more advanced than with carcinomas of the uterus.

There is no official clinical staging system for sarcomas of the uterus, but the following is that most commonly applied, whatever the histopathologic type. It correlates well with prognosis.[2]

- *Stage I:* Sarcomas confined to the uterus.
- *Stage II:* Sarcomas involving the corpus and cervix.
- *Stage III:* Sarcomas extending outside the uterus, but confined to the pelvis.
- *Stage IV:* Sarcomas extending beyond the true pelvis.

It should be noted that Stage I includes those patients whose tumors are confined to the uterine corpus whether the uterus is enlarged or not. This appears to be the only practical method of clinical staging, despite the fact that enlargement from sarcoma would obviously carry a much worse prognosis than enlargement from associated leiomyomas. Needless to say, this form of staging is surgical and retrospective, because most sarcomas are discovered incidentally after sectioning a uterus which has been removed for benign disease. It would be an error to consider prognosis in sarcomas of the uterus as being related only to the clinical stage of the disease, because it is now clear that different histopathologic types require different treatment and vary markedly with regard to prognosis.

CLASSIFICATION

An accurate histopathologic diagnosis is essential before an intelligent decision can be made with regard to the treatment of any tumor. If sarcomas of dissimilar origin and clinical behavior are grouped together, the results of treatment will be very difficult to evaluate. As pointed out by Kempson and Bari,[3] establishing accurate diagnostic criteria for uterine sarcomas has been especially difficult because of the large variety of histopathologic patterns that occur, and because of the difficulty in separating malignant from benign mesenchymal neoplasms. Several different classifications of uterine sarcomas have been proposed, but none of these has been universally accepted.[4-6]

Kempson and Bari[3] have proposed a modification of Ober's classification that is both histogenetically correct and clinically applicable (Table 1.)

Using the classification of Kempson and Bari, the pathologic diagnosis correlates well with patient survival and provides the clinician with a logical basis for management.

In this classification "pure" sarcomas contain a single recognizable sarcomatous element, whereas "mixed" sarcomas contain two or more different malignant elements. The malignant cells in *homologous* tumors are recognizable as being derived from mesenchymal tissue normally present in the uterus. *Heterologous* tumors, on the other hand, contain cells differentiated into mesenchymal structures not normally present in the uterus, such as striated muscle, cartilage, or bone. Thus, a pure sarcoma, such as leiomyosarcoma, is composed of a single cell type found in the normal uterus. A pure heterologous tumor, such as a chondrosarcoma or rhabdomyosarcoma, contains a single type of heterologous sarcoma cell. The mixed sarcomas contain tumor cells that have differentiated into at least two types of homologous or heterologous sarcoma without evidence of epithelial features, such as sarcomas containing mixtures of stromal sarcoma and leiomyosarcoma, or stromal sarcoma and rhabdomyosarcoma.

Malignant mixed Müllerian tumors (mixed mesodermal tumor) are uterine sarcomas mixed with carcinoma. The carcinoma may be squamous carcinoma, adenocarcinoma, undifferentiated carcinoma, or any combination of these. If the sarcomatous element is homologous, it is often referred to as "carcinosarcoma." If it is heterologous, it is usually called "mixed mesodermal tumor."

TABLE 1. CLASSIFICATION OF UTERINE SARCOMAS

I. Pure sarcomas
   A. Pure homologous
      1. Leiomyosarcoma
      2. Stromal sarcoma
      3. Endometrial stromatosis (endolymphatic stromal myosis)
      4. Angiosarcoma
      5. Fibrosarcoma
   B. Pure heterologous
      1. Rhabdomyosarcoma (including sarcoma botryoides)
      2. Chondrosarcoma
      3. Osteosarcoma
      4. Liposarcoma
II. Mixed sarcomas
   A. Mixed homologous
   B. Mixed heterologous with or without homologous elements
III. Malignant mixed Müllerian tumors (mixed mesodermal tumors)
   A. Malignant mixed Müllerian tumor, homologous type. Carcinoma plus leiomyosarcoma, stromal sarcoma, or fibrosarcoma, or mixtures of these sarcomas
   B. Malignant mixed Müllerian tumor, heterologous type. Carcinoma plus heterologous sarcoma with or without homologous sarcoma
IV. Sarcomas, unclassified
V. Malignant lymphoma

(From Kempson RL, Bari W: Hum Pathol 1:331, 1970, with permission.)[3]

Some sarcomas are composed mainly of undifferentiated cells and defy classification, even with the use of histochemical stains. These fall into the group of "unclassified sarcomas." The malignant lymphoma has also to be considered as a separate group. Thus, a large variety of tumors falls within the category of uterine sarcomas, but the most important are the leiomyosarcomas, the endometrial stromal sarcomas, the mixed homologous sarcomas, and the mixed heterologous sarcomas. Other types are rarely encountered, and so the Gynecologic Oncology Group (GOG) has endorsed a simplified classification which identifies these four histologic types and "other uterine sarcomas," in an effort to expedite the accumulation of data.

PURE SARCOMAS

Pure Homologous Sarcomas

Included in this group of tumors are leiomyosarcomas, endometrial stromal sarcomas, endometrial stromatosis (endolymphatic stromal myosis), fibrosarcomas, and angiosarcomas.

Leiomyosarcoma. Leiomyosarcoma is usually thought to be the most common malignant nonepithelial tumor of the uterus. It is difficult to differentiate from a benign cellular myoma. Some differentiate the malignant from the benign tumor on the basis of atypism[7] while others[3,8] require a certain number of mitotic figures per unit area of tumor. Still others[9,10] require evidence of invasion before the diagnosis of leiomyosarcoma is made. With these variations in diagnostic criteria, it is not surprising that sarcomatous change has been reported in the literature as from 0.13 to 6 percent[8,9] and the 5-year survival rate from 0 to 68 percent.[11] Also from 0[8] to 91 percent[12] of leiomyosarcomas have been considered to originate in preexisting leiomyosarcomas.

Clinical Picture. In reviewing some of the larger reported series some differences are noted, but a general pattern emerges.[5-8,11,13]

- *Age:* The usual age range is from 30 to 80 years but the modal age is in the 40 to 60 range. Thus, the patients are generally older than the peak age for benign leiomyoma, but below the peak age for endometrial carcinoma.
- *Race:* Although a preponderance of black patients is noted in some of the series, this generally reflects the general patient population treated in the institution.[13] It is interesting that there is apparently no racial predilection for the leiomyosarcoma despite the fact that leiomyomas are common in black women.
- *Parity:* Parity does not appear to play a role in this particular group of sarcomas.
- *History:* In the past, a history of previous irradiation has been related to the development of uterine sarcomas. However, Taylor and Norris[8] have reported that none of their 39 patients with leiomyosarcoma gave a history of irradiation. In reviewing the series of Silverberg,[13] Aaro and coworkers,[5] Montague and coworkers,[14] and Evans,[15] 12 of 254 (4.8 percent) patients with leiomyosarcoma gave a history of previous irradiation.
- *Symptoms:* Abnormal vaginal bleeding is by far the most common complaint. A few complain of abdominal or pelvic pain. Only a few complain of pressure symptoms, backache, or weight loss. Significant osteal pain and cough suggest the possibility of metastases. Not uncommonly the patients are asymptomatic.
- *Physical findings:* In the majority of cases, a pelvic mass is present which is easily detectable on pelvic or rectovaginal examination. Cervical ulceration or a necrotic "fibroid" may be noted on speculum examination. If a patient has been followed by the same gynecologist in successive pelvic examinations, an increase in the size of the uterus may be detected. However, it must be emphasized that this is uncommon, and in only 3 of 105 cases reported by Aaro and coworkers[5] was there a history of rapid growth of an apparent leiomyoma.
- *Pathology:* Leiomyosarcomas of the uterine wall may arise de novo from myometrial fibers of the uterine wall or from the smooth muscle fibers of a leiomyoma.

- *Gross appearance:* Most leiomyosarcomas have grown to a considerable size by the time they are diagnosed and removed. They are usually described as being soft and yellow or tan, and are separated with some difficulty from the surrounding myometrium.

In contrast, a benign leiomyoma is usually described as being firm and showing a prominent whorled pattern on section. However, as pointed out by Silverberg,[13] the distinction is often not so easily made and more than two-thirds of the leiomyosarcomas in his series were diagnosed before and after operation as benign leiomyomas. The uterus may contain one or more leiomyomas, whereas most leiomyosarcomas are solitary tumors. Origin from a preexisting leiomyoma probably occurs, but is sometimes difficult to prove. Aaro and coworkers[5] were able to demonstrate such a relationship in 22 of 105 leiomyosarcomas, with 11 of these being entirely encompassed by the outer "capsule" of an apparently benign leiomyoma. In Silverberg's[13] series of 26 of 34, and in Stearns and Sneeden's[12] series 35 of 57 patients with leiomyosarcoma also harbored leiomyomas in the same uterus. However, Taylor and Norris[8] reported this in only 13 of 39 patients, and these authors challenged the concept that malignant change ever develops in a leiomyoma. The explanation for the difference in opinion may lie in the fact that Taylor and Norris diagnosed leiomyosarcoma only when the number of mitotic figures was 10 or more per 10 high-power fields (hpf). In microscopic appearance, well-differentiated leiomyosarcomas retain the general orderly pattern of a leiomyoma (Fig. 1). The tumor cells are somewhat more plump, the nuclei are larger and darker, and there is a greater variation in size and in the density of nuclear staining.[16] Mitoses are usually numerous and may have an abnormal appearance.

Many anaplastic leiomyosarcomas are more cellular and pleomorphic. Some have an alveolar pattern. "Strap cells" similar to those seen in rhabdomyosarcomas are found in some very poorly differentiated tumors. They are characterized by an eccentrically placed nucleus and abundance of eosinophilic cytoplasm. For the pathologist, the most difficult microscopic differential diagnosis is between a cellular leiomyoma and a well-differentiated leiomyosarcoma. A well-differentiated leiomyosarcoma which shows few mitoses, does not invade blood vessels or muscle, is confined to the uterus, is removed intact, and is unlikely to recur or to metastasize. Tumors entirely confined within a leiomyoma have a better prognosis. In the series reported by Aaro and coworkers, 7 of the 11 patients in this category survived 5 years.[5]

Taylor and Norris[8] reported that the finding of more than 10 mitoses in 10 hpf provided the most accurate basis for the diagnosis of leiomyosarcoma. These authors also stated that "the lesions with fewer than 10 mitoses in 10 hpf proved benign on follow-up regardless of the degree of pathologic atypism." However, Kempson and Bari[3] noted that 9 of 12 patients who had tumors with 10 or more mitoses per 10 hpf were dead of tumor or alive with metastases, as were 5 of 6 patients who had tumors with mitoses of 5 to 9 per

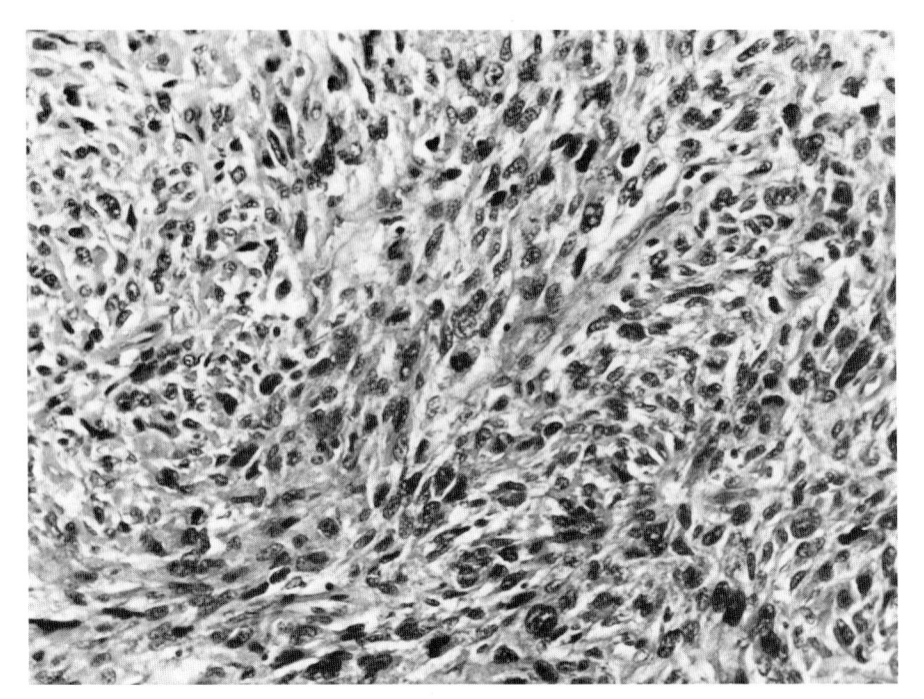

Figure 1. Grade 2 leiomyosarcoma. Note evidence of anaplasia such as difference in size, shape and chromatin pattern of nuclei. Most important, note the presence of mitotic figures. H&E. ×250.

10 hpf. Aaro and coworkers stated that mitotic atypia was the most important single factor in establishing a uterine tumor as malignant, and they accepted as few as 1 mitosis per 10 to 20 hpf and graded all tumors on the basis of mitotic rate.[5] Thus, while it may be regarded as a guide, the counting of mitotic figures is certainly not the answer because as shown by the report of Silverberg,[17] when the same ten microscopic slides were sent to six different, experienced pathologists, there was anything but unanimity on the number of mitotic figures per hpf. There is general agreement that tumor grade is important.

Some authors have demanded evidence of vascular or other invasion,[6,9,10,12,18] but this is impractical because almost all of such tumors are lethal. Also, this criterion for malignancy will fail to identify a small number of patients who will ultimately die of their disease. The presence or absence of giant cells is now thought to be of no significance. Large tumors that have invaded the urinary bladder or rectum have a poor prognosis. Women with well-differentiated leiomyosarcoma have a relatively good prognosis. On the other hand, patients with moderately anaplastic tumors have a relatively poor prognosis; only 5 of 19 patients with such lesions survived 5 years in the series reported by Spiro and Koss.[7]

In the pretreatment investigation of any patient admitted with suspected carcinoma or sarcoma of the uterus, examination under anesthesia and a fractional curettage should be performed. This does not often give a diagnosis of sarcoma. Any perimenopausal or postmenopausal woman in whom no malignancy is detected at curettage, and who continues to bleed, should be prepared for a hysterectomy.

In addition to the usual routine admittance studies, a liver profile, an x-ray of the chest, a sonogram of the pelvis, and an intravenous pyelogram (IVP) should be obtained. If there is any history of a bowel upset, a sigmoidoscopy and barium enema should be performed. If there is a history of dyspepsia, an upper gastrointestinal investigation is merited. If the patient has a history of hematuria, a cystoscopy should be performed.

Management. The keystone of management in leiomyosarcoma is total abdominal hysterectomy with bilateral salpingo-oophorectomy. In a younger patient, the ovaries may be preserved if they appear normal and there is no extension of the disease beyond the uterus. Belgrad and colleagues[19] reported the cumulative 2-year survival rates from four institutions and found them to be 59 percent for surgery, 41 percent for surgery and radiotherapy, and 8 percent for radiotherapy alone. Aaro and coworkers[5] reported a 55 percent 5-year survival rate in those patients treated with abdominal hysterectomy. Radiotherapy appears to have little or no value in the management of leiomyosarcomas, even in the form of adjuvant or palliative therapy.[20]

Chemotherapy has not had an adequate trial in the management of leiomyosarcoma. Gottlieb and coworkers[20] have reported remissions in 6 of 16 patients with leiomyosarcoma. The regimen used was adriamycin, 60 mg per square meter (60 mg/m^2) given intravenously on first day, and dimethyl-triazino imidazole carboxamide (DTIC), 250 mg/m^2 intravenously on first through fifth days, with the entire regimen being repeated every 21 days. Smith[21] reported on eight patients with leiomyosarcoma who received radiation therapy combined with vincristine in a dose of 1.5 mg/m^2 of body surface at weekly intervals for 10 to 12 weeks. When the radiation was completed, the patients received the "VAC" regimen for 2 years in the following manner: vincristine, 1.5 mg/m^2 intravenously for 1 day every 4 weeks, actinomycin D 0.5 mg per day intravenously for 5 days every 4 weeks, cyclophosphamide 5 to 7 mg/kg/day intravenously for 5 days every 4 weeks. This course of treatment was repeated every 4 weeks as tolerated for up to 2 years. Of the eight patients with leiomyosarcomas of the uterus, seven were alive and without evidence of disease 10 to 40 months after treatment. Thus, there may be a place for chemotherapy in the management of leiomyosarcoma.

Hormonal therapy in the form of estrogens may be indicated, although no controlled study has been undertaken to our knowledge. It is interesting that only 2 of the 18 premenopausal patients in Silverberg's[13] series died, and the third patient developed metastasis but is living at 9 years. These three patients had grade 3 or 4 tumors with vascular invasion. Two of them had extensive tumors in which a diagnosis of malignancy was made at gross inspection, and one had more than 10 mitoses per 10 hpf. However, these findings were also present in some of the premenopausal patients who are long-term survivors. Thus, the prognosis appears to be very good in premenopausal women without vascular invasion, and it would appear that it would be worthwhile to run a controlled study on the effects of estrogen therapy postoperatively in postmenopausal women with leiomyosarcoma.

Endometrial Stromal Sarcoma. Endometrial stromal sarcomas arise from the endometrial stroma and represent 0.2 percent or less of uterine sarcomas.[22] This is an aggressive tumor, which infiltrates the myometrium, frequently metastasizes and, carries a high mortality. These sarcomas may occur at any age, but the model age is similar to that for leiomyosarcoma. Neither race nor parity plays a significant part in predisposing the patient to this tumor.

Clinical Picture. Abnormal vaginal bleeding is the presenting symptom in over 70 percent of the patients with endometrial stromal sarcomas. Other complaints such as a foul discharge or pelvic pain are less common. Approximately 60 percent of the patients have an enlarged uterus, and in about 20 percent a mass is visible in the cervical canal on vaginal speculum examination.

Histopathology
Gross. Tumors are usually poorly defined and have polypoid elevations of soft consistency. They are often yellow to gray in color and often contain areas of necrosis and hemorrhage. The tumors tend to bulge into the uterine cavity and infiltrate the myometrium (Fig. 2).
Microscopic. The cells are arranged in a predominantly uniform fashion (Fig. 3). No heterologous elements are observed in the tumor. Lymphatic permeation can be seen and may simulate the more benign lesion called endolymphatic stromal myosis. As pointed out by Kempson and Bari,[3] sheets of cells with basophilic nuclei and indistinct cytoplasm are the most striking feature. Strands of tumor cells separating the smooth muscle fibers of the myometrium and fine strands of reticulin surrounding individual tumor cells, or clumps of tumor cells, can be demonstrated using silver stains. As is pointed out by Norris and Taylor,[23] infiltrating stromal sarcomas with large numbers of mitoses are aggressive and metastasize frequently. They set the dividing line between the mitotic activity of stromal sarcomas and endolymphatic stromal myosis at 10 mitoses per 10 hpf. In a series reported by Kempson and Bari,[3] even more emphasis was placed on mitotic rate, because all the stromal sarcomas contained more than 20 mitoses per 10 hpf, while the endolymphatic stromal myosis tumors had 5 or fewer per 10 hpf.

Management. The treatment of choice is abdominal hysterectomy with bilateral salpingo-oophorectomy and radiotherapy. Belgrad and coworkers[19] reported the cumulative total of survival rates from 4 series of patients to be 6 of 16 (37 percent) with surgery alone, 12 of 21 (57 percent) with surgery and

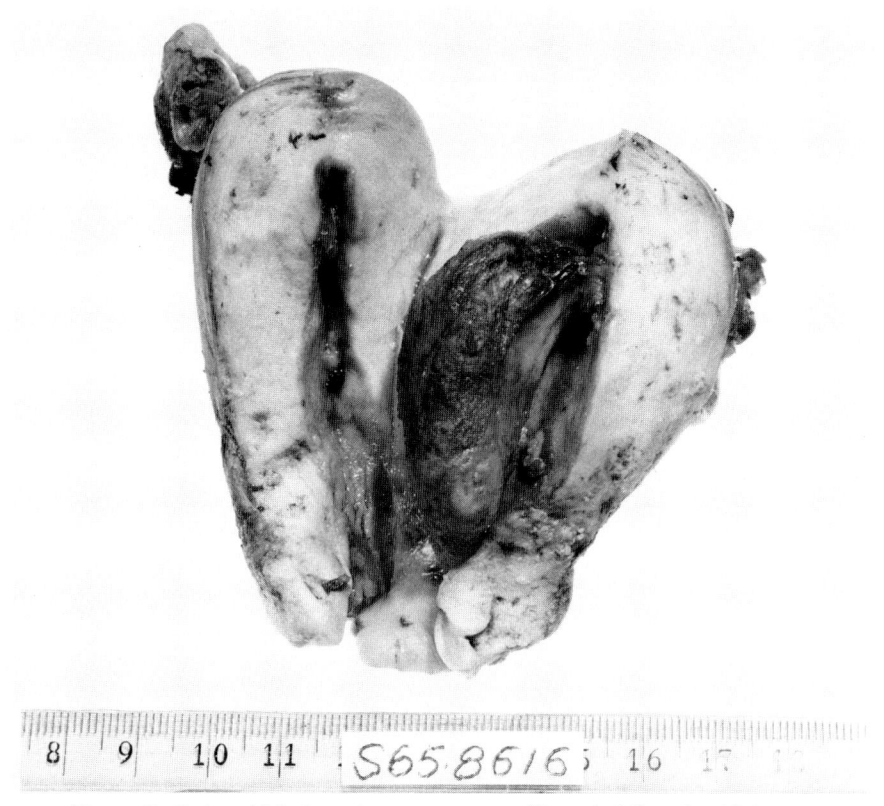

Figure 2. Endometrial stromal sarcoma, pure. Characteristic polypoid, hemorrhagic, partially necrotic tumor is seen.

radiotherapy, and 2 of 13 (15 percent) with radiotherapy alone. Pelvic recurrences may occur with this tumor, but it may also invade veins and lymphatics and produce distant metastases. These are most commonly pulmonary or osseous. In a series of cases reported by Park,[24] 6 percent had pulmonary metastasis, and spread to the vagina, broad ligaments, lymph nodes, and abdominal cavity was noted in another 8 percent. A similar distribution of metastatic lesions was described by Norris and Taylor in their review of 53 cases.[23]

As pointed out by Gilbert and associates,[25] if a diagnosis of endometrial stromal sarcoma is made preoperatively, then preoperative pelvic irradiation is probably worthwhile. Postoperative pelvic irradiation should be used in addition to surgery. They also stated that postoperative radiation should be used if the diagnosis is not made until the uterus is removed. The best results with this type of therapy, of course, would be expected with clinical Stage I disease. The gravity of the disease, however, is readily appreciated when it is noted that in their series of 17 patients with Stage I endometrial stromal

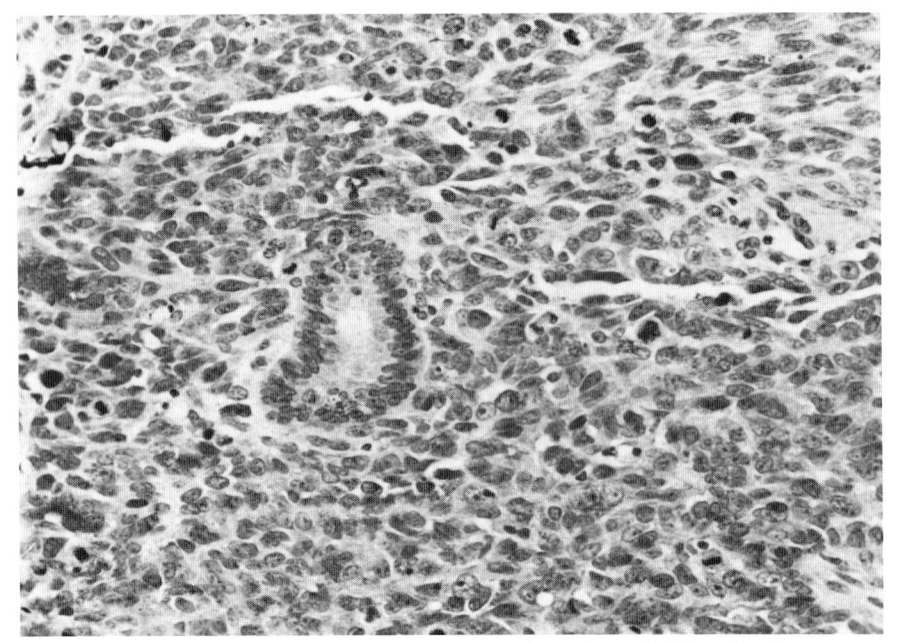

Figure 3. Endometrial stromal sarcoma, pure. Note the well-differentiated sarcomatous stromal cells, abutting against a benign gland at periphery of the base of tumor in Figure 2. H&E. ×250.

sarcoma, 13 had recurrences, and of the 4 that did not, 2 had tumors arising in polyps. Even minimal muscle invasion was found to be a poor prognostic sign. The median survival time of the 13 patients who had recurrences was 19 months, and the 4 patients without recurrence were alive without disease from 2 to 16 years later. There were two patients with clinical Stage II endometrial stromal sarcoma that recurred in the pelvis, abdomen, and elsewhere within 1 year. Five patients had Stage IV disease and these presented with distant metastases in liver, lung, or both. None of these patients was ever free of disease, and treatment failed to control the disease in the abdomen, pelvis, or elsewhere. The survival was from 1 month to 3 years with an average survival of 5 months.

Kempson and Bari[3] reported that all of their patients died within 2.5 years, and that all of their stromal sarcomas contained more than 20 mitoses per 10 hpf. On the other hand, Norris and Taylor[23] reported a 26 percent 5-year survival rate for patients with stromal sarcomas in which the mitotic counts were greater than 10 per 10 hpf. However, the survivors in their series had small tumors confined to the uterus. It is possible that tumors with counts of 6 to 20 per 10 hpf may be of low-grade malignancy, compared to tumors with mitotic counts greater than 20 per 10 hpf, but it seems more likely that other factors, such as the extent of myometrial invasion, play a more important part.

Treatment of endometrial stromal sarcomas with chemotherapeutic agents has been generally discouraging.[26-28] However, Hoovis[22] and Smith[21] have sounded a more encouraging note. As in the case of radiotherapy, it may be helpful if chemotherapy was given prior to surgery, as well as postoperatively, for optimal results.

Endometrial Stromatosis (Endolymphatic Stromal Myosis). The report by Hart and Yoonessi[29] details the clinical and pathologic features of patients with endometrial stromatosis of the uterus. This low-grade tumor may give risk to local recurrences following surgery, but may also produce pulmonary metastases. Although much less aggressive than endometrial stromal sarcoma, this tumor is by no means benign (Figs. 4, 5). In contrast to the endometrial stromal sarcomas, which have high mitotic rates (exceeding 10 to 20 mitoses per 10 hpf), in endometrial stromatosis there are usually fewer than 5 to 6 mitosis per 10 hpf.[3,23]

Clinical Course. The clinical course of patients with stromatosis is much more favorable than those with endometrial stromal sarcoma. Norris and Taylor[23] recorded a 5-year survival rate of 100 percent for 19 patients with endometrial stromatosis, which they designated as endolymphatic stromal my-

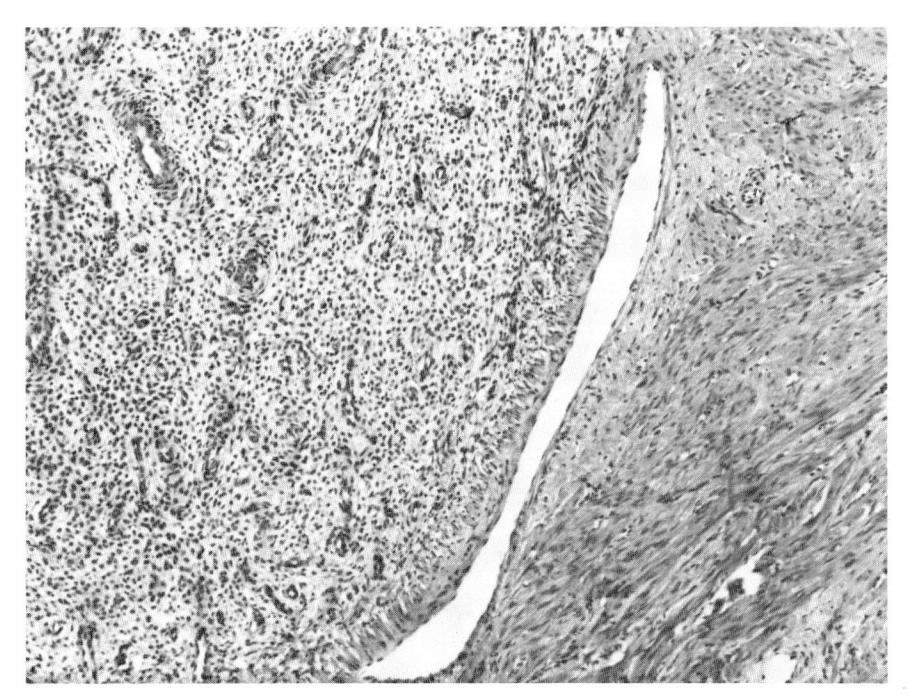

Figure 4. Endometrial stromatosis. A tongue of endometrial stroma, without glands, deep in the myometrium, is seen bulging into the wall of a lymphatic space. H&E. ×40.

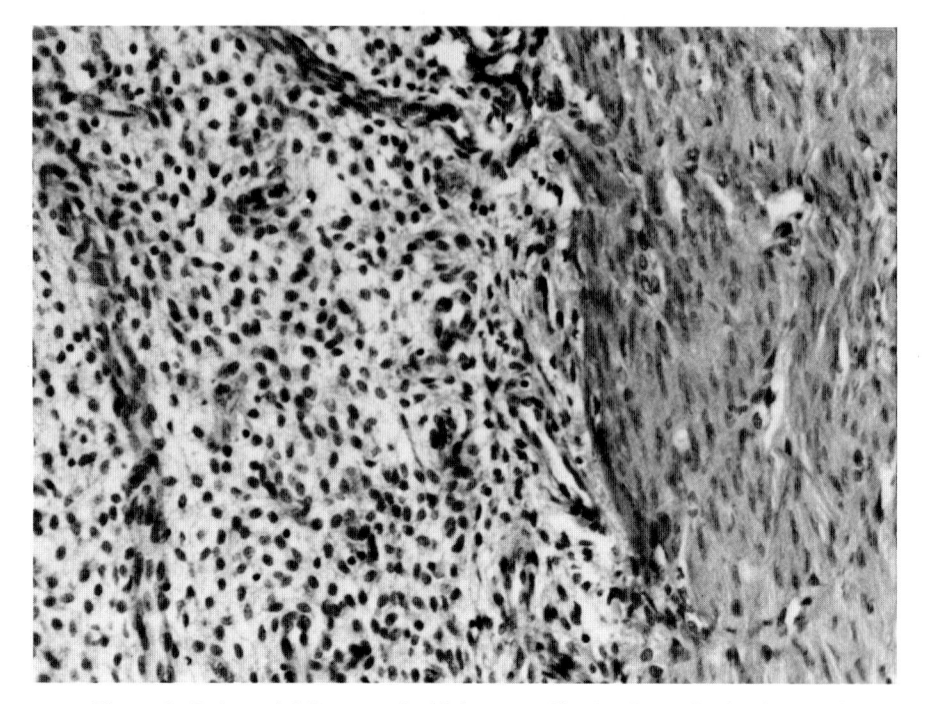

Figure 5. Endometrial Stromatosis. Higher magnification illustrating benign, monotonous appearance of stromal nuclei in a delicate fibrillar matrix. H&E. ×95.

osis. Only one of their patients died as a result of stromatosis, 12.7 years after the initial treatment. Six patients were alive with tumor at 3.5 to 19 years after diagnosis, even though there was evidence of pulmonary metastases in two of them. Kempson and Bari[3] described seven patients with stromatosis alive 3 to 15 years after treatment without recurrence or metastases. All of their patients were found to have tumors that were confined to the uterus. Baggish and Woodruff[30] described 12 patients with stromatosis, 8 of whom developed tumor recurrences and 3 of whom died of tumor. Hart and Yoonessi[29] reported recurrent or persistent stromatosis in seven patients after postoperative intervals of 3 to 14 years, despite the fact that four of these patients were thought to have tumor confined to the uterus at the time of surgery. Four of their patients eventually died from tumor within 3.8 to 9.4 years after the initial surgery, but only two deaths were directly attributable to the stromatosis.

Management. Total abdominal hysterectomy should be the minimal treatment. Because of the tendency to intravascular extension into the parametrium with spread to the broad ligament and to the adnexal structures, bilateral salpingo-oophorectomy should also be performed. Conservation of the ovaries may be justified in a young patient if the uterine wall is only superficially involved and vascular penetration is minimal. Recurrent and metastatic lesions are amenable to surgical excision.[30-33] Radiotherapy may be beneficial for recurrent or metastatic lesions.[23,33] The roles of adjunctive hormonal therapy, chemotherapy, and radiotherapy remain speculative. Radiotherapy should probably be reserved for recurrent lesions. Chemotherapy has no established place at this time. Progestational hormonal therapy has been reported to be of value.[30,34,35]

MIXED MESODERMAL TUMORS

Mixed mesodermal tumors are uterine sarcomas mixed with various types of carcinoma. They are composed of mesodermal elements arising from the endometrial stromal cells, and epithelial elements arising from the cells of the endometrial glands. Ober[4] separated the mesenchymal sarcoma into homologous and heterologous tumors of the uterus. Homologous mixed mesodermal tumors are tumors with nonspecific sarcomatous elements and carcinomatous elements; they are often referred to as "carcinosarcomas." Heterologous mixed mesodermal tumors are those tumors having a combination of carcinomatous and heterologous sarcomatous elements such as striated muscle cell, cartilage, osteoid, bone, or fat.

Several authors have shown a significant difference in prognosis between those tumors. Norris and Taylor[36] believe that carcinosarcoma has a better prognosis than mixed mesodermal tumor. However, this difference has not been confirmed by others.[5,37-42] Chuang and colleagues[37] suggested that for practical purposes they can be considered in the same category and managed in the same way.

Age. The median age of patients is 65 years with a range of 44 to 91 years.[36,37,43] Almost all patients are postmenopausal.

Race. Norris and Taylor[36] reported that 7 of 21 patients were blacks, the remainder were white. This supports the view of Steinberg[44] and others[41,45] that these tumors occur more frequently in blacks. In contrast, however, Chuang and colleagues[37] reported the incidence in blacks to be only 2 percent.

Parity. With known parity, 12 to 40 percent are nulliparous.[37,43,46]

Predisposing Factors. The incidence of prior radiation therapy ranges from 12 to 37 percent.[5,43,45,46] Norris and coworkers reported that 9 of 31 patients had a history of pelvic irradiation from 7 to 26 years prior to the discovery of the tumor,[46] and it is suggested as a possible causative agent.[47] Paloucek and associates[48] in their study of 5797 women treated for uterine bleeding, stated that those who had had irradiation developed more pelvic cancer than those who received no radiation. Corscaden and colleagues[9] believed that the underlying cause for which the irradiation was required was a more important factor in etiology than the irradiation itself. Symmonds and Dockerty[49] suggested that patients who have menometrorrhagia sufficiently severe to require radiation are those with an inherent tendency to develop sarcoma and other uterine cancers. As in patients with endometrial carcinoma, hypertension and obesity are prevalent in women with mixed mesodermal tumors.

Cause and Histogenesis. Formerly, mixed mesodermal tumors were thought to have originated from embryonic cell rests.[4,44] However, most authors now believe that these tumors originate from undifferentiated stromal cells that have the capacity to differentiate into both epithelium and stroma.[18,23,44]

Incidence. Mixed mesodermal tumors are reported to account for about 20 percent of the uterine sarcomas,[18] but in recent years the disease appears to be increasing.

Clinical Picture. The most common complaints are abnormal bleeding, vaginal discharge, pelvic pressure, and pelvic pain, symptoms referable to urinary tract, or intestine, and abdominal enlargement. Some patients give a history of having passed large fragments of necrotic tissue, and patients with extensive disease may complain of weakness, lassitude, and anorexia. Only a few patients are asymptomatic. Pelvic examination may reveal enlargement of the uterus or prolapse of polypoid masses out of the vagina. The irregularity produced by the tumor may be mistaken for leiomyoma. Parametrial extension may cause thickening or nodularity. Metastases to the external genitalia are rare. Some patients have no abnormal pelvic findings upon examination.[46] The diagnosis is often made only after curettage. Chuang and colleagues[37] reported that on the basis of curettings, the initial diagnosis was correct in 75 percent of the cases. The diagnosis was also made on occasion by biopsy of a cervical tumor, but sometimes the diagnosis was not made until after hysterectomy. Haynes and Kosasky[50] reported two of the nine patients with suspicious cells in routine Papanicolaou smears.

Histopathology. Mixed mesodermal tumors are not dependent on the cell type. They are typically soft and usually they arise as a large polypoid mass,[46] apparently from the uterine lining and not from the myometrial wall (Figs. 6–8). Presumably they arise from the mesenchyme between the endometrium and myometrium. Sometimes large tumors fill and distend the uterine cavity, with prolapse of some malignant polyps through the cervix. The tumor is usually attached to the posterior wall rather than the anterior wall.[51] Hemorrhage is quite frequent. On cross-section the tumors often appear to be shiny and gelatinous in contrast to the granular apearance of adenocarcinoma, and myometrial invasion is quite common.[46]

The basic cellular component of these neoplasms is a mesenchymal

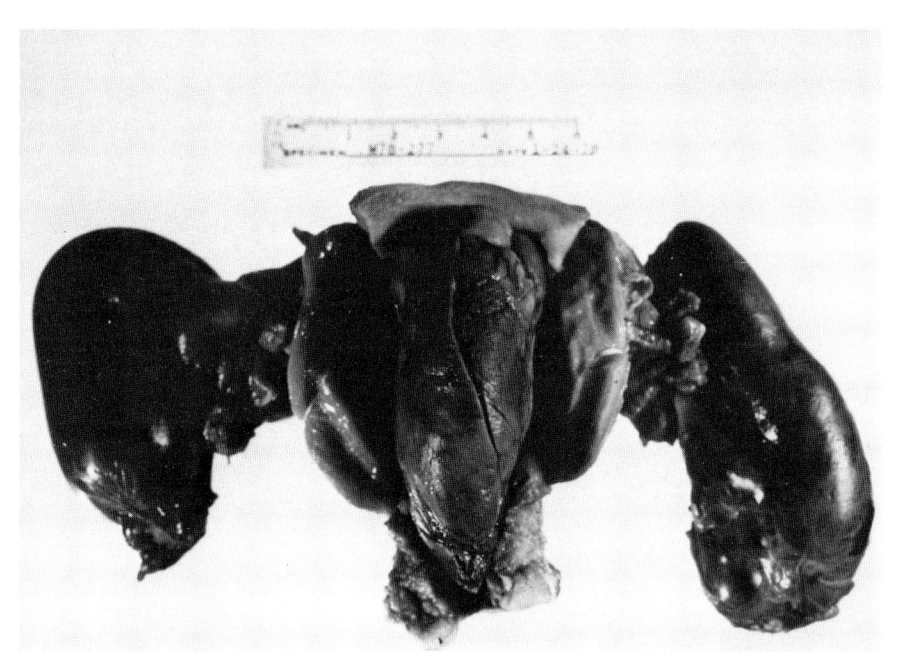

Figure 6. Malignant mixed Müllerian tumor, heterologous type. A polypoid, hemorrhagic, partially necrotic tumor is seen filling and dilating the endometrial cavity, effacing the cervix, and attempting to "deliver." Bilateral hematosalpinges are seen.

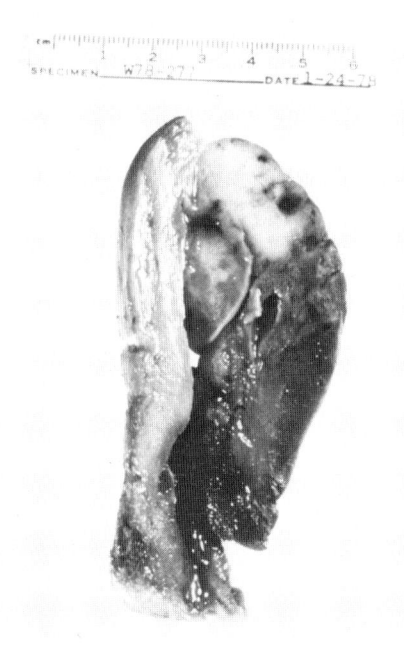

Figure 7. Malignant mixed Müllerian tumor, heterologous type. Sagittal section of tumor seen in Figure 6. Base of tumor appears to be at fundus and grossly not invading the myometrium.

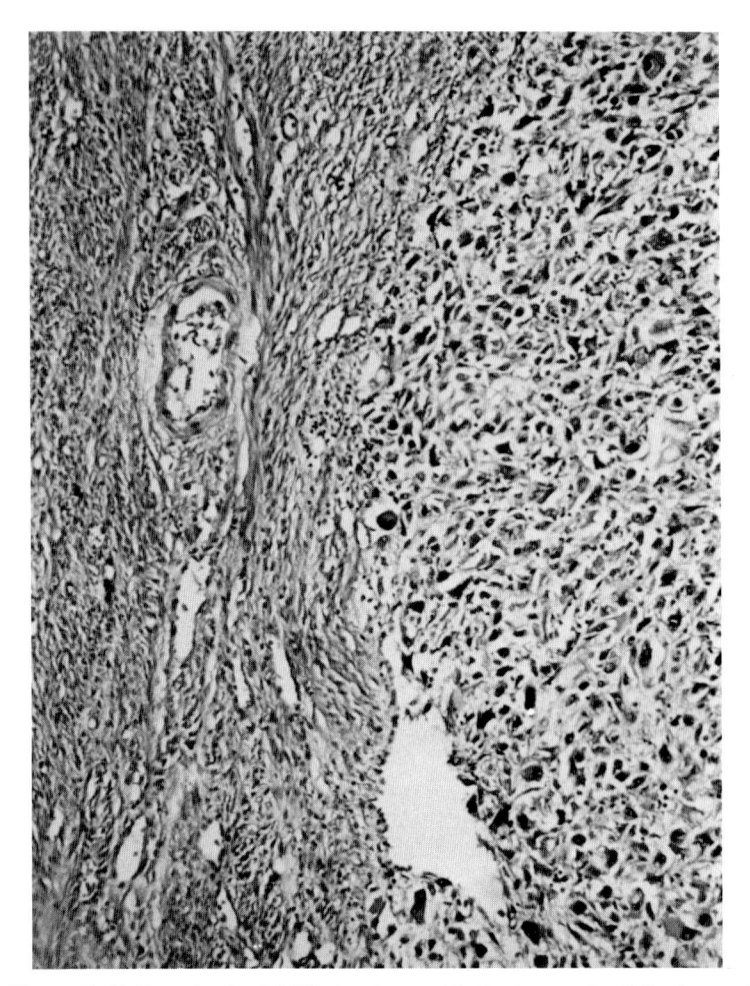

Figure 8. Malignant mixed Müllerian tumor. Photomicrograph of the base of tumor as seen in Figure 7 also appears to be noninfiltrating. H&E. ×95.

sarcoma that is composed of fusiform cells as described by Ober and Tovell.[52] This lesion has been called fibromyxosarcoma,[49] endometrial sarcoma,[44] and undifferentiated sarcoma.[53] Giant cells are frequently found.[46] The heterologous mesenchymal elements commonly include striated and immature myoblasts, osteogenic sarcoma and chondrosarcoma (Figs. 9, 10). Rhabdomyosarcomatous and chondrosarcomatous components are the most common heterologous elements. Immature rhabdomyoblasts, either with or without cross-striations, are sufficiently characteristic to confirm the presence of rhabdomyosarcoma. There are often only small foci of recognizable patterns with extensive areas of undifferentiated epithelium. Careful histologic examination of the operative specimens has often demonstrated the

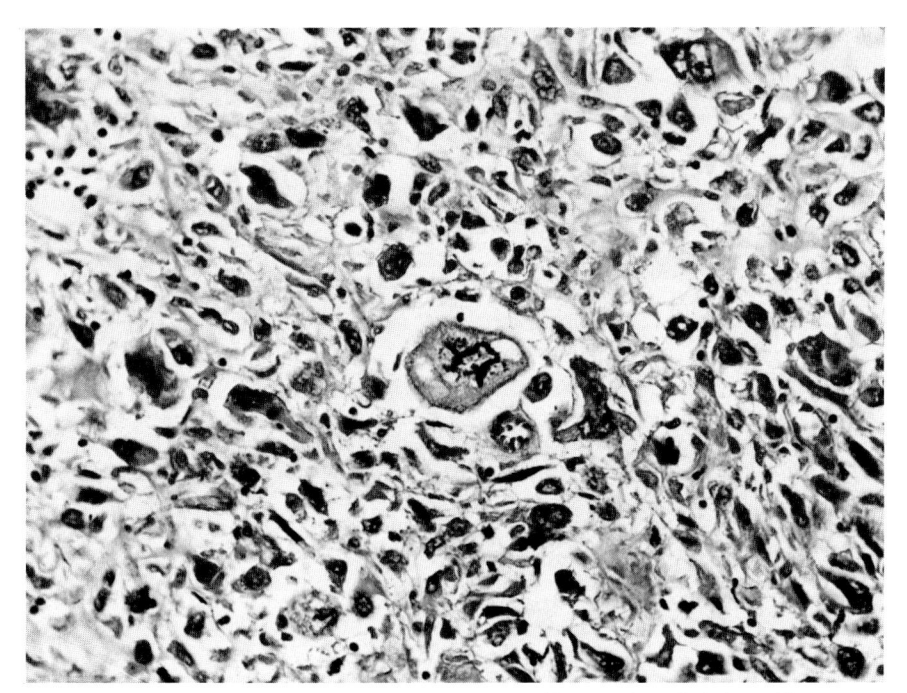

Figure 9. Malignant mixed Müllerian tumor. Malignant giant rhabdomyoblasts with eosinophilic granular cytoplasm, abnormal mitotic figures, bizarre cytoplasmic configurations. Careful study of "strap cells," especially with Mallory-Heidenhain stain, may demonstrate cross-striations. H&E. ×250.

presence of heterologous elements and reclassification of the tumor.[44,49,54] The epithelial elements include adenocarcinoma and less frequently are squamous metaplasia and squamous carcinoma. Microscopic examination of the metastatic lesion may reveal pure sarcoma and pure carcinoma or a combination of both types.

Electron microscopic studies have revealed cells similar to adenocarcinoma cells, sarcomatous cells with increased numbers of microvesicles, and an intermediate cell.[55] Growth of carcinosarcoma in tissue culture has revealed sarcomatous and carcinomatous cell types but no evidence of intermediate or transitional cells.[56]

Treatment. Treatment includes surgery, radiation therapy, and chemotherapy. The most common surgery performed is total abdominal hysterectomy and bilateral salpingo-oophorectomy. More radical surgery such as radical hysterectomy with pelvic lymphadenectomy, and pelvic exenteration has not been proved to increase the survival rate significantly. Radical hysterectomy with pelvic lymphadenectomy may be considered if the cervix is invaded by the tumor. Exenteration might have a place in selected cases where the tumor is centrally localized in the pelvis.[37] On the other hand, inadequate excision

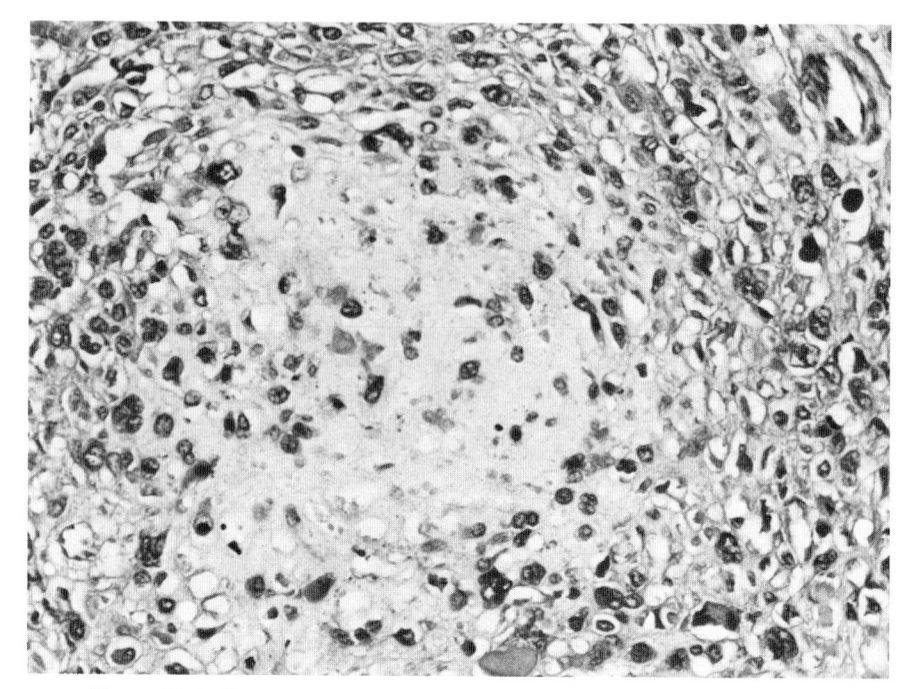

Figure 10. Malignant mixed Müllerian tumor, heterologous. Same tumor as Figures 6–9, demonstrating chondroid matrix, another manifestation of heterologous elements. H&E. ×250.

almost invariably results in prompt recurrence and death, regardless of the adequacy of subsequent attempts at resection.[49] Local removal of a necrotic, prolapsing tumor is advised by Symmonds and Dockerty[49] to rid the inoperable patient of offensive drainage, to control bleeding, and also to prepare operable patients for more definitive procedures.

Methods of radiation therapy used have included external radiation, radium implantation, and radioisotope perfusion.[57] Most early reports support the view that radiotherapy appears to offer very little in the control of this neoplasm,[5,44-46,58] and Chuang and colleagues[37] have reported that preoperative and postoperative radiation do not improve the 5-year survival rate. However, some more recent reports, including that of Rachmaninoff and Clinic,[59] suggest that the disease is better controlled with a combination of surgery and 5000 rads to the whole pelvis (Table 2). Salazar and associates[60] have reported on 63 patients with Stage I mixed mesodermal sarcoma with 5-year survival being 52 percent with surgery alone, 48 percent with surgery and radiotherapy, and 29 percent with radiotherapy alone. In patients with Stages II, III, and IV disease the 5-year survival was 5 percent with surgery, 16 percent with surgery and radiotherapy, and there were no survivors with radiotherapy alone. At this time it appears that while adjunctive radiotherapy may give better local control radiotherapy alone gives a poor survival rate. When the

TABLE 2. EFFECT OF DIFFERENT THERAPIES ON SURVIVAL

Authors	Total Patients	Alive 5 Yr	Treatment Provided Survivors		
			Surg.	Radiat.	S+R
Rachmaninoff and Clinic	30	6	2	1	3
Norris et al.	31	6	2	0	4
Norris and Taylor	31	8	5	1	2
DiSaia et al.	94	21	2	2	17
Chuang et al.	49	6	5	0	1
Masterson and Kremper	25	4	0	0	4
Edwards et al.	8	2	1	0	1
Symmonds et al.	19	5	2	0	3
Total	287	57	19	4	35
Percent		20%	33%	7%	60%

tumor is confined to the uterus, total abdominal hysterectomy, bilateral salpingo-oophorectomy with selective para-aortic and pelvic lymphadenectomy is recommended.

Chemotherapy has been employed as a supplement to surgery, radiation or both with some good results.[61] Masterson and Kremper[43] reported a case of rectal recurrence 3 years after the primary treatment, which was controlled by cyclophosphamide alone, but doxorubicin has been reported to be the most effective single agent. Omura and Blessing[62] reported a 27 percent response (complete or partial) with adriamycin, and the addition of DTIC did not increase response. However, in a GOG study, in which adriamycin was compared with no adjuvant treatment in postoperative patients with mixed Müllerian tumor, no benefit was evident, and further entry of these patients was discontinued. Another popular 5-day regimen is a combination of

- Vincristine 1mg/m^2 IV on days 1 and 5,
- Adriamycin 40 mg/m^2 IV on day 2,
- Cytoxan 400 mg/m^2 IV on day 2,
- DTIC 200 mg IV daily for 5 days.

This course is repeated every 4 weeks depending upon the CBC and platelet count, and the severity of other side effects, such as peripheral neuritis and obstipation. However, until controlled studies are available, this regimen is not of proved efficacy. In 1983, Hannigan, Freedman, and Rutledge[63] reported on their experience with adjuvant chemotherapy in early uterine sarcoma. In addition to hysterectomy and radiotherapy, 34 patients received adjunctive chemotherapy and 67 patients received no adjunctive chemotherapy. Seventeen patients who received chemotherapy received combination vincristine, 1.5 mg/m^2 weekly; actinomycin D, 0.5 mg intravenously on days 1 to 5; and cyclophosphamide, 300 mg intravenously on days 1 to 5. Seventeen other patients received adriamycin either alone at a dose of 50 mg/m^2 BSA/month or in combination with vincristine and cyclophosphamide. Neither the

TABLE 3. EFFECT OF EXTRAUTERINE DISEASE ON SURVIVAL

	Uterine Disease		Extrauterine Disease		
Authors	No. of Patients	Alive After 5 yr	No. of Patients	Alive After 5 yr	Total Survivors
Norris and Taylor	19	8	12	0	8
Norris et al.	17	6	14	0	6
Masterson and Kremper	15	3	10	1	4
Aaro et al.	29	15	24	2	17
DiSaia et al.	34	18	41	3	21
Chuang et al.	20	6	22	0	6
Haynes et al.	4	0	4	0	0
Total	138	56	127	6	62
Percent		41%		5%	23%

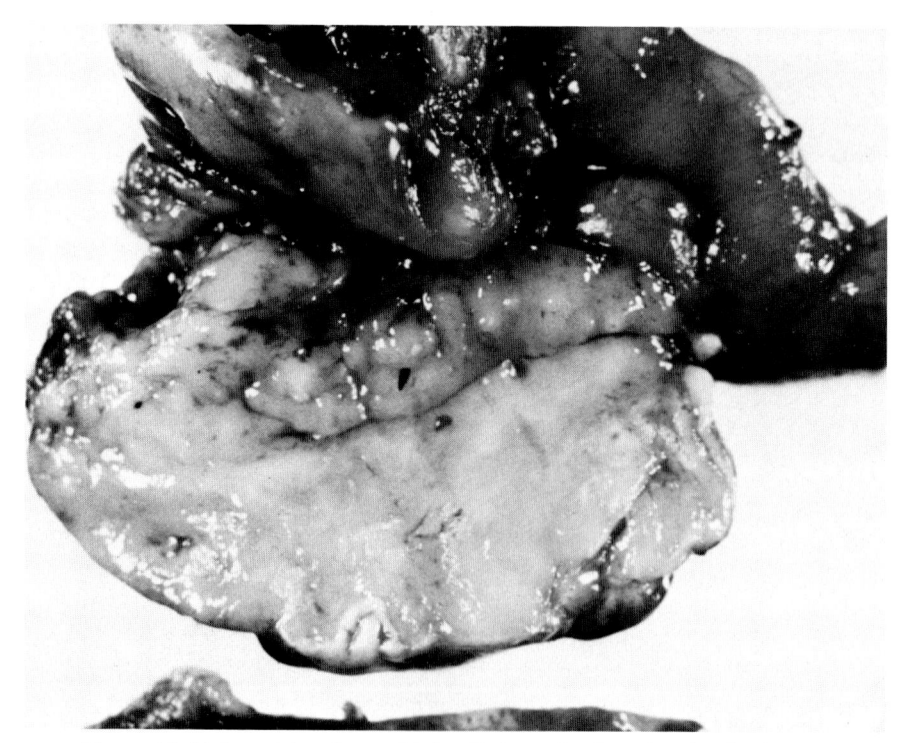

Figure 11. Malignant lymphoma, histiocytic type. Section of an involved ovary removed at the time of a staging procedure for a primary lymphoma of the uterus. "Fish-flesh" is the typical appearance, with gross obliteration of normal organ structure.

probability of survival nor the disease-free interval was improved by the addition of adjuvant chemotherapy. One thing seems clear, as in the case of other uterine sarcomas, surgery is the keystone of management.

Prognosis. Patients with mixed mesodermal tumors have a poor prognosis.[39,42,43,59,61,63,64] However, the outlook is more favorable if the tumor is confined to the uterus at the time of treatment.[42,65] The approximate 5-year survival for patients with a tumor limited to the uterus is 43 percent, but this drops to about 5 percent when there is extrauterine disease.[46] Norris and colleagues suggested that the presence of cartilage within mixed mesodermal tumors is associated with a favorable prognosis,[46] but it becomes unfavorable if the tumors contain striated muscle.[7] Symmonds and Dockerty[49] believed the presence of rhabdomyosarcoma per se does not indicate a hopeless prognosis, provided there is no serosal or other extrauterine extension of the tumor. Chuang and coworkers,[37] on the other hand, reported that the presence of different elements in a tumor did not modify the outcome significantly. They also stated that the number of mitoses in mixed mesodermal tumors did not correlate with survival rate. The survivors tended to have a tumor less than 5 cm in diameter, fewer symptoms, and no extension beyond the uterus. In the final analysis early diagnosis probably plays the most significant role in patient survival (Table 3).

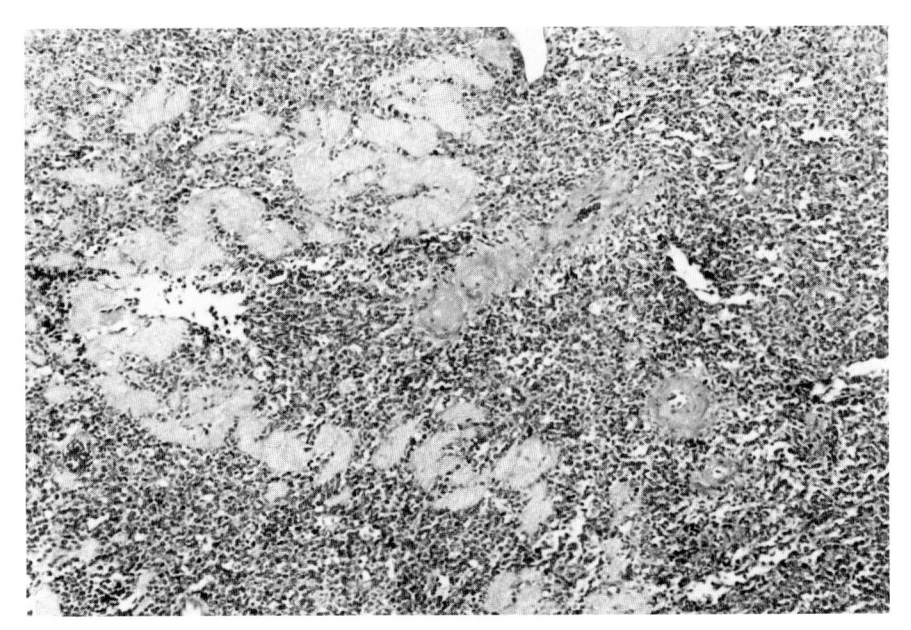

Figure 12. Malignant lymphoma, histiocytic type. Unlike carcinoma, which invades and destroys normal structures, lymphoma cells here are seen around and through an old corpus albicans, leaving it morphologically intact. H&E. ×40.

The majority of recurrences occur within a year, although some are not seen until 3 to 5 years have elapsed. The pelvic cavity and the vagina were often involved in recurrent disease. At postmortem examination, the most frequent sites of metastasis are the rectum, bladder, and pelvic and para-aortic lymph nodes.[43] Metastases to the omentum and mesentery and to the lung and pleura have also been reported.[37]

SARCOMA BOTRYOIDES

This is a tumor closely related to mixed mesodermal tumors in that it may also contain heterologous elements. However, it occurs with rare exceptions in a different age group and location than do mixed mesodermal tumors.[4,40] The distribution of metastatic lesions is also similar in these two neoplasms.[57] The mixed mesodermal tumors appear to have less propensity for "blood borne" metastasis.[41]

MALIGNANT LYMPHOMA

Aaro and coworkers[5] reported 3 cases of lymphosarcoma among 177 patients with sarcoma of the uterus. In two of the three patients, the tumors originated

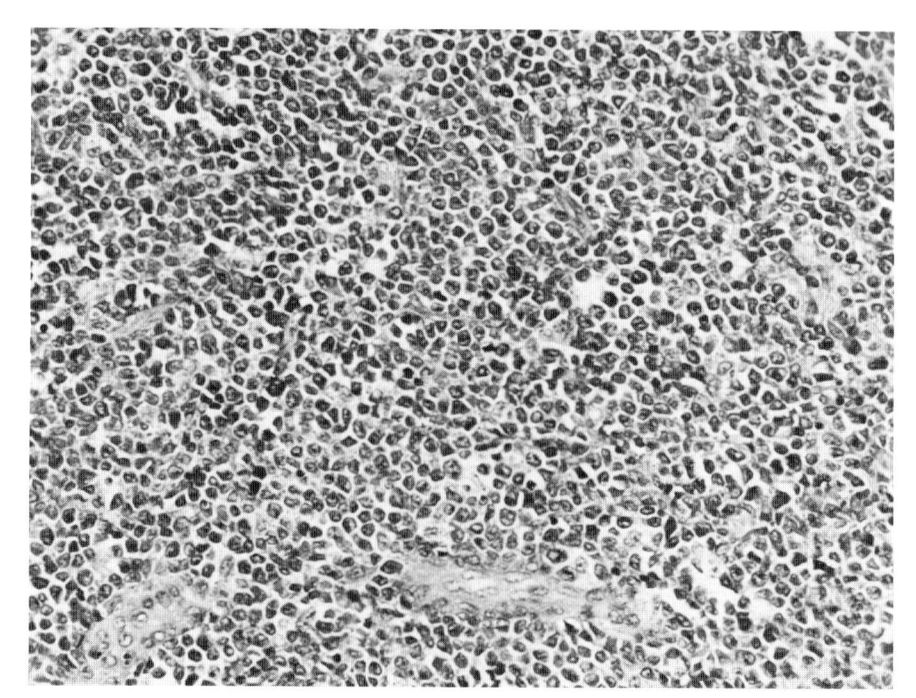

Figure 13. Malignant lymphoma, histiocytic type. Same tumor as Figures 11 and 12, demonstrating a monotonous sheet of noncohesive cells with vesicular nuclei, indented, lobulated, and with prominent nucleoli. H&E. ×250.

in the cervix and were of reticulum cell-type. The remaining patient had involvement of both endometrium and cervix with lymphoblastic lymphosarcoma.

The first patient was a 40-year-old woman treated by total abdominal hysterectomy and right salpingo-oophorectomy with postoperative radiotherapy. She had no evidence of disease 6.5 years after treatment. The second was a 63-year-old woman who was treated with a total hysterectomy and bilateral salpingo-oophorectomy and the removal of an enlarged pelvic lymph node. This patient showed no evidence of recurrence 8 years later. The third patient was a 49-year-old woman who was complaining of postmenopausal bleeding. Cervical biopsies and endometrial curettage revealed lymphosarcoma. The patient was treated with radiotherapy as usually given for a squamous cell carcinoma of the cervix. She showed no evidence of recurrence 12.5 years after treatment.

Although these tumors are rare and may carry a good prognosis as indicated above, others presenting, even as an exophytic cervical tumor, may be associated with widespread disease. In one patient recently encountered, the diagnosis was made on cervical biopsy, but exploratory laparotomy revealed widespread intraabdominal disease (Figs. 11–13).

UNCLASSIFIED SARCOMAS

Some uterine sarcomas are composed mainly of undifferentiated cells and despite the use of special stains and the cutting of multiple sections, they defy classification. These very poorly differentiated tumors carry a very poor prognosis.

REFERENCES

1. Virchow R: Die Krankhaften Geschwülste (Vol. 1). Berlin, August Hirschwald, 1964, p 182
2. Vongtama V, Karlan JR, Piver SM, et al: Treatment, results, and prognostic factors in Stage I and Stage II sarcomas of the corpus uteri. Am J Roentgenol 126:139, 1976
3. Kempson RL, Bari W: Uterine sarcomas. Classification, diagnosis and prognosis. Hum Pathol 1:331, 1970
4. Ober WB: Uterine sarcoma: histogenesis and taxonomy. Ann NY Acad Sci 75:568, 1959
5. Aaro LA, Symmonds RE, Dockerty MB: Sarcoma of the uterus: A clinical and pathological study of 177 cases. Am J Obstet Gynecol 94:101, 1966
6. Barstick EG, Bowe ET, Moore JG: Leiomyosarcoma of the uterus. A 50 year review of 42 cases. Obstet Gynecol 32:101, 1968
7. Spiro RH, Koss LG: Myosarcoma of the uterus: A clinicopathological study. Cancer 18:571, 1965

8. Taylor HB, Norris HJ: Mesenchymal tumors of the uterus. IV. Diagnosis and prognosis of leiomyosarcomas. Arch Pathol 82:40, 1966
9. Corscaden JA, Singh BP: Leiomyosarcoma of the uterus. Am J Obstet Gynecol 75:149, 1958
10. Gudgeon DH: Leiomyosarcoma of the uterus. Obstet Gynecol 32:96, 1968
11. Christopherson WM, Williamson EO, Gray LA: Leiomyosarcoma of the uterus Cancer 29:1512, 1972
12. Stearns HC, Sneeden VD: Leiomyosarcoma of the uterus. Am J Obstet Gynecol 95:374, 1966
13. Silverberg SG: Leiomyosarcoma of the uterus. A clinicopathological study. Obstet Gynecol 38:613, 1971
14. Montague ACW, Swartz DP, Woodruff JD: Sarcoma arising in a leiomyoma of the uterus. Am J Obstet Gynecol 92:421, 1965
15. Evans N: Malignant myomata and related tumors of the uterus. Surg Gynecol Obstet 30:225, 1920
16. Krause FT: Gynecologic Pathology. St. Louis: Mosby, 1967
17. Silverberg SG: Reproducility of the mitosis count in the histological diagnosis of smooth muscle tumors of the uterus. Hum Pathol 7:451, 1976
18. Norris HJ, Taylor HB: Postradiation sarcoma of the uterus. Obstet Gynecol 26:689, 1965
19. Belgrad R, Elbadawi N, Rubin P: Uterine sarcoma. Radiology 114:181, 1975
20. Gottlieb JA, Baker LH, Quagliana JM, et al: Chemotherapy of sarcomas with a combination of Adriamycin and dimethyl triazino imidazole carboxamide. Cancer 30:1632, 1972
21. Smith JP: Chemotherapy in gynecologic cancer. Clin Obstet Gynecol 18:109, 1975
22. Hoovis ML: Response of endometrial stromal sarcoma to cyclophosphamide. Am J Obstet Gynecol 108:1117, 1970
23. Norris HJ, Taylor HB: Mesenchymal tumors of the uterus. I. A clinical and pathologic study of 53 endometrial stromal tumors. Cancer 19:755, 1966
24. Park WW: Stromatous endometriosis. A report of five cases. J Obstet Gynaecol Br Emp 56:755, 1949
25. Gilbert HA, Kagan AR, Lagasse L, et al: The value of radiation therapy in uterine sarcoma. Obstet Gynecol 45:84, 1975
26. Malkasian GD Jr, Mussey E, Decker DG, Johnson CE: Chemotherapy of gynecologic sarcomas. Cancer Chemother Rep 51:507, 1968
27. Hreshchyshyn MM: Experiences with chemotherapy in gynecologic cancer. NY J Med 64:2431, 1964
28. White TH, Clover JS, Peete CH Jr, Parker RY: A 34-year clinical study of uterine sarcoma, including experience with chemotherapy. Obstet Gynecol 25:657, 1965
29. Hart WR, Yoonessi M: Endometrial stromatosis of the uterus. Obstet Gynecol 49:393, 1977
30. Baggish MS, Woodruff JD: Uterine stromatosis. Clinicopathologic features and hormone dependency. Obstet Gynecol 40:487, 1972
31. Hunter WC: Uterine stromal endometriosis (stromatosis). Am J Obstet Gynecol 83:1564, 1962
32. Hunter WC, Nohlgren JE, Lancefield SN: Stromal endometriosis or endometrial sarcoma. A re-evaluation of old and new cases, with special reference to duration, recurrences and metastases. Am J Obstet Gynecol 72:1072, 1956

33. Koss LG, Spiro RH, Brunschwig A: Endometrial stromal sarcoma. Surg Gynecol Obstet 121:531, 1965
34. Krumholz BA, Lobovksy FY, Halitsky V: Endolymphatic stromal myosis with pulmonary metastases. Remission with progestin therapy. Report of a case. J Reprod Med 10:85, 1973
35. Pellillo D: Proliferative stromatosis of the uterus with pulmonary metastasis. Remission following treatment with a long-acting progestin: A case report. Obstet Gynecol 31:33, 1968
36. Norris HJ, Taylor HB: Mesenchymal tumors of the uterus. III. A clinical and pathologic study of 31 carcinosarcomas. Cancer 19:1459, 1966
37. Chuang JT, Van Velden DJJ, Graham JB: Carcinosarcoma and mixed mesodermal tumors of the uterine corpus: A review of 49 cases. Obstet Gynecol 35:769, 1970
38. Taylor CW: Müllerian mixed tumor. Acta Pathol Microbiol Scand 80 (suppl 23):48, 1972
39. Hayes D: Mixed Müllerian tumor of the corpus uteri. J Obstet Gynaecol Br Commonw 81:160, 1974
40. Williams TJ, Woodruff JD: Similarities in malignant mixed mesenchymal tumors of the endometrium. Obstet Gynecol Surv 17:1, 1962
41. Williamson EO, Christopherson WM: Malignant mixed Müllerian tumors of the uterus. Cancer 29:585, 1972
42. DiSaia PJ, Castro JR, Rutledge FN: Mixed mesodermal sarcoma of the uterus. Am J Roentgenol Radium Ther Nucl Med 117:632, 1973
43. Masterson JG, Kremper J: Mixed mesodermal tumors. Am J Obstet Gynecol 104:693, 1969
44. Sternberg WH, Clark WH, Smith RC: Malignant mixed Müllerian tumors (mixed mesodermal tumors of the uterus): A study of twenty-one cases. Cancer 7:704, 1954
45. Krupp PJ, Sternberg WH, Clark WH, et al: Malignant mixed Müllerian neoplasms (mixed mesodermal tumors). Am J Obstet Gynecol 81:958, 1961
46. Norris HJ, Roth E, Taylor HB: Mesenchymal tumors of the uterus. II. A clinical and pathological study of 31 mixed mesodermal tumors. Obstet Gynecol 28:57, 1966
47. Klein J: Carcinosarcoma of the endometrium. Am J Obstet Gynecol 65:121, 1953
48. Paloucek FB, Randall CL, Graham JB, Graham S: Cancer and its relation to abnormal vaginal bleeding and radiation. Obstet Gynecol 21:530, 1963
49. Symmonds RE, Dockerty MB: Sarcoma and sarcoma-like proliferation of the endometrial stroma. I. A clinicopathologic study of 19 mixed mesodermal tumors. Surg Gynecol Obstet 100:232, 1955
50. Haynes DM, Kosasky HJ: Mixed mesodermal tumors of the uterus. South Med J 58:292, 1965
51. Taylor CW: Mesodermal mixed tumor of the female genital tract. J Obstet Gynaecol Br Emp 2:177, 1958
52. Ober WB, Tovell HMM: Mesenchymal sarcomas of the uterus. Am J Obstet Gynecol 77:246, 1959
53. Alznauer RL: Mixed mesenchymal sarcoma of the corpus uteri. AMA Arch Pathol 60:329, 1955
54. Liebow AA, Tennant R: Mesodermal mixed tumors of the body of the uterus. Am J Pathol 17:1, 1941
55. Silverberg S: Malignant mixed mesodermal tumor of the uterus: An ultra structural study. Am J Obstet Gynecol 110:702, 1971

56. Rubin A: The histogenesis of carcinosarcoma (mixed mesodermal tumor) of the uterus as revealed by tissue culture studies. Am J Obstet Gynecol 77:269, 1959
57. Edwards DL, Sterling LN, Keller RH, Nolan JF: Mixed heterologous mesenchymal sarcomas (mixed mesodermal sarcomas) of the uterus. Am J Obstet Gynecol 85:1002, 1963
58. Bartsich EG, O'Leary JA, Moore JG: Carcinosarcoma of the uterus: A 50 year review of 32 cases (1917–1966) Obstet Gynecol 30:518, 1967
59. Rachmaninoff N, Clinic ARW: Mixed mesodermal tumors of the uterus. Cancer 19:1705, 1966
60. Salazar OM, Bonfiglio TA, Patten SF, et al: Uterine sarcomas: natural history, treamtent and prognosis. Cancer 42:1152, 1978
61. Smith JP, Rutledge F, Delclos L, Sutow W: Combined irradiation and chemotherapy for sarcoma of the pelvic in females. Am J Roentgenol Radium Ther Nucl Med 123:571, 1975
62. Omura GA, Blessing JA: Chemotherapy of Stage III, IV, and recurrent uterine sarcomas: A randomized trial of Adriamycin versus Adriamycin and DTIC. AACR Abst. No. 103, Proceedings of AACR/ASCO, April 1978
63. Hannigan EV, Freedman RS, Rutledge FN: Adjuvant chemotherapy in early uterine sarcoma. Gynecol Oncol 15:56, 1983
64. Mortel R, Nedwich A, Lewis GC, Brady L: Malignant mixed Müllerian tumors of the uterine corpus. Obstet Gynecol 35:468, 1970
65. Mortel R, Koss KG, Lewis JL, D'Urso JR: Mesodermal mixed tumors of the uterine corpus. Obstet Gynecol 43:248, 1974

CHAPTER 6
Cancer of the Fallopian Tube

Cancer of the fallopian tube is one of the most uncommon primary cancers of the genital tract.

PRIMARY CARCINOMA OF THE TUBE

The reported incidence of tubal carcinoma is 0.3 to 1.1 percent of all gynecologic malignancies.[1] Approximately 1100 cases have been reported in the literature,[2] and a busy gynecologist would expect to see one case in a professional lifetime. As a result of the relative rarity of the disease, experience with diagnosis and management is based on collected small series from various institutions,[2-5] and even single case reports from the literature.[6-9]

Epidemiology

The cause of cancer of the fallopian tube is unknown. Indeed, it is interesting that the tube is so prone to infection but is so resistant to neoplasia. Although atypical epithelial proliferations and carcinoma in situ of the tube have been reported, progression to invasive carcinoma has not been documented.[10] The disease may occur at any age, ranging in the literature from 21 to 82, with a mean age of 53 years.[2,4] The tube, like the uterus, is of Müllerian origin, but the cancer appears to occur at a slightly earlier age than endometrial cancer.

Pathology
The most common form of cancer of the tube arises from the mucosa and is an adenocarcinoma. Adenocanthoma[2] and endometrioid carcinoma have also been reported.

Gross Pathology
The mass is usually located in the ampullary portion of the fallopian tube, and is unilateral in approximately 80 percent of the patients. The affected tube has the appearance of a hydrosalpinx, except that the adhesions which are so common with pelvic inflammatory disease are absent. Bleeding into the tube results in a hematosalpinx, with spillage into the peritoneal cavity being occasionally seen. The routes of spread are similar to those for ovarian carcinoma, but lymph nodes are involved in up to 53 percent of cases, with para-aortic nodes being involved in up to 33 percent.[1]

Histology
The typical microscopic pattern shows a tall abnormal tubal epithelium with three main pictures: grade 1—a papillary pattern; grade 2—a papillary-alveolar pattern; grade 3—an alveolar-medullary pattern.[4] A typical tubal carcinoma is shown in Figure 1.

Differentiation from a serous cystadenocarcinoma of the ovary may be difficult. The criteria for identification of a primary tubal carcinoma were laid down by Finn and Javert in 1949.[11] These are:

1. The epithelium of the endosalpinx is replaced in whole or part by adenocarcinoma.
2. The histologic character of the cells resembles the epithelium of the endosalpinx.
3. The endometrium and ovaries are normal; affected by a benign lesion; or contain a malignant lesion that, by its small size, distribution, and histologic characteristics, appears to be metastatic to the tube.
4. The prime involvement is in the endosalpinx and perisalpinx; the lymphatics of the muscularis and mesosalpinx are rarely involved.
5. Tuberculosis should be carefully excluded.

As pointed out by Johnson and associates in 1978,[12] electron microscopy can be helpful when the diagnosis is in doubt, and in differentiating ciliary cell origin from interciliary cell origin.

Clinical Picture
Many patients with cancer of the tube will present with perimenopausal or postmenopausal bleeding. Abdominal discomfort is not uncommon. On abdominal examination, some distention may be found, and rarely, an umbilical nodule.[9] On pelvic examination, a tubal mass suggestive of a hydrosalpinx may be palpated, but the presence of this in the postmenopausal woman should alert the physician. Occasionally, the patient complains of a gush of

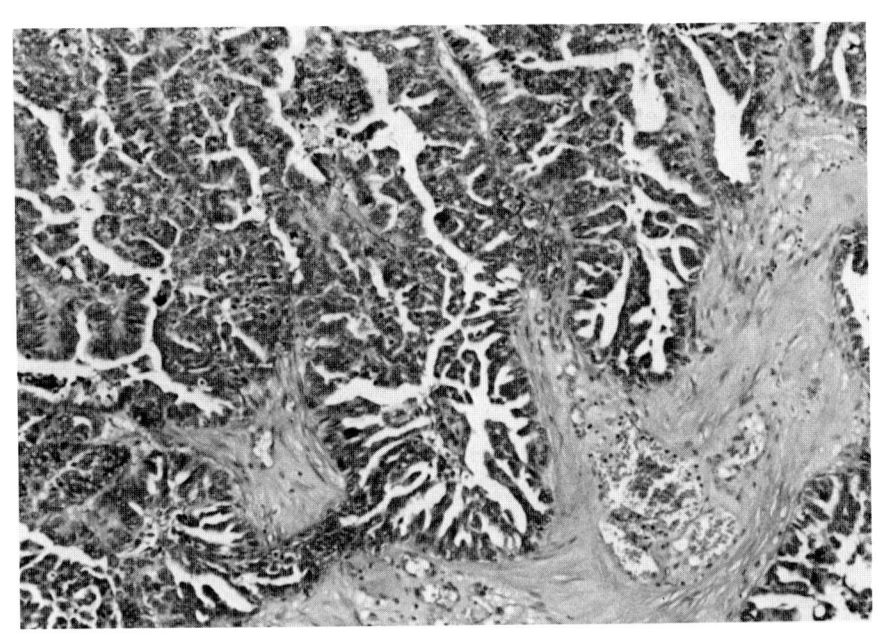

Figure 1. Papillary adenocarcinoma of the tube, the most common type. Delicate papillary fronds forming an endophytic mass which is histologically identical to the papillary serous cystadenocarcinoma of the ovary.

fluid coming from the cervix and this is often bloodstained. Only about 10 percent of the patients have a positive Papanicolaou smear,[4] but a positive smear in the presence of a negative fractional curettage should alert the gynecologist. The diagnosis should also be kept in mind in any patient with perimenopausal or postmenopausal bleeding in whom a fractional curettage is negative and in whom bleeding persists. A correct preoperative diagnosis is made in only about 2 percent of patients. Ancillary methods are no substitute for clinical alertness.[7,8] The conditions most likely to lead to an accurate diagnosis are:

1. A symptom complex of bleeding, pain, and watery discharge.
2. The presence of a pelvic mass which, on compression, appears to become smaller in association with an increase in watery discharge through the cervix (hydrops tubae profluens).
3. Persistently positive Papanicolaou smears with a negative fractional curettage and a normal appearing cervix.
4. A flat film of the abdomen showing a pelvic mass.
5. Ultrasonography showing the presence of a pelvic mass of fusiform shape in the adnexal area.
6. A computed tomography (CT) scan showing a fusiform adnexal mass.
7. Hysterosalpingography may demonstrate the lesion, but it may spread the malignant cells into the peritoneal cavity and so is generally undesirable.

Clinical Staging

Although there is no official staging classification for cancer of the fallopian tube, most authorities favor a staging system based on the FIGO classification for ovarian cancer.[1,4]

- Stage I A: Growth limited to one tube; no ascites. No tumor on the external surface and capsule intact. Tumor present on the external surface and/or capsule ruptured.
- Stage I B: Growth limited to both tubes; no ascites. No tumor on the external surface and capsule intact. Tumors present on the external surface and/or capsule ruptured.
- Stage I C: Tumor either Stage I A or Stage I B, but with ascites present, or with positive peritoneal washings.
- Stage II: Growth involving one or both types with pelvic extension.
- Stage II A: Extension and/or metastases to the uterus and/or ovaries.
- Stage II B: Extension to other pelvic tissues.
- Stage II C: Tumor either Stage II A or Stage II B, but with ascites and positive peritoneal washings.
- Stage III: Growth involving one or both tubes with intraperitoneal nodes or both. Tumor limited to the true pelvis with histologically proved malignant extension to the small bowel or omentum.
- Stage IV: Growth involving one or both tubes with distant metastases. If pleural effusion is present, there must be positive cytology to allot a case to Stage IV. Parenchymal liver metastases indicates Stage IV.

Using this unofficial FIGO staging system, Sedlis[13] calculated 3 years' survival figures by stage as Stage I—60 percent, Stage II—40 percent, Stage III—10 percent, Stage IV—0 percent. However, the exact effect of the treatment method on survival is difficult to evaluate.[2]

Management

The management of carcinoma of the tube is essentially the same as that for carcinoma of the ovary. The patient should be explored through a vertical incision. The entire abdomen is carefully assessed after ascitic fluid or saline washings have been obtained for cytologic examination. The standard treatment at this time is total abdominal hysterectomy, bilateral salpingo-oophorectomy, omentectomy, and debulking as in ovarian carcinoma. Para-aortic lymphadenectomy and bilateral pelvic node sampling is useful prognostically if not therapeutically. If the disease is apparently limited to the tube and ovary, some authors prefer to use radioactive chromium phosphate (^{32}P). Radiation therapy has been commonly used in the management of these patients. As in the case of ovarian carcinoma, the entire abdomen usually has to be treated. The role of chemotherapy is not established at this time because no controlled studies are available. *Cis*-platinum, doxorubicin, and cyclophosphamide may be useful,[14] but they are not without risk.[15] It would appear to be logical to use a progestational agent, such as megesterol acetate 40 mg twice daily for 3 weeks, alternating with tamoxifen 10 mg twice daily for 3 weeks. However, in view of the absence of hard data, the patients should be told that no definite benefit can be expected from chemotherapy at this time.

Prognosis

The 5-year survival rate for tubal carcinoma is approximately 40 percent.[1,13] As with ovarian carcinoma, the earlier the stage of disease, the better will be the prognosis. As with carcinoma of the ovary, it is hoped that refinements in ultrasonography and CT scanning may result in earlier diagnosis in the future. Meanwhile, the main way results can be improved is by gynecologists having a high index of suspicion for this disease.

METASTATIC CANCER OF THE FALLOPIAN TUBE

This is not uncommon. The most likely primary origins are ovary, breast, and gastrointestinal tract. The treatment is that of the primary carcinoma, with removal of the metastatic tumor if it is resectable. The prognosis is almost uniformly poor. Adenomatoid tumors, the most frequent benign tubal tumors, must not be mistaken for metastatic adenocarcinoma of the tube. This tumor

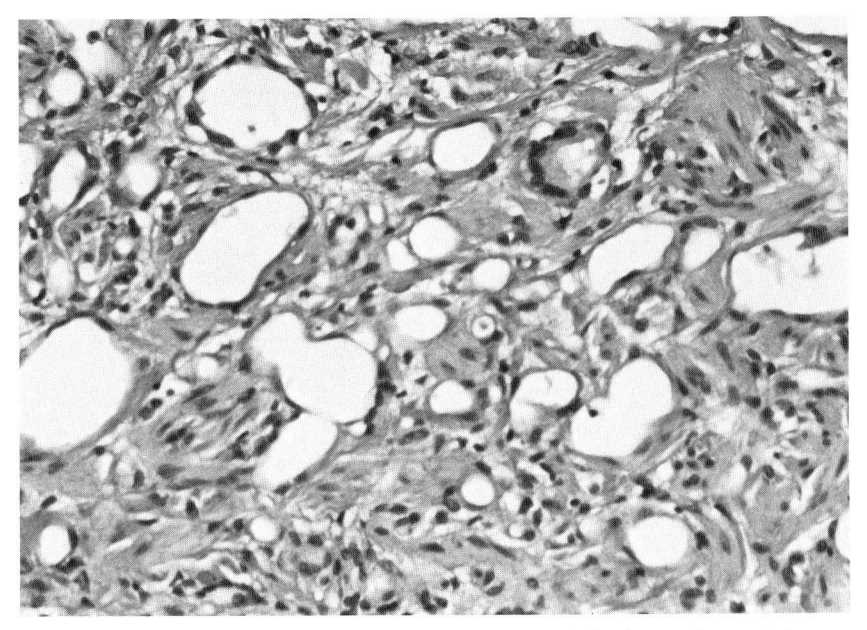

Figure 2. Adenomatoid tumor. Within a smooth muscle background are tubuloglandular elements lined by vacuolated flat to cuboidal epithelium. Lymphocytes are seen sprinkled throughout the tumor.

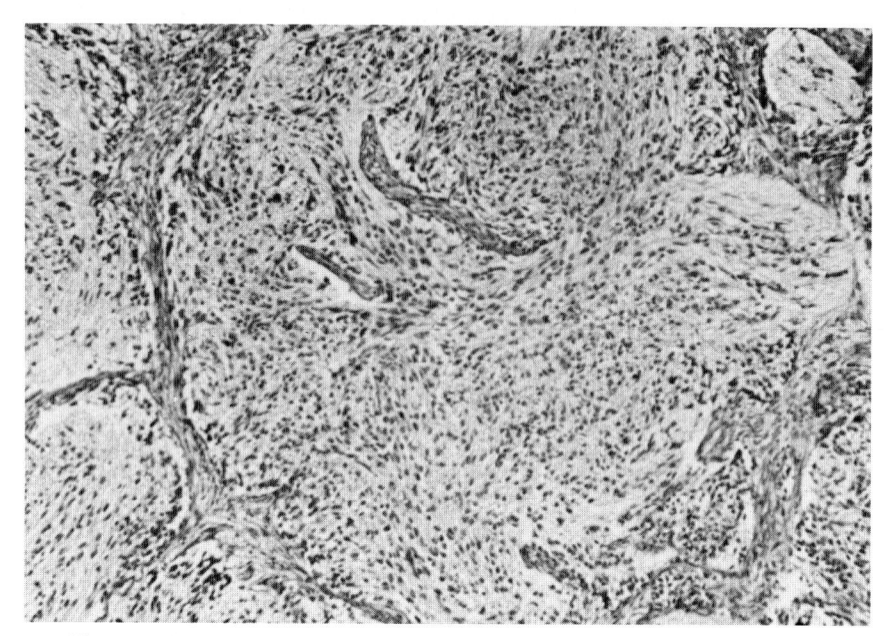

Figure 3. Immature teratoma of the tube. In this portion of the tumor, field after field of primitive neuroectodermal tissue was present.

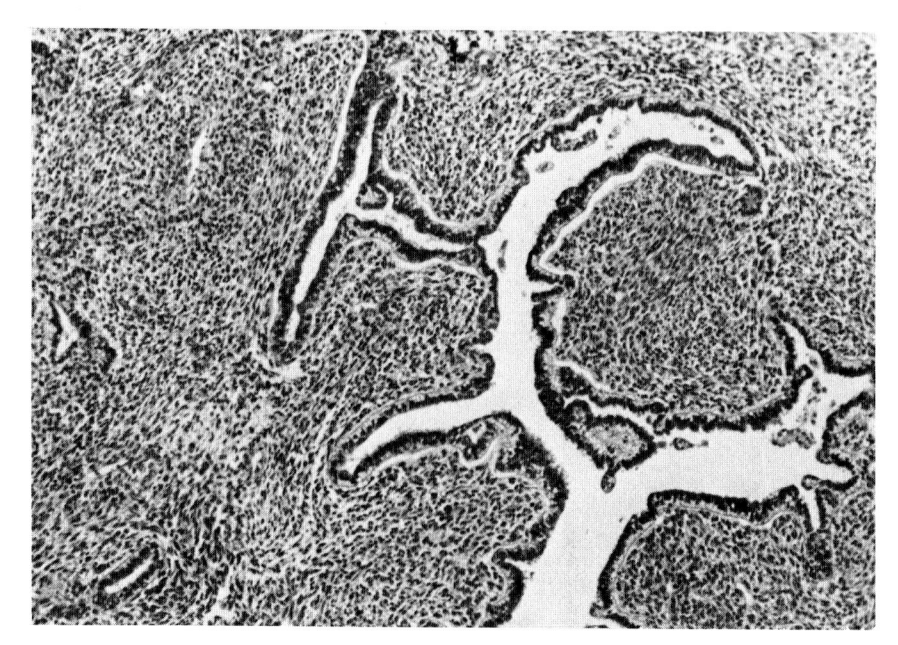

Figure 4. Immature teratoma of the tube. Embryonal endodermal structures are present in a background of rhabdomyoblasts representing a mesodermal component.

is made up of tubular and glandular-like spaces lined by vacuolated, flat, or cuboidal epithelial-like cells, which seem to penetrate bundles of smooth muscle forming an ill-defined mass (Fig. 2). A sprinkling of lymphocytes is also a noticeable feature.

Electron microscopic and histochemical studies confirm that these structures are of mesothelial origin rather than being epithelial in nature, and therefore the term benign mesothelioma has been offered as being more appropriate.

SARCOMA OF THE FALLOPIAN TUBE

A few sarcomas of the fallopian tube have been recorded. Leiomyosarcoma, reticulum cell sarcoma, and lymphoma have been reported. In addition, approximately 25 cases of mixed Müllerian tumor of the tube have been reported.[16,17] The surgical and radiotherapeutic treatment is as for carcinoma of the tube, and chemotherapy as for sarcomas of the uterus would appear to be indicated postoperatively. Pulmonary metastases are common and the outlook is generally very poor.

Choriocarcinoma of the Tube

This is extremely rare, but may follow an ectopic or intrauterine pregnancy. The condition may be expected in a patient with an elevation in the serum beta human chorionic gonadotropin (hCG), in whom the uterus is found to be empty at the time of dilation and curettage. The treatment is total abdominal hysterectomy with bilateral salpingo-oophorectomy and chemotherapy as for gestational trophoblastic neoplasia.

Malignant Teratoma of the Tube

Only one case of malignant or immature teratoma has been described[18] prior to a case recently encountered by the authors (Figs. 3, 4). Considering the lack of any experience with this unique tumor, management should most probably be that of immature teratoma of the ovary.[19]

REFERENCES

1. Tamimi HK, Figge DC: Adenocarcinoma of the uterine tube: Potential for lymph node metastases. Am J Obstet Gynecol 141:132, 1981
2. Hershey DW, Fennell RH, Major FJ: Primary carcinoma of the fallopian tube. Obstet Gynecol 57:367, 1981
3. Sieck UV: Primary adenocarcinoma of the fallopian tube. Aust NZ J Obstet Gynaecol 18:147, 1978
4. Yoonessi M: Carcinoma of the fallopian tube. Obstet Gynecol Survey 34:257, 1979
5. Roberts JA, Lifshitz S: Primary adenocarcinoma of the fallopian tube. Gynecol Oncol 13:301, 1982

6. Gaffney EF, Cornog J: Endometrioid carcinoma of the fallopian tube. Obstet Gynecol 52:34S, 1978
7. Starr AJ, Ruffolo EH, Shenoy BV, Marston BR: Primary carcinoma of the fallopian tube. A surprise finding in a postpartum tubal ligation. Am J Obstet Gynecol 132:344, 1978
8. Schinfeld JS, Winston HG: Primary tubal carcinoma in pregnancy. Am J Obstet Gynecol 137:512, 1980
9. Galle PC, Jobson VW, Homesley HD: Umbilical metastasis from gynecologic malignancies: A primary carcinoma of the fallopian tube. Obstet Gynecol 57:531, 1981
10. Stern J, Buscema J, Parmley T, et al: Atypical epithelial proliferations in the fallopian tube. Am J Obstet Gynecol 140:309, 1981
11. Finn WF, Javert CT: Primary and metastatic cancer of the fallopian tubes. Cancer 2:803, 1949
12. Johnson L, Diamond I, Jolly G: Ultrastructure of fallopian tube carcinoma. Cancer 42:1291, 1978
13. Sedlis A: Carcinoma of the fallopian tube. Surg Clin North Am 58:121, 1978
14. Deppe G, Bruckner HW, Cohen CJ: Combination chemotherapy for advanced carcinoma of the fallopian tube. Obstet Gynecol 56:530, 1980
15. Diamond SB, Rudolph SH, Lubicz SS, et al: Cerebral blindness in association with *cis*-platinum chemotherapy for advanced carcinoma of the fallopian tube. Obstet Gynecol 59:84S, 1982
16. Hanjani P, Petersen RO, Bonnell SA: Malignant mixed Müllerian tumor of the fallopian tube. Gynecol Oncol 9:381, 1980
17. Kahanpaa KV, Laine R, Saksela E: Malignant mixed Müllerian tumor of the fallopian tube: Report of a case with 5-year survival. Gynecol Oncol 16:144, 1983
18. Sweet RL, Selinger HE, McKay DG: Malignant teratoma of the uterine tube. Obstet Gynecol 45:553, 1975
19. Norris HJ, Zirkin HJ, Benson WL: Immature (malignant) teratoma of the ovary. Cancer 37:2359, 1976

CHAPTER 7
Epithelial Carcinoma of the Ovary

INTRODUCTION

No organ in the human body is the site of origin or metastasis for a greater range of tumors than the ovary. One reason is the variety of cell types in the ovary, including some which, given appropriate stimuli, can develop into any tissue in the body. This mixture of cells is subjected throughout reproductive life to the trauma of repeated cycles of follicle growth and rupture followed by corpus luteum growth and regression. The ovary is in close proximity to a route of rapid access for a variety of natural and unnatural irritants from the outside world via the patent genital tract. Finally, the vasculature and anatomic position of the ovaries predispose them to metastasis from genital and nongenital tumors.

The range of primary malignancies that can arise in the ovary is frequently cited as a reason why their etiology is so unclear: ". . . rather like taking all the tumors of the head and lumping them together. . . ." in search for an etiology.[1] The range of tumors possible and their uncertain etiology are often used to rationalize the poor prognosis and to lend support to what Smith has called the "indifference still too prevalent in the treatment of ovarian cancer.[2] Such arguments ignore the fact that approximately 85 percent of primary ovarian malignancies are of epithelial origin, and these predominantly of the serous type, and that little more is known of the etiology of other genital tract malignancies even though the results of treatment are better.

Discussions usually open with the sad statistics of the disease: approximately 18,000 new cases in the United States in 1982, with 11,400 deaths for a diagnosis to death ratio of 1.6:1 (Table 1),[3] approximately 60 percent of

TABLE 1. ESTIMATED DIAGNOSIS AND DEATH RATES FOR VARIOUS CARCINOMAS IN THE FEMALE IN THE UNITED STATES, 1984

	New Cases	Death	Diagnosis/Death Ratio
Lung	38,000	31,000	1.2:1
Large bowel	63,000	29,500	2.1:1
Breast	115,000	37,000	3:1
Cervix (invasive)	16,000	7100	2.3:1
Corpus	39,000	3000	13:1
Ovary	18,300	11,500	1.6:1

(Data from American Cancer Society: Cancer Facts and Figures. New York, 1984, with permission.)[3]

patients with disease outside the pelvis at presentation,[4] and overall 5-year survival rates of the order of 30 percent, virtually unchanged for a quarter of a century (Table 2).[5,6]

It cannot be disputed that these facts are correct, and that because approximately 1 in every 70 newborn females in the United States will live to develop ovarian cancer,[7] we will all too frequently be faced with the tragic end point of the disease, which, as Woodruff points out, has changed little since T. Spencer Wells described it a century ago: ". . . as the end approaches, we have the symptoms of failure, first of one power then of another . . . step by step Death is felt to be advancing. The patient watches his approach as keenly as we. . . . We come . . . day by day to be idle spectators of a sad ceremony and leave . . . humbled by the consciousness of the narrow limits which circumscribe the resources of our art."[8]

But it is well known to practicing gynecologic oncologists that present day knowledge, applied appropriately, can achieve a degree of palliation and prolongation of useful life not previously attainable, even if total survival is not increased. Furthermore, we are all aware of a large number of patients whose prognosis is significantly worsened by a failure to use current techniques and knowledge appropriately. Not only are 25 percent of patients with ovarian cancer initially treated by specialists other than gynecologists,[9] but among the gynecologists the least experienced surgeon will often have the first (and best) opportunity to resect the tumor.[10] The attitude of hopelessness that is so common among those treating patients with ovarian malignancy, and which is the

TABLE 2. 5-YEAR SURVIVAL RATES FROM COLLECTED SERIES OF OVARIAN CANCER PATIENTS

	No. of Patients	5-Year Survival
Stage I	751	61%
Stage II	401	40%
Stage III	539	5%
Stage IV	101	3%

(Modified from Tobias JS, Griffiths CT: N Engl J Med 294:877, 1976, with permission.)[5]

basis for much of the apparent indifference mentioned earlier is further compounded by misinterpretation of knowledge by prominent surgeons as demonstrated by this comment on one of the articles quoted previously:

> Once something is published, it becomes medical fact, and whereas bloodletting may no longer be fashionable, one may now have to have a sterilized ruler to pare down each metastasis to 1.6 cm if one is to cure the patient with ovarian cancer.[11]

While we would be the last to suggest that application of current knowledge and techniques would revolutionize ovarian cancer statistics, we do believe that it could improve the lot of a large number of women each year, and lead toward the more satisfactory therapy of the disease in the future. It is to this end that we have prepared this chapter.

ETIOLOGY

The etiology of epithelial cancers of the ovary remains obscure despite a wide range of experimental, demographic, and epidemiologic studies. This discussion summarizes the more relevant data and theories from the perspective of gynecologic oncologists managing the condition on a daily basis.

Geographic and Racial Factors

It is well known that ovarian cancer is seen with markedly different frequency in various parts of the world (Table 3).[3] The highest incidence rates are reported from the Scandinavian countries, with the United States falling in about the middle, and the Asian countries reporting the lowest incidence. While it is recognized that there are marked variations in the availability and quality of diagnostic, therapeutic, and data collection facilities from one country to another, it is generally accepted that the figures represent real and

TABLE 3. AGE-STANDARDIZED OVARIAN CANCER DEATH RATES, 1970–1971

	Death Rate per 100,000 Population
Denmark	12.9
Sweden	9.6
Norway	9.5
England and Wales	9.1
Scotland	8.5
United States	7.3
Ireland	5.8
Italy	3.3
Japan	2.1

(Data from American Cancer Society: Cancer Facts and Figures. New York, 1982, with permission.)[3]

significant differences in incidence rates. Support for this contention comes from studies of the Israeli population published in 1968, which showed ovarian cancer to be three times more common in women of European and North American origin than among those of Asian and African origin.[12] Because of the patterns of migration to Israel and the fact that ovarian cancer is most commonly diagnosed among older women, this difference reflects the transplanted incidence rates of the countries of origin of the women.

Country of residence is shown to be of greater importance than race by studies of migrant populations from Asian countries to the United States. Ovarian cancer rates for first- and second-generation Chinese migrants to the United States approach those of white Americans, but are at least twice as high as for Chinese in Singapore and Hong Kong.[13] Similarly, the mortality rate for ovarian cancer among first- and second-generation Japanese residing in the United States rises from the very low rates seen in Japan to be comparable to that of native Americans.[14] The average annual incidence rates of various cancers among populations of different racial origins in various areas of the Pacific basin illustrates this point (Table 4).[15]

Retrospective Studies

Incidence rates of ovarian carcinoma do not only vary geographically: it appears that they have changed with time. Woodruff points out that there was an extremely low incidence of malignancy among the ovarian tumors reported by the Atlee brothers in 1852 (none in 219 cases), Spencer Wells in 1872 (7 malignancies among 500 ovarian tumors), and Emmett in 1880 (none in over 100 tumors).[8] Although operative and follow-up notes may have been deficient, cancer was a well-known condition at this time and it is inconceivable that surgeons would have failed to recognize it. Even with shorter life expectancy, one would anticipate many more cases if roughly 10 percent of ovarian

TABLE 4. CANCER INCIDENCE RATES PER 100,000 FOR WOMEN OF DIFFERENT RACIAL ORIGINS IN THE PACIFIC BASIN FOR VARIOUS PERIODS BETWEEN 1968–1976

Site	Racial Origin	Osaka	Hong Kong	Hawaii	Los Angeles
Ovary	Japanese	3.2	—	6.9	7.5
	Chinese	—	4.6	5.8	11.1
	European	—	—	13.7	13.6
Breast	Japanese	13.7	—	44.2	56.6
	Chinese	—	28.6	54.2	40.9
	European	—	—	80.3	86.1
Corpus	Japanese	7.7	—	15.6	19.9
	Chinese	—	4.0	19.7	7.9
	European	—	—	28.8	35.9
Cervix	Japanese	17.7	—	7.6	9.6
	Chinese	—	28.5	13.1	12.2
	European	—	—	13.1	10.5

(Modified from Menck MR, Henderson BE: Natl Cancer Inst Monogr 53:119, 1979, with permission.)[15]

tumors in women under 40 years of age were malignant as they are in 1984. In England and Wales, the age-standardized mortality rates for ovarian cancer have more than doubled since 1931,[16] and similar changes have been noted in the United States.[7] These changes are not explicable in terms of improved diagnostic techniques or population aging.

Epidemiologic studies therefore show ovarian cancer to be a disease of the present century, most common in the Western countries. Studies of migrants indicate a very strong environmental effect on the incidence, while the low incidence in Japan tends to suggest that the degree of industrialization of a country is not a major factor.

Fertility and Family Size

Beral and colleagues demonstrated a clear inverse relationship between completed family size and ovarian cancer incidence in Britain, the United States, and 18 other countries.[16] In the widely different populations studied, they could find no other common factor that was highly correlated with average family size yet was unrelated to childbearing that could predispose to ovarian cancer. Furthermore, relative risks, calculated on the basis of their assumptions concerning such a relationship agreed closely with the findings of retrospective studies. Although they conclude that it is pregnancy itself which protects against ovarian cancer, they were unable to say whether the protection comes from suppression of ovulation, hormonal or immunologic changes, or some other effect. Fraumeni and coworkers[17] found a higher frequency of ovarian cancer among Catholic nuns than the general population. Breast, endometrial, and bowel cancer rates were also raised. The authors suggested that nulliparity and possibly hormonal factors might be implicated. McGowan and associates[18] also found a significantly lower pregnancy rate among women with ovarian cancers.

"Incessant Ovulation"

Drawing on information from a range of animal and human studies, Fathalla proposed that "the extravagant and mostly purposeless ovulations" seen in women are a major causative factor of ovarian malignancy.[19] Briefly stated, he argues that ovulatory cycles occur in women almost continuously from puberty to menopause at a rate of roughly 13 per year, whereas in other mammals ovulation is either confined to a breeding season or occurs after the act of coitus and so will most frequently be followed by pregnancy. Although examples of all ovarian tumor types seen in humans have been described in animals, the overall incidence of ovarian cancer is low, chiefly because of the extreme rarity of epithelial ovarian tumors in animals. Egg production in domestic hens can be markedly increased by changing light-dark cycles, but the higher productivity is accompanied by an equally dramatic increase in the incidence of epithelial ovarian tumors. Studies in the rat and mare show a sharp increase in mitotic activity in the epithelial cells of the ovary in relationship to the ovulatory follicle, and in mares where ovulation repeatedly occurs from the same "ovulatory fossa," it is a common site of origin of epithelial ovarian cysts. He also points out that before puberty and in women who do not ovulate, such as those with gonadal dysgenesis, there is a paucity of ovarian tumors, whereas in nuns and infertile women there is a higher incidence. Finally, he draws attention to the rough correspondence of ovarian cancer rates to those of multiple ovulation evidenced by binovular twinning around the world. Although Fathalla's arguments are simple and compelling, there has not been general acceptance of this hypothesis.

Peritoneal Irritants
Woodruff believes the increasing incidence of ovarian carcinomas in the present century is due to some agent entering the peritoneal cavity through the vagina, uterus, and tubes.[8] Certainly, particulate matter can pass from the upper vagina to the peritoneal cavity in less than 30 minutes.[20] Using special preparation techniques and electron microscopy, Henderson and colleagues found talc granules in 10 of 13 ovarian epithelial tumors.[21] Keal showed a tenfold increase in the incidence of ovarian cancer among women working in asbestos-related industries,[22] though Newhouse and coworkers have so far been unable to demonstrate such a relationship in a prospective study.[23] Talc and asbestos are closely related. Until recently, condoms and contraceptive diaphragms were stored in or dusted with talc, offering an explanation for the relationship between decreased family size and ovarian carcinoma. Changes in toilet habits and increasing use of talc on the vulvar area could explain both increasing incidence rates of ovarian cancer, and the changes in rates seen among Asian migrants to the United States.

Oral Contraception
If "incessant ovulation" is causally related to ovarian malignancy then use of oral contraceptives should lower the incidence. Case control studies by Newhouse and coworkers[23] and Casagrande and associates[24] showed that ovarian cancer risk was decreased by use of oral contraceptives. The former group suggested that each 12 months of oral contraceptive use had the same protective effect as 1 pregnancy. McGowan and associates[18] found that women with ovarian cancer used oral contraceptives significantly less often than controls. However, their ovarian cancer patients also reported more difficulty conceiving than controls, which could explain the lower oral contraceptive usage. Similarly, Joly and colleagues[25] found a history of greater difficulty in conceiving and more spontaneous abortions in ovarian cancer patients. A more recent study seeking to clarify the relationship between oral contraceptive use and ovarian cancer failed to resolve the issue, mainly because of the predominantly young group of women studied.[26]

Endogenous Hormone Levels
While exogenous hormones may play a role in the etiology of ovarian cancer, other studies suggest the possible role of endogenous hormones. Wynder and coworkers[27] correlated the standardized mortality rates for breast and ovarian cancers in various countries and found a significant correlation, for which they

invoked a possible common endocrine etiology. Fox and Langley[28] applied similar statistical data to incidence rates and found a highly significant correlation between rates for breast and ovarian cancers in different countries. Cholesterol is a precursor of steroid hormones and it has been postulated that dietary factors may explain both the varying incidence around the world, and the changing incidences among migrants. Dairy product and fat consumption is relatively low in Asian countries, but relatively high in the West, and in particular in the Scandinavian countries. But although hormonal and dietary manipulations produce nonepithelial tumors in animals, they do not lead to epithelial tumors. For example, it is possible to produce granulosa cell tumors by transplanting the ovaries of mice to their spleens, a procedure that raises the circulating levels of follicle stimulating hormone (FSH),[29] or by oophorectomy in one of a pair of parabiotic rats.[30]

These studies do not explain a possible hormonal influence on the epithelial tumors. In an attempt to provide the necessary link, Gondos[31] pointed out that at the time when the interstitial cells of the fetal ovary develop the ultrastructural and histochemical properties of steroid secretion, the surface epithelium undergoes diffuse proliferation with marked nuclear irregularity and pleomorphism, producing appearances similar to those seen in the common epithelial tumors of adult life. After about the fifth month of gestation, the epithelium reverts to an apparently inactive layer. It has, nevertheless, shown the ability to respond to hormonal stimuli with changes similar to neoplasia, an ability which Gondos[31] postulates may be retained for life. This hypothesis gains support from recent reports documenting the presence of estrogen and progesterone receptors in at least a proportion of epithelial ovarian cancers.[32,33]

The Pluripotential "Secondary Müllerian System"

Common to most theories regarding the etiology of ovarian carcinoma is the assumption that the surface epithelium of the ovary retains through life its potential to develop along many different pathways, given appropriate stimuli. Lauchlan[34] refers to the concept of a "secondary Müllerian system," a term used to describe cells of similar embryologic origins to those which, in fetal life, form the linings of the uterus, tubes, and endocervical canal, but which have remained in an undifferentiated state, and are situated external to the cavities of the original Müllerian ducts.[34] The "germinal epithelium" of the ovary, so named because it was once thought to be the origin of germ cells, is the best example of secondary Müllerian tissue. In the embryo and fetus, the cells of this layer bear a close resemblance to tubal epithelium but by birth the cilia are lost and they are visually similar to the rest of the celomic peritoneum. However, Lauchlan[34] cites a great deal of evidence that given appropriate stimulation, this secondary Müllerian tissue can differentiate into tubal, endometrial, and endocervical epithelium, as seen in epithelial tumors of the ovary. Groups of these pluripotential cells may be found scattered throughout the pelvic peritoneum, the general peritoneal cavity, and even in lymph nodes.[35] This is evidenced by the frequency with which glandular inclusion cysts lined with Müllerian-type epithelium are seen in the pelvic peritoneum and elsewhere in the abdomen. These could arise from stimulation of several portions of the secondary Müllerian system by a common agent. Cells of this type on the ovarian surface may become buried in the ovarian stroma by ovulation, or the retraction of corpora lutea and atretic follicles.[36] These benign lesions may be stimulated to increasing degrees of mitotic activity up to frank malignancy by some exogenous or endogenous stimulus, and due to their potential to develop into any of the Müllerian tissues could form one of the common epithelial neoplasms.

Endometriosis is seen as a benign example of activation of the secondary Müllerian system. Although it has been clearly demonstrated that the cells of the menstrual effluent are viable on transplantation,[37] it has also been shown that degenerating endometrium, rendered cell-free by passage through a millipore filter will lead to cellular differentiation and proliferation of the secondary Müllerian system.[38] This is in essence the theory of Novak on the genesis of endometriosis.[39] Woodruff believes that most, if not all, ovarian malignancies are mesotheliomas of the peritoneal cavity, most likely resulting from stimulation of cells of the secondary Müllerian system by "proliferating agents" entering the peritoneal cavity via the cervix, uterine cavity, and fallopian tubes.[8,40] Inclusion cysts may hold such agents in proximity to the pluripotent epithelium for long periods of time allowing the maximal possible exposure to their oncogenic effects.

Other Factors

A number of other pertinent observations relating to the epidemiology of ovarian cancer should be mentioned. West[41] noted that women with ovarian cancer reported a history of mumps significantly less often than control patients. This was interpreted as indicating either that mumps infection protected against ovarian cancer, or that a factor protecting a woman from mumps infection predisposes her to ovarian cancer. Although the known affinity of the mumps virus for the gonads made this an attractive theory, other authors have been unable to substantiate the relationship.[18,42] Osbourne and DiGeorge[43] showed an increased incidence of epithelial ovarian cancers and metastatic ovarian tumors in women with blood Group A. Several studies have shown familial incidences of ovarian cancers but such cases seem to be the exception rather than the rule.[44-48]

McGowan and associates[18] concluded that the woman most at risk for ovarian cancer has a family history of gynecologic cancer, has been exposed to rubella in the peripubertal period, is of low parity or nulliparous, has experienced difficulty in conceiving, has exacerbated premenstrual symptoms, and has had a surgical menopause less commonly than controls. Szamborski and coworkers[49] found that the three most common high-risk factors in patients with epithelial cancers of the ovary were late menarche (over 14 years), early menopause (under 45 years), and infertility. All of these factors suggest inadequate ovarian function, and we are left with the conclusion that this may be one of the most important basic factors predisposing to carcinoma of the ovary.

CLINICAL PICTURE

Regardless of the etiology of ovarian cancers we are poor at diagnosing them in their early stages. Data pooled by Tobias and Griffiths[5] from 5 studies involving over 1100 patients show that only 26 percent of ovarian cancers are diagnosed while they are confined to the ovaries, and in 53 percent of cases extrapelvic spread is present at the time of diagnosis (Table 5, Fig. 1).

In fact, of all common cancers studied by Cutler and colleagues[50] ovarian cancer rates a poor eighth in terms of the proportion of cases diagnosed with localized disease, exceeded only by stomach, lung, and pancreas. The end results evaluation program shows the 5-year survival for localized ovarian cancer to be 76 percent, for disease with regional spread 32 percent, and with distant spread 12 percent; and pooled data from other studies show an even worse prognosis for advanced disease (Table 2).[5] It is clear that if the prognosis is to improve, early diagnosis is essential.

Symptomatology of Early Disease

In its early stages ovarian carcinoma is a notoriously silent disease. Abdominal pain, swelling, and a palpable mass, though all too commonly seen, are manifestations of advanced disease. The most common symptoms reported by 638 patients with ovarian cancer are shown in Table 6.[51]

Barber[52] describes the "generally insidious" signs of early ovarian cancer as being a feeling of abdominal distention and vague discomfort, associated with flatulence and eructations, and a loss of appetite with a sense of bloating after meals. Such symptoms are so vague and nonspecific that they may not lead the patient to seek help and, if they do, the physician needs to be especially astute to recognize their cause. Furthermore, the nature of the symptoms are such that a family physician or internist is most likely to be consulted. Consequently, all physicians must be aware of the possible significance of persistent gastrointestinal symptoms in women over the age of 40 with a history of ovarian dysfunction.

TABLE 5. EXTENT OF DISEASE AT TIME OF DIAGNOSIS IN COMBINED SERIES TOTALLING 1121 PATIENTS

Stage I	Confined to ovaries	26%
Stage II	Intrapelvic spread	21%
Stage III	Intraabdominal, extrapelvic spread, excluding liver parenchyma	37%
Stage IV	Parenchymal liver involvement or extra-abdominal spread	16%

(Modified from Tobias JS, Griffiths CT: N Engl J Med 294:877, 1976, with permission.)[5]

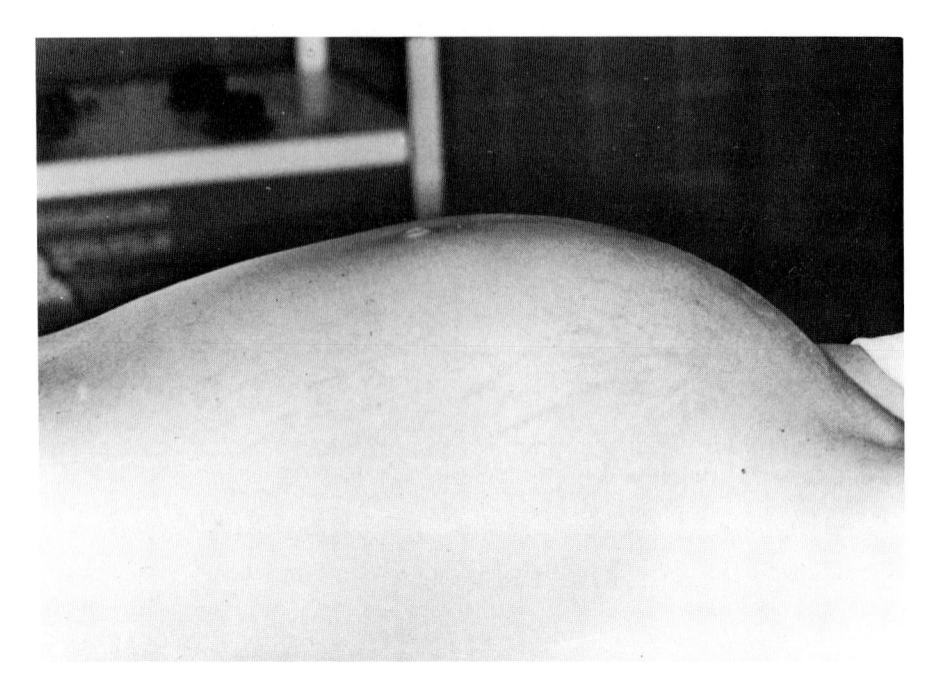

Figure 1A. The all too common appearance of the abdomen in a patient with a large ovarian tumor. The enlargement may be due to ascites, tumor mass, or both.

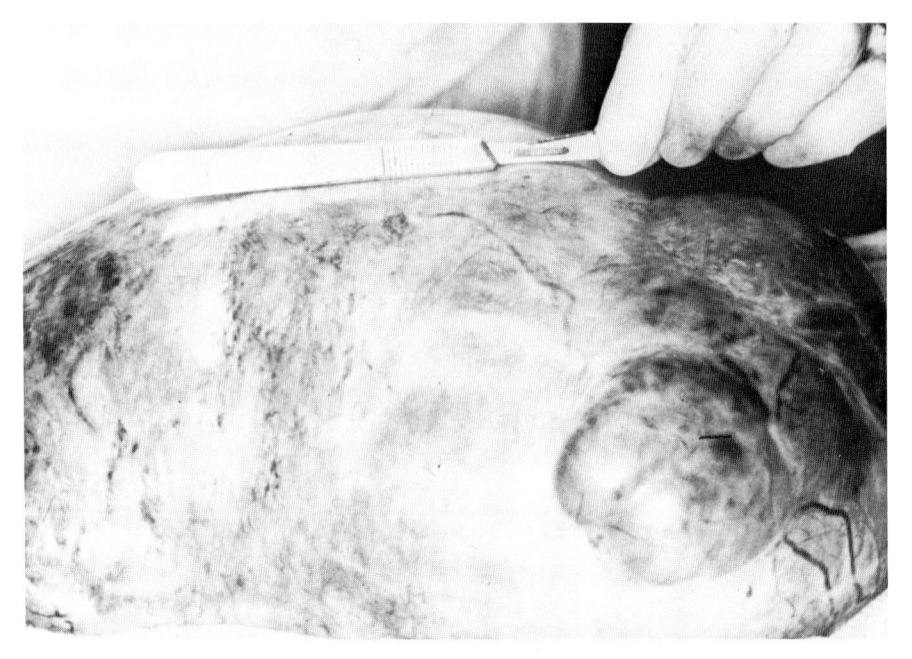

Figure 1B. In this case it was due to a massive benign mucinous cystadenoma.

TABLE 6. PRESENTING COMPLAINTS IN 638 CASES OF OVARIAN CANCER

Abdominal distention	36%	Menstrual abnormality	9%
Chronic abdominal pain	30%	Weight loss abnormality	5%
Postmenopausal bleeding	9%	Inguinal node enlargement	2%
Acute abdominal pain	9%		

(Modified from Rutledge F, et al: Gynecologic Oncology, New York, Wiley, 1976, with permission.)[51]

The importance of symptoms pointing to pelvic disease in improving the survival of patients is well illustrated by the study of Stone and associates,[53] where 5-year survivals were approximately 45 percent when the presenting symptom was bleeding, 20 percent when it was abdominal pain, 15 percent when gastrointestinal symptoms led to consultation, and less than 10 percent when ascites or a mass was present. Bleeding is not common with ovarian cancer, and the tumors that may cause it are uncommon. We believe that in the majority of cases, bleeding, indicating the need for pelvic examination, allowed the fortuitous discovery of an ovarian tumor at an earlier stage.

The importance of early diagnosis is emphasized by the dismal median survival times for patients with ovarian carcinoma (Table 7). Unfortunately, as Barber points out, a tumor volume of one ml, which is about the smallest clinically detectable, contains about a billion cancer cells and may already be associated with widespread intraabdominal seeding.[52]

Screening for Ovarian Cancer

Unfortunately, there are no simple or reliable cytologic, biochemical, or immunologic screening tests for early ovarian cancer. Vaginal cytology will detect only between 10 and 15 percent of advanced ovarian cancers.[54,55] Although useful for follow-up of some of the rarer germ cell tumors, carcinoembryonic antigen, alpha-fetoprotein, and human chorionic gonadotropin are of no help in the diagnosis and management of the common epithelial tumors.[7,56] Many other tumor-associated antigens have been investigated but so far have proved to be of little value for general use.[57]

We must rely on the annual medical examination, and in particular on

TABLE 7. MEDIAN SURVIVAL TIME FOR OVARIAN CANCER

Age	Median Survival (Years)
All ages	1.4
Under 45	5.4
45–54	1.8
55–64	1.3
65–74	0.9
75 and over	0.8

(Data from Barber HRK: American Cancer Society, Ca—A Cancer Journal for Clinicians 29:341, 1979, with permission.)[52]

the pelvic examination, for detecting ovarian cancer. The authors strongly believe that annual "mini-screening" examinations of the breasts, abdomen, and pelvis, utilizing cytology and vaginal and rectal examinations are an essential part of any program designed to reduce cancer morbidity and mortality in women. With reference to ovarian cancer we are in full agreement with Barlow,[58] who summed up the opinions of a discussion group on the early diagnosis of ovarian cancer:

> We all recognize the limitations of the pelvic examination (but) there is no doubt that, if more careful and more frequent pelvic examinations were done on more women on a regular basis, and the finding of adnexal enlargement was appropriately acted upon, more early ovarian cancers would be detected.

When ovaries are palpated on pelvic examination, one must consider whether they are normal or abnormal. The roughly walnut-sized ovaries of the reproductive years are not normal for the postmenopausal woman. Barber and Graber[59] drew attention to the fact that within 3 to 5 years of the menopause the ovary atrophies and becomes impalpable on vaginal examination. Approximately 10 percent of postmenopausal women with palpable ovaries will have an ovarian neoplasm. In fact, palpable ovaries more than 1 year before the menarche or in the postmenopausal woman are abnormal, and the possibility of neoplasia must be considered. In the postmenopausal woman with palpable ovaries the correct management is examination under anesthesia and if the finding is confirmed, total hysterectomy and bilateral salpingo-oophorectomy with the other staging procedures as described later in this chapter.

It is absolutely essential that all physicians recognize that "in the 40 to 60 age group, quibbling about centimeters is illogical. Any tumor that grows in the ovary in this age group is pathologic."[60]

It should also be remembered that ovaries palpable premenopausally by an inexperienced examiner, or in an obese woman, may well be pathologically enlarged.

Ovarian Enlargement in the Reproductive Years

During the reproductive years the possibility that an ovarian enlargement is benign or functional is greater. Nonetheless, it is wise to remember that in the age group 20 to 44 years, approximately 10 percent of ovarian tumors will be malignant, and in the over 45 age group almost 40 percent.[61] Where there is any suggestion of malignancy, exploration is mandatory. In addition, any symptomatic mass, bilateral masses, those bound down or adherent, or masses larger than 5 cm diameter constitute an indication for exploration. Where a small, freely mobile, smooth-surfaced cyst is felt to be functional, a short period of observation is acceptable. To hasten regression of functional cysts Spanos[62] advised the suppression of gonadotropins, which can be most conveniently performed by use of oral contraceptives for two cycles. Of 286 patients studied, such treatment led to the disappearance of the masses in all but 81 of the patients over a period of 6 weeks. When the patients with persistent masses were explored, none had physiologic cysts and five had malignant ovarian tumors. This approach is certainly reasonable, but it cannot be emphasized strongly enough that the penalty for overlooking an early ovarian carcinoma may be very great for the patient concerned. "To wait until one feels a solid tumor mass of 5 cm and then to expect a cure is an exercise in fancy and futility."[7]

Some Guidelines for Differentiating Ovarian from Nonovarian Masses

There are many conditions other than ovarian carcinoma that may produce adnexal masses. Some simple rules will help in deciding the management.

1. As a guide to size, remember that a tennis ball is 7 cm in diameter.
2. Remember the need for an empty bladder and rectum to allow proper examination. In some cases a catheterization or an enema may be needed to ensure adequate emptying.
3. If the conditions in the differential diagnosis are normally treated surgically, then exploration is reasonable.
4. Do not allow the known presence of benign disease to delay the recognition of malignancy; for example, women with known myomas of the uterus may still get ovarian carcinoma. Similarly, the demonstration of diverticular disease on a barium enema does not mean that a pelvic mass is not an ovarian carcinoma. Myomas do not enlarge spontaneously after the menopause.
5. Examination under anesthesia still has an important place in assessing dubious lesions.
6. Laparoscopy, because it does not allow palpation of visible lesions and structures that appear normal, has only a limited role.
7. Laparotomy is the final arbiter and, when one is considering such a lethal disease as ovarian carcinoma, it must be employed freely.

Noninvasive Tests

Noninvasive tests have so far proved to be of little value in the diagnosis and differential diagnosis of ovarian tumors. In our experience, ultrasound has not been reliable in the detection or identification of ovarian masses and has, on several occasions, led to totally false conclusions. We are sure that with modern techniques and skillful operators the most optimistic reports of their value, with diagnostic accuracy of the order of 80 to 90 percent for masses over 2 cm will be fulfilled,[63,64] but our experience has led us to agree with Donald's comments regarding the diagnosis of ovarian tumors: "Sonar will do little better as a diagnostic tool than the trained hands and eyes of a gynecological surgeon. . . ."[65]

Similarly, our personal experience with the use of computerized axial tomography (CT scanning) has been disappointing, and clearly the technology is not readily available to all, while the expense is considerable. CT scanning is certainly no substitute for exploratory laparotomy.[66]

Preoperative Assessment

These comments should not be interpreted as indicating an attitude of diagnostic nihilism and surgery at all costs. The study of Piver and coworkers[67] of 100 consecutive patients referred for further treatment after surgical diagnosis of ovarian cancer shows that such an attitude does exist; of the patients studied, only one-third had received any investigation beyond routine physical examination and preoperative laboratory work and 11 percent had not had a pelvic examination before surgery. The intraoperative evaluation was equally deficient. This is the antithesis of good care. The critical point is to use clinical judgment to select investigations and management that will most accurately and effectively allow the safe treatment of the patient.

We advise the following preoperative assessment in all patients with suspected ovarian malignancy:

1. A complete history and physical examination including cervical cytology and rectovaginal examination.
2. Complete blood count, serology, serum electrolytes, and renal and liver profiles.
3. Chest x-ray.
4. Urinalysis and, if the patient is in the reproductive age group, pregnancy tests.
5. If pregnancy has been ruled out, an intravenous pyelogram (IVP). This is especially important to exclude a pelvic kidney, or ureteral compression, displacement, or duplication.
6. Barium enema, upper GI series, liver scans, and endoscopic bowel examinations may be indicated by findings on history and physical examination. Recently double contrast enemas (DCE) have been suggested to help ascertain the extent of tumor spread.[68]
7. Enlarged groin or supraclavicular nodes should be biopsied.
8. In the child or adolescent, or when a pregnancy has occurred recently, serum alpha-fetoprotein and beta-hCG estimations may be indicated.
9. If a pleural effusion is present, thoracentesis for cytologic examination is indicated.
10. Preoperative abdominal paracentesis or culdocentesis is discouraged because fluid is more safely and easily removed at surgery.
11. Ultrasonography, CT scanning, and lymphograms are rarely of significant value.
12. It cannot be overemphasized that, at the present time, the most definitive diagnostic procedure for ovarian masses is laparotomy, and it is likely to remain so for a very long time.

Prime Indications for Laparotomy

1. An adnexal mass in a woman of any age that enlarges progressively beyond 5 cm while under observation.
2. Any symptomatic ovarian tumor, regardless of size.
3. Any adnexal mass greater than 10 cm in diameter.
4. Any pelvic mass first discovered after the menopause, or enlarging after the menopause.
5. Ovaries that are readily palpable in the postmenopausal woman.

PATHOLOGY

The currently accepted histologic classification of ovarian tumors is that of the World Health Organization, published in 1974.[69] In this chapter we are concerned only with epithelial ovarian tumors and the classification of this group is

TABLE 8. HISTOLOGIC CLASSIFICATION OF EPITHELIAL OVARIAN TUMORS (WHO)

A. Serous tumors
 1. Benign
  a. Cystadenoma and papillary cystadenoma
  b. Surface papilloma
  c. Adenofibroma and cystadenofibroma
 2. Of borderline malignancy (carcinomas of low malignant potential)
  a. Cystadenoma and papillary cystadenoma
  b. Surface papilloma
  c. Adenofibroma and cystadenofibroma
 3. Malignant
  a. Adenocarcinoma, papillary adenocarcinoma, and papillary cystadenocarcinoma
  b. Surface papillary carcinoma
  c. Malignant adenofibroma and cystadenofibroma
B. Mucinous tumors
 1. Benign
  a. Cystadenoma
  b. Adenofibroma and cystadenofibroma
 2. Of borderline malignancy (carcinomas of low malignant potential)
  a. Cystadenoma
  b. Adenofibroma and cystadenofibroma
 3. Malignant
  a. Adenocarcinoma and cystadenocarcinoma
  b. Malignant adenofibroma and cystadenofibroma

C. Endometrioid tumors
 1. Benign
  a. Adenoma and cystadenoma
  b. Adenofibroma and cystadenofibroma
 2. Of borderline malignancy (carcinomas of low malignant potential)
  a. Adenoma and cystadenoma
  b. Adenofibroma and cystadenofibroma
 3. Malignant
  a. Carcinoma
   i. Adenocarcinoma
   ii. Adenoacanthoma
   iii. Malignant adenofibroma and cystadenofibroma
  b. Endometrioid stromal sarcomas
  c. Mesodermal (Müllerian) mixed tumors, homologous and heterologous
D. Clear cell (mesonephroid) tumors
 1. Benign: adenofibroma
 2. Of borderline malignancy (carcinomas of low malignant potential)
 3. Malignant: carcinoma and adenocarcinoma
E. Brenner tumors
 1. Benign
 2. Of borderline malignancy (proliferating)
 3. Malignant
F. Mixed epithelial tumors
 1. Benign
 2. Of borderline malignancy
 3. Malignant
G. Undifferentiated carcinoma
H. Unclassified epithelial tumors

shown in Table 8. The tumors are classified according to the predominant cell types and the relative amounts of glandular and fibrous elements. In each subgroup tumors are classified as benign, "borderline," or malignant (Figs. 2–6).

Some general points relating to this classification merit attention. "Borderline" tumors are defined by the World Health Organization as those tumors that, while not showing invasion of the adjacent stroma, have some of the morphologic features of cancer. These include varying combinations of epithelial cell stratification, detachment of cell clusters from their sites of origin, and mitotic activity and nuclear abnormalities intermediate between benign and frankly malignant. It is our preference to call these "tumors of low malignant potential" rather than "borderline" because their course is clearly malignant, albeit over a prolonged interval.

Stromal invasion is usually easily recognized in serous tumors, but may be more difficult to assess in mesonephroid and endometrioid tumors. Furthermore, both light and electron microscopic studies have demonstrated the coexistence of areas of benign, "borderline," and frankly malignant tissues

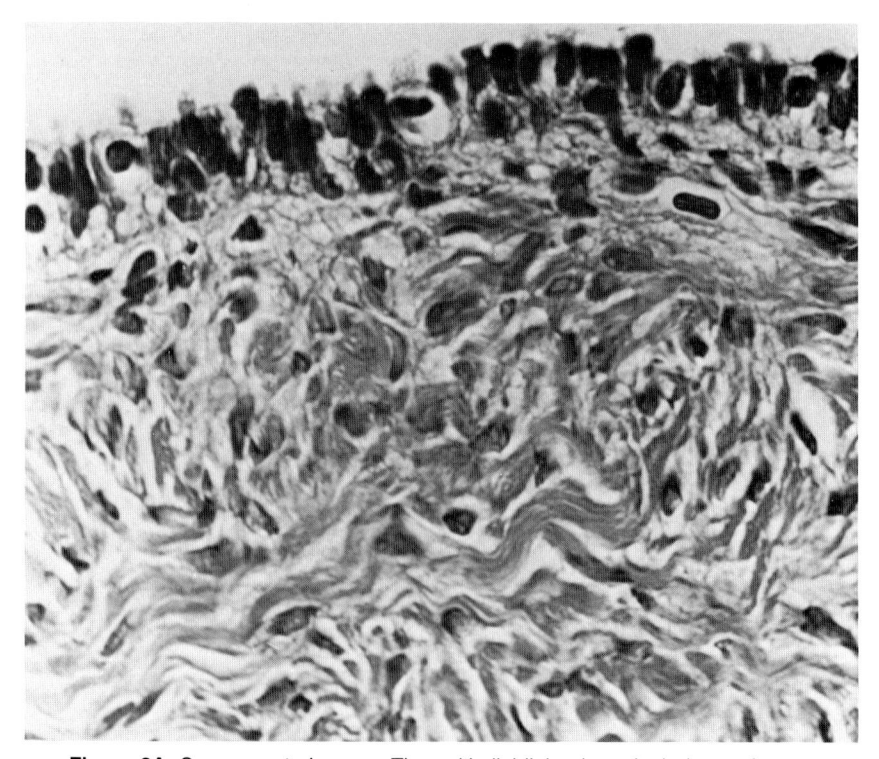

Figure 2A. Serous cystadenoma. The epithelial lining is a single layer of pseudostratified cells, which include ciliated, clear, and columnar varieties. This is identical to the epithelial lining of the normal fallopian tube. H&E. Original magnification ×200.

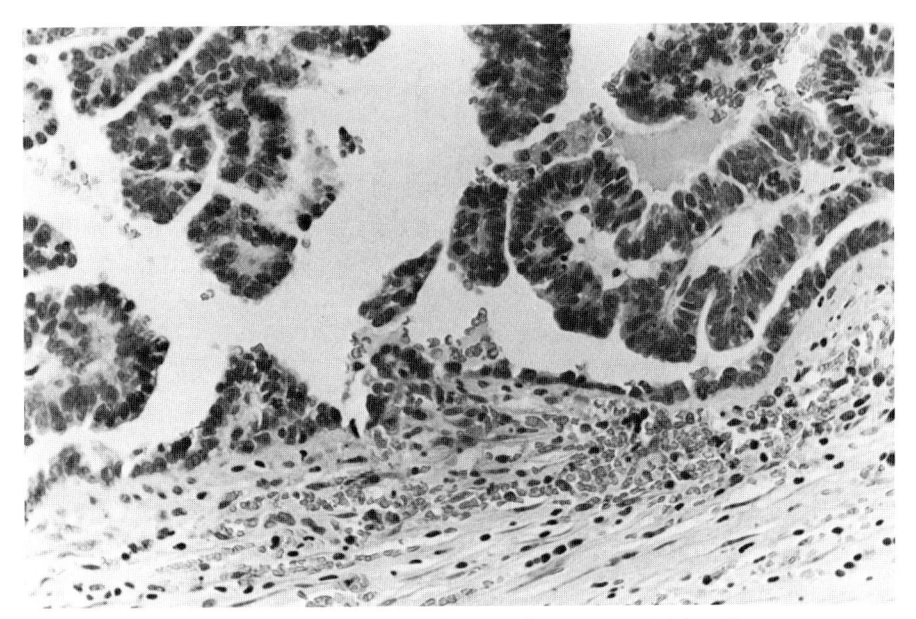

Figure 2B. Papillary serous tumor of low malignant potential (papillary serous cystadenoma of borderline malignancy). The serous epithelium is papillary, and stratified, has cytologic malignant criteria, and is shedding clusters of malignant cells into the lumen. There is, however, no evidence of invasion into the underlying ovarian cortical stroma. H&E. Original magnification ×80.

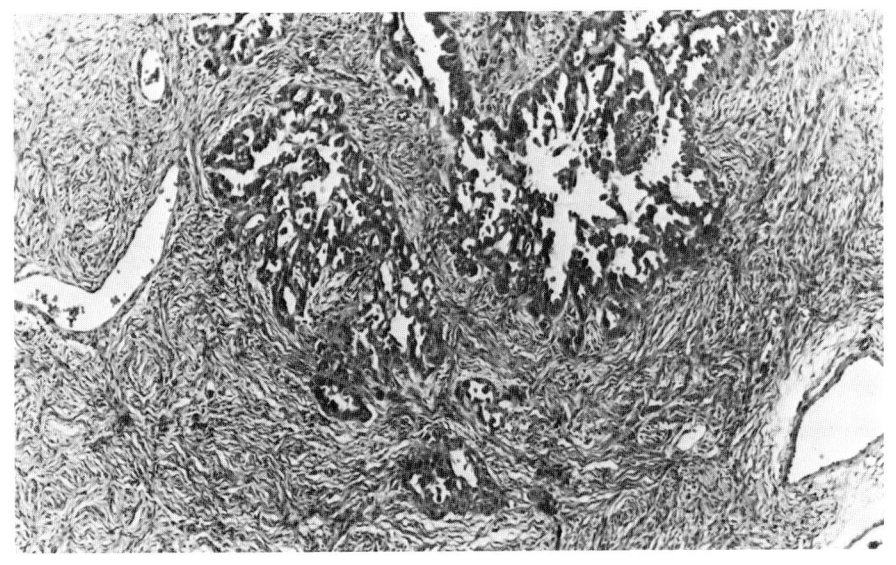

Figure 2C. Papillary serous cystadenocarcinoma. There is frank invasion by cytologically malignant papillary and acinar neoplasm into the ovarian cortical stroma. Psammoma bodies (calcospherites) are usually present in the more differentiated tumors. H&E. Original magnification ×30.

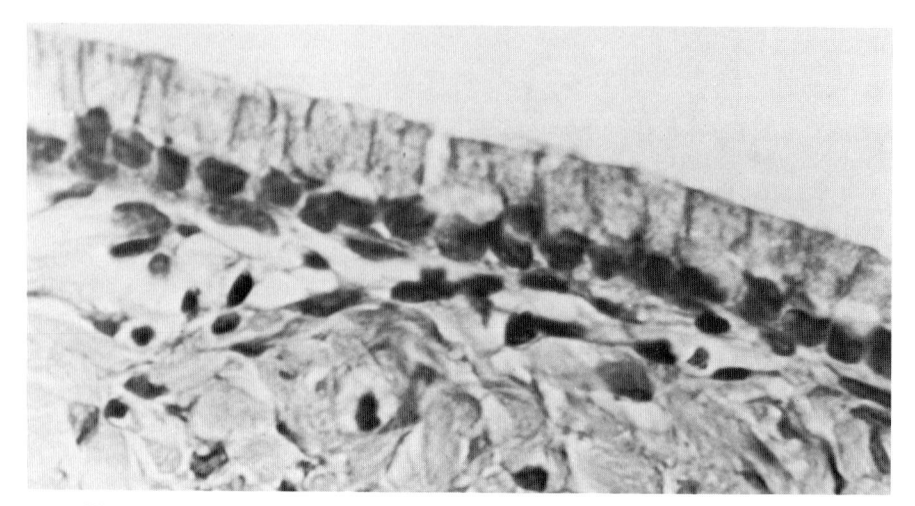

Figure 3A. Mucinous cystadenoma. A single layer of epithelium lines the cyst and is characterized by columnar cells with basal nuclei, the overlying cytoplasm containing and distended by mucus. This is identical to the epithelium of the endocervix, again reflecting the pluripotentiality of the ovarian germinal epithelium. H&E. Original magnification ×200.

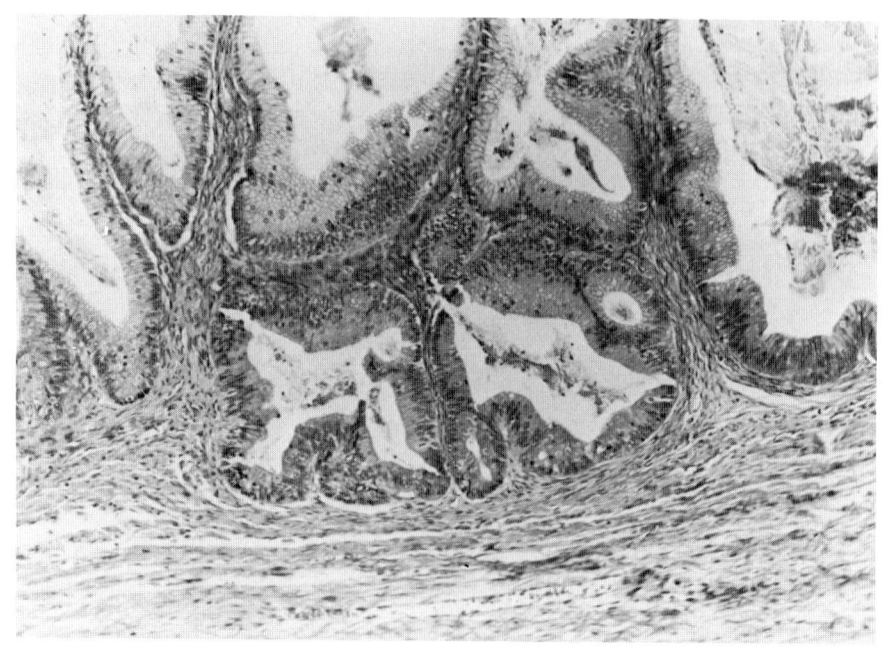

Figure 3B. Papillary mucinous carcinoma of low malignant potential (mucinous cystadenoma of borderline malignancy). The epithelium is thrown up into papillary folds, with minor stratification and cellular atypia. As in the borderline serous tumor, there is no invasion of ovarian stroma, but rather an impression of pushing into the stroma. H&E. Original magnification ×80.

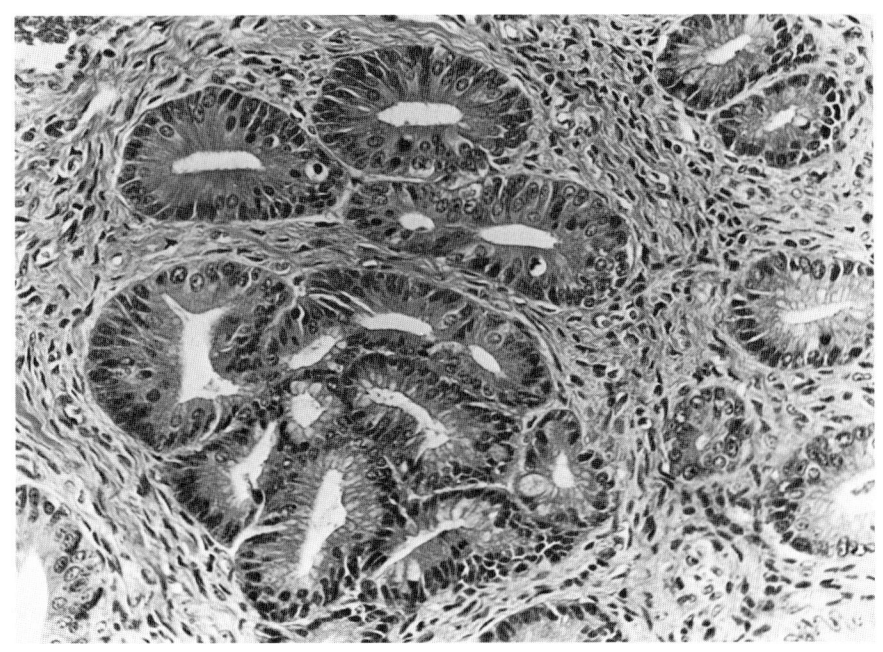

Figure 3C. Well-differentiated mucinous adenocarcinoma. Mucin-producing acinar structures, cytologically malignant, unequivocally invading the stroma surrounding a papillary mucinous cystic tumor. The cells feature an increased nuclear/cytoplasmic ratio, loss of polarity, and stratification, and chromatin characteristics of malignancy. H&E. Original magnification ×80.

within a single tumor. Because the clinical behavior is equated to the most malignant portion of the tumor, the importance of examination of multiple sections before making a final diagnosis is obvious. Among serous tumors a subgroup of surface papillomas is defined because they metastasize earlier than encapsulated tumors of the same stage.

The multilocular nature of mucinous tumors may make it difficult to be sure whether glandular structures within the stroma are invasive, or merely buds from other glands. It may be necessary to take into account histologic grading, nuclear activity, and stromal response to diagnose invasion in mucinous tumors. Epithelium four or more cell layers thick is generally considered to be malignant in this group.

Pathologic Considerations in Management Planning

Four factors are generally assumed to be important in determining the prognosis for any patient with ovarian malignancy. They are the histologic type of tumor, the stage, the histologic grade, and the host response. We will examine each of these factors individually.

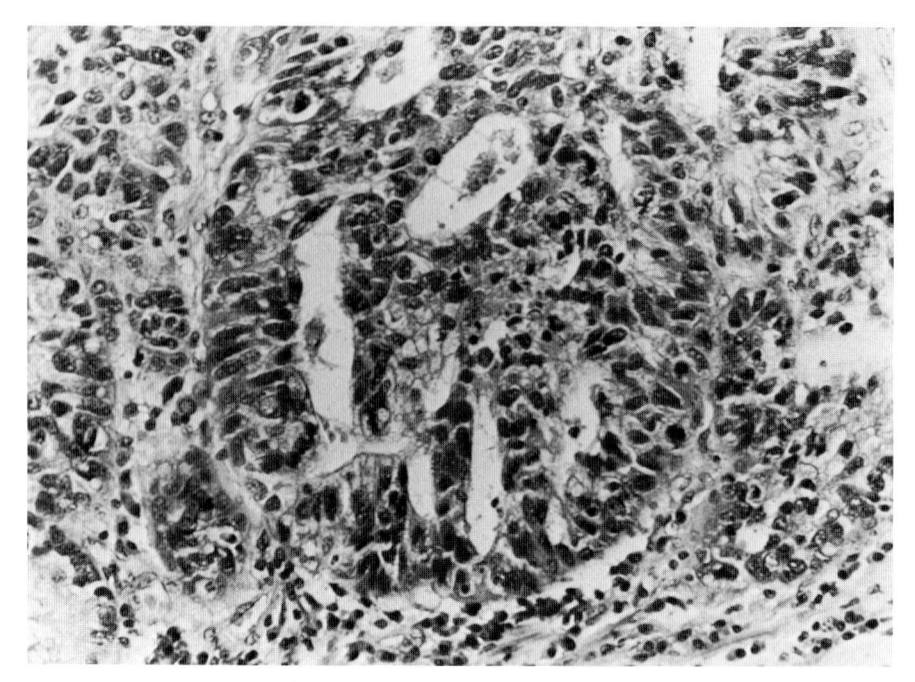

Figure 4. Endometrioid carcinoma of the ovary. Although identical to its endometrial counterpart, this is primary, arising also from the ovarian germinal epithelium. The back-to-back neoplastic acini with "cribiform appearance" are characteristic. A significant number, perhaps 30 percent, may be seen arising from benign ovarian endometriosis; however, it is usually a de novo phenomenon. H&E. Original magnification ×80.

Histologic Tumor Type. The relative frequencies of the most common types of primary ovarian malignancies are shown in Table 9.[56] Clearly epithelial tumors are the most important type of ovarian cancer in terms of numbers diagnosed. The relative proportion of each cell type varies widely from one study to another, probably reflecting variations in both patient populations and histologic criteria. Institutions seeing predominantly patients referred for treatment of advanced stage disease may have a very different distribution of tumor types than those reporting all ovarian tumors diagnosed over a period of time. Ozols and colleagues[70] found the distribution to be 40 percent serous, 3 percent mucinous, 3 percent endometrioid, 8 percent mixed, and 46 percent undifferentiated among a group of patients referred with Stages III and IV disease. Decker and associates[71] reported on over 700 patients where roughly one-third of the patients had Stage I disease; 68 percent had serous tumors, 21 percent mucinous, 5 percent endometrioid, and 6 percent solid tumors. This distribution was roughly the same for each stage except that the proportion of mucinous tumors was higher among Stage I lesions.

It has generally been accepted that among epithelial tumors of the ovary there is a simple relationship between histologic type and outcome, with

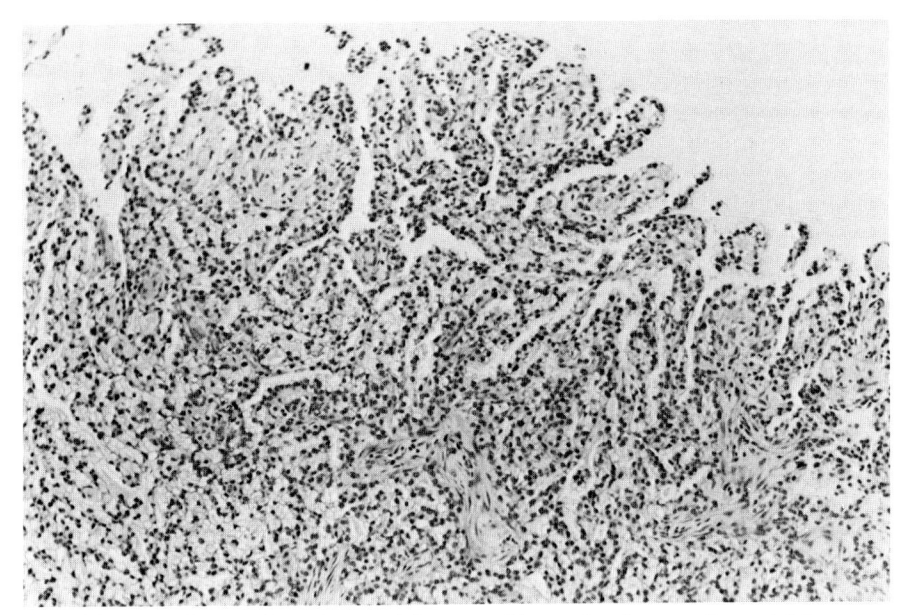

Figure 5. Clear cell carcinoma of the ovary. These clear tumor cells, containing glycogen, form sheets, tuboalveolar, and papillary structures. It is Müllerian in origin rather than mesonephric as originally described. This epithelial tumor arises in identical histologic appearance from the ovarian germinal epithelium, as well as in the uterus and vagina. H&E. Original magnification ×30.

serous tumors having a poor prognosis, mucinous tumors a relatively good prognosis, and endometrioid tumors a prognosis intermediate between the others. Gallager[72] points out that many factors conspire to make such a relationship difficult to substantiate. Ovarian tumors commonly have mixed patterns, but with large tumors only small areas are normally sampled histologically. Many tumors are undifferentiated and difficult to classify accurately, and subvariants of great prognostic significance may be found in small foci within otherwise classifiable large tumors. He concludes that great effort is needed to standardize concepts, criteria for interpretation, and terminology before any firm conclusions can be drawn on the effects of the cell type of prognosis. What we do know, however, is that more serous tumors are seen than mucinous, at all stages, and that the majority of mucinous tumors will be in the earlier stages of the disease and will have lower histologic grades. It appears, however, that epithelial tumors of all histologic types are equally lethal when compared by stage and grade.[71] This emphasizes the critical importance of staging. Cell type among the epithelial tumors has one other important relationship—the propensity for the coexistance of endometrioid tumors of the ovary and carcinoma of the endometrium. Ovarian endometrioid carcinomas have been found in association with an endometrial carcinoma in 5 to 29 percent of cases, and with endometrial hyperplasia in 12 to 20 percent (Fig. 7).[28]

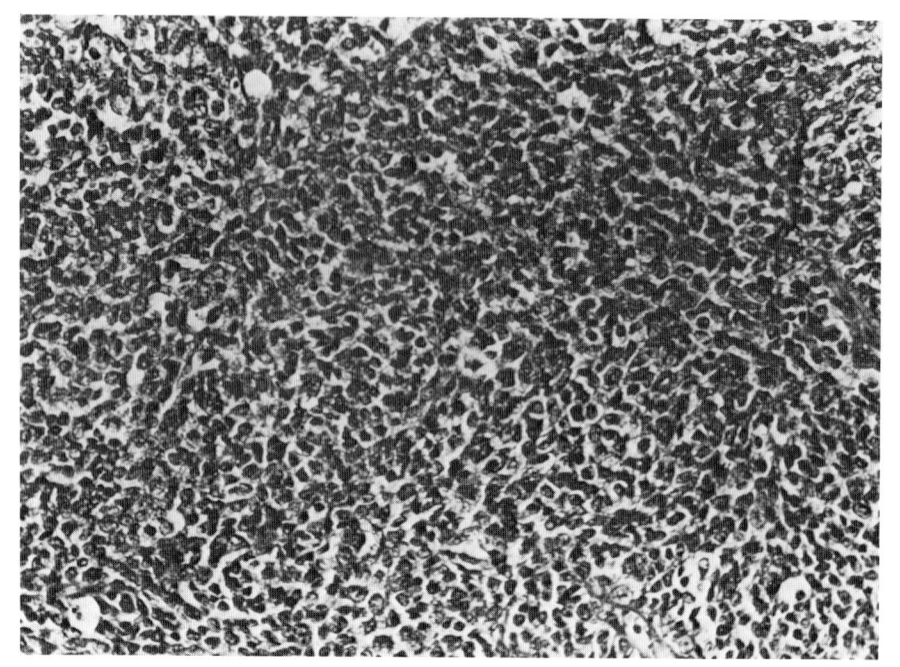

Figure 6. Small cell carcinoma of the ovary, associated with hypercalcemia. This is a highly lethal tumor, most often found in younger women and associated with hypercalcemia, which subsides with removal of the tumor and reappears with recurrence. Studies, including electron microscopy and histochemistry, strongly suggest an epithelial origin. The histology of this diffuse small cell anaplastic tumor may be confused with lymphoma. A reticulin stain is helpful in the differential diagnosis. H&E. Original magnification ×80.

Although the majority of primary ovarian malignancies are epithelial, a small proportion are of gonadal stromal origin or are germ cell tumors. The proportion of nonepithelial tumors is much higher in children and adolescents than in older women. These tumors present special problems and will be further considered in Chapter 8.

TABLE 9. CLASSIFICATION AND APPROXIMATE DISTRIBUTION OF HISTOLOGIC TYPES OF PRIMARY OVARIAN MALIGNANCIES

Tumor Type	Proportion of Cases
Common epithelial	85%
Sex cord (gonadal stromal)	5%
Germ cell	6%
Soft tissue, not specific to ovary	3%

(Data from McGowan L: Gynecologic Oncology. New York, Appleton-Century-Crofts, 1978, with permission.) [56]

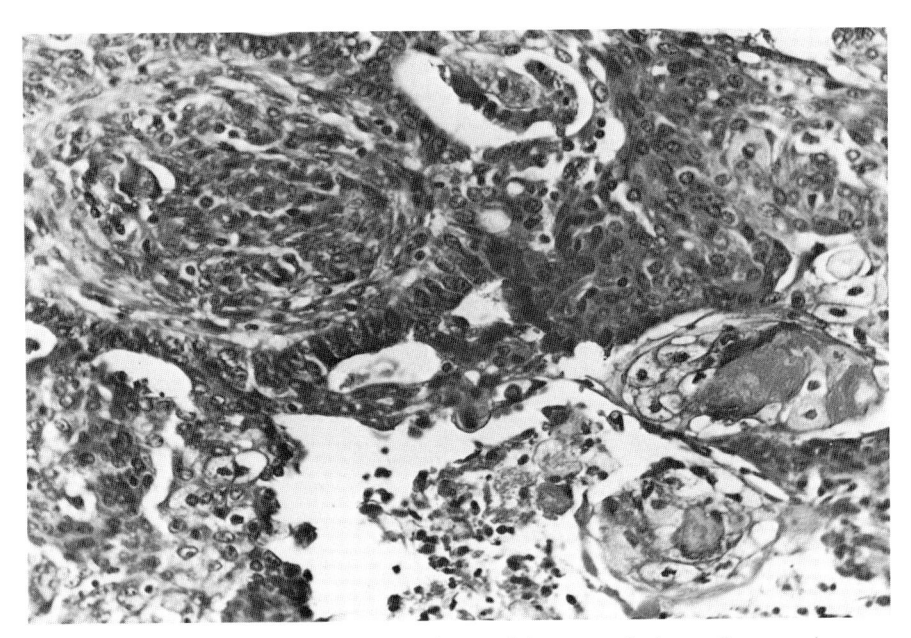

Figure 7A. Endometrioid adenoacanthoma of the ovary. As is so often seen in well-differentiated endometrial adenocarcinoma, there occur areas of benign squamous metaplasia, either as "morules" in the upper right corner, or actual squamous keratin pearls as present in the lower right. H&E. Original magnification ×80.

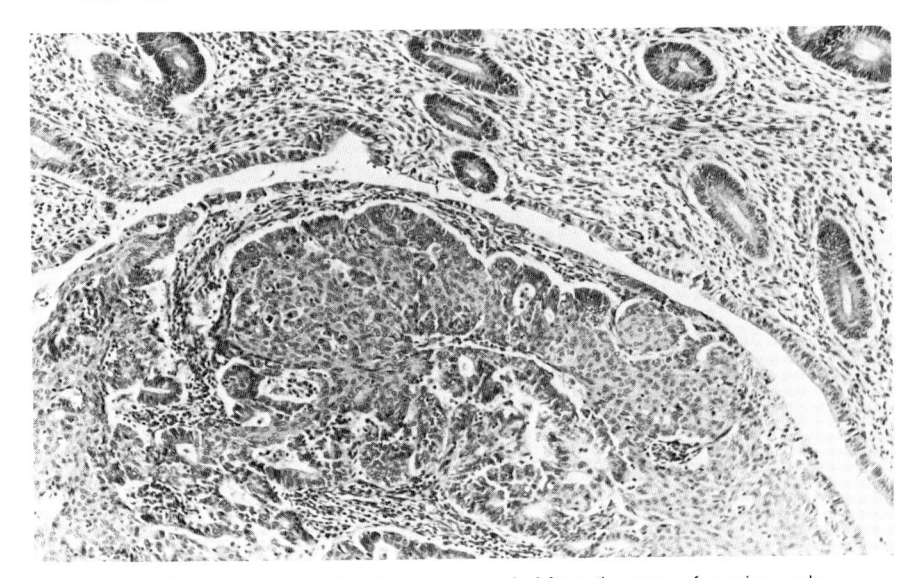

Figure 7B. This is the endometrium as sampled from the case of ovarian endometrioid adenoacanthoma (Fig. 7A). In a very significant number of these cases (about 30 percent) one finds a concomitant endometrial adenoacanthoma, also well-differentiated, usually small and without myometrial invasion. H&E. Original magnification ×30.

The role of the pathologist in diagnosing the cell type of ovarian tumors also involves recognizing secondary tumors and indicating their most likely origin. The frequency with which metastatic tumors are found in the ovary is variable. Johansson[73] suggested that between 30 and 50 percent of malignant ovarian tumors were metastatic, and others have agreed with this.[74] Bennington and coworkers[61] found that 25 percent of malignant tumors in their series were metastatic. Figures tend to be inflated when patients with advanced lesions of the breast, which are known to metastasize to the ovaries, have oophorectomies as part of their treatment and the metastases are found incidentally. Fox and Langley[28] believe that about 30 percent of women dying with carcinoma will have ovarian metastases, but in a large proportion these will only be detectable microscopically. The most common sites of primary tumors producing ovarian metastases are the breast, colon, stomach, and endometrium. Thus, it is essential that both surgeons and pathologists consider the possibility that any ovarian tumor may be metastatic (Fig. 8).

The Pathologist's Role in Staging. Accurate staging of ovarian carcinoma may often depend heavily on the pathologist. The advantages of the ready availability of reliable frozen section reports for identifying tumor type and confirming malignancy is obvious, but the value of such a service for staging may be considerable. This is especially so when conservative therapy is considered

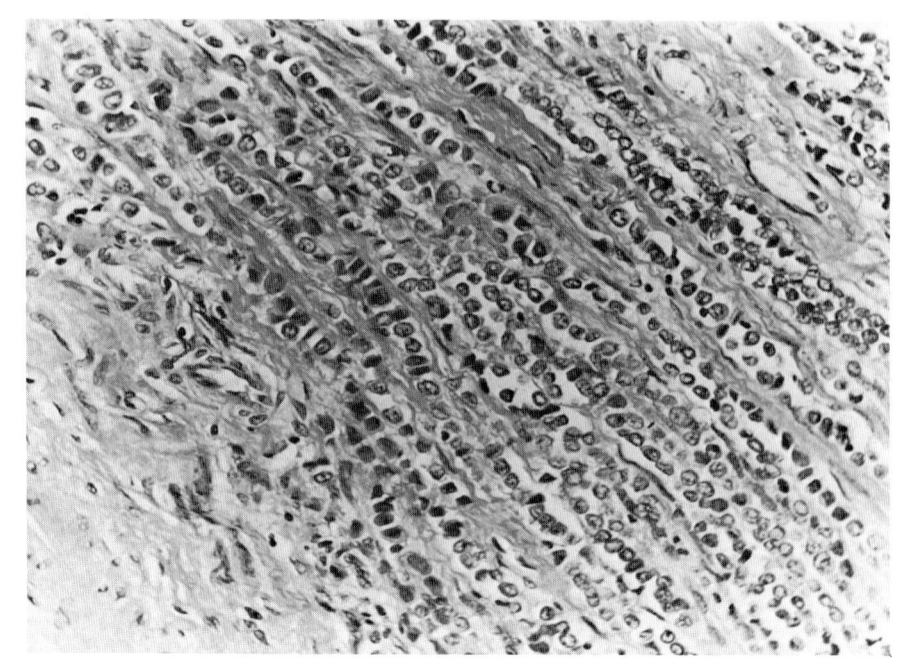

Figure 8. Metastatic adenocarcinoma to the ovary from a primary breast tumor. The very characteristic "Indian file" arrangement of tumor cells in a fibrous stroma is practically diagnostic of this tumor. H&E. Original magnification ×80.

for tumors assumed to be Stage I A. Without frozen sections one must be prepared to accept a high chance of reoperation on patients treated conservatively when biopsy results become available.

The microscopic examination of multiple sections of the omentum, nodes, and tissues sampled because of suspicious characteristics, or as random biopsies, is a critical part of accurate staging. Rubin[75] emphasizes the fact that ovarian cancer frequently has an occult spread that far exceeds that apparent to the naked eye. He refers to a "conversion rate," which is the difference between the clinical stage and the stage present when all tissues are analyzed pathologically (Fig. 9).

Histologic Grading. Several systems of histologic grading of tumors have been described that attempt to indicate relative degrees of malignancy and prognosis. Broders[76] developed a system of classifying carcinoma according to the percentage of undifferentiated cells present. Grade 1 is the most differentiated and grade 4 the least. Ewing[77] developed a system using only three grades, with Broders' grades 3 and 4 combined. The basis of the classification is the degree of uniformity of cells, nuclear regularity, the nuclear-cytoplasmic ratio, the number and size of the nucleoli, and mitotic activity. The

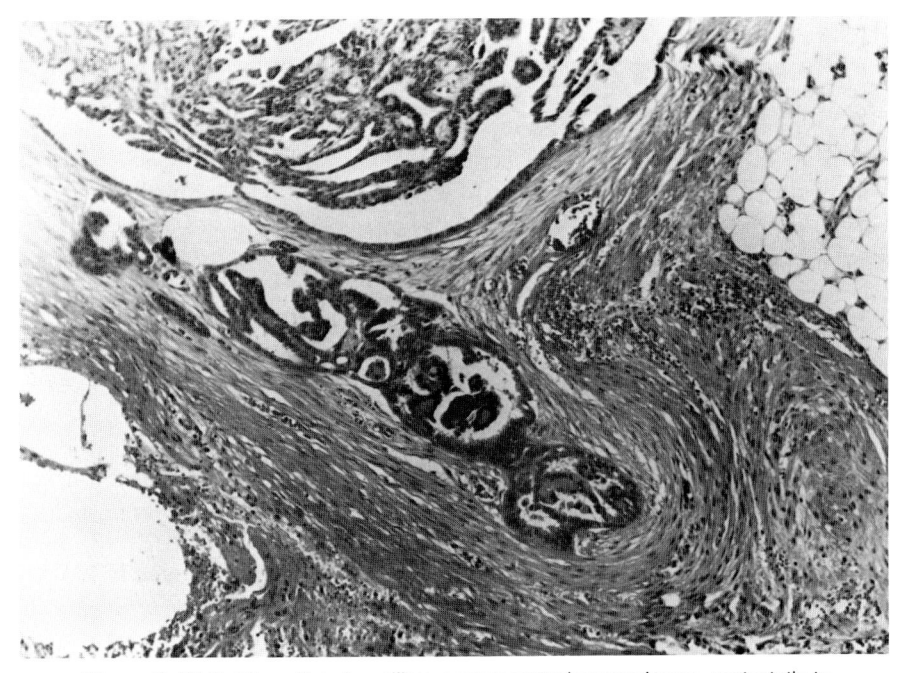

Figure 9. Well-differentiated papillary serous cystadenocarcinoma, metastatic to the omentum. The numerous psammoma bodies, as seen in the center, are responsible for the gritty or calcified nature of these omental nodules. H&E. Original magnification ×30.

Ewing system of classification is the most widely used today, but it is essential that clinicians know which system is in use by their pathologist.

Decker and colleagues[71] have shown that within any given stage of ovarian cancer the prognosis is directly related to the grade of tumor, regardless of the cell type. There is a broad correlation between stage and grade, and because fewer mucinous tumors are found in advanced stages there is a higher proportion of mucinous tumors in lower grades, and hence, the apparent better prognosis of mucinous tumors. Dyson and associates[78] found that most of their patients with mucinous tumors had grade 1 lesions, while the serous tumors were most frequently grades 2 and 3. They reported that in a group of 319 patients those with grade 1 lesions had a 79 percent 5-year survival with treatment, those with grade 2 lesions 39 percent, and those with grade 3 lesions 12 percent. Similar figures are provided by Day and coworkers.[79] This concept is very important because patients with late-stage lesions of low grade do well with appropriate treatment, and those with early-stage high grade lesions do very poorly unless very aggressively treated.

Host Response to the Tumor. An area where the pathologist may be able to provide help of prognostic value is in assessing the host resistance to the tumor. Barber and colleagues[80] investigated the host response as judged by the lymphocytic and plasma cell infiltration around ovarian tumors. In Stage I tumors there was minimal cellular response, but as the stage and volume of disease increased it became greater. This led Barber to conclude that there may be a critical volume required to stimulate tissue response. The significance of these findings is uncertain. Nalick and associates[81] showed a definite reduction in immunocompetence among patients with ovarian cancer, which bore a direct relationship to both the presence and extent of the disease. However, at the present time estimates of host response to ovarian cancers do not aid in management.

"Borderline" Tumors, or Tumors of Low Malignant Potential. As mentioned earlier, we favor the latter designation because these tumors are undoubtedly malignant, but have a course that is very prolonged compared with other ovarian cancers. These tumors histologically show a picture that is intermediate between benign and frankly malignant. They may on occasion be of considerable size, with diffuse intraabdominal spread and have associated ascites. The stage and prognosis in a series of 64 cases of serous tumors of low malignant potential reported by Julian and Woodruff are shown in Table 10.[82]

Although this subgroup was first described in serous tumors it is now recognized to occur in association with all of the epithelial cell types. Hart and Norris[83] reported a corrected 10-year survival of 96 percent for mucinous tumors of low malignant potential. The relative proportions of tumors of each cell type that were of low malignant potential among 990 epithelial tumors of the ovary reported by Aure and coworkers is shown in Table 11.[84] These tumors are more common in younger women.

TABLE 10. STAGE AND PROGNOSIS FOR SEROUS OVARIAN CARCINOMAS OF LOW MALIGNANT POTENTIAL

Stage	Percentage	Relative 5-Year Survival
I A	39	100%
I B	14	100%
II A	11	100%
II B	11	86%
III	17	82%
IV	8	80%

(Data from Julian CG, Woodruff JD: Obstet Gynecol 40:860, 1972, with permission.)[82]

With sufficient follow-up, between 15 and 25 percent of patients with these tumors die from them.[84] We agree with Creasman and coworkers[85] that conservative therapy for tumors of low malignant potential should be reserved for true Stage I A lesions, as detailed later. There is no cause for complacency when this type of tumor is found.

Several factors are relevant, however. First, even though of advanced stage, these lesions are often relatively easy to resect, and the prognosis is good. Many a surgeon has pronounced a tumor unresectable, and told the patient and her relatives that death is near at hand, only to be faced with the very slow and unpleasant progression of disease over a period of many years during which time the nature of the lesion becomes painfully obvious. This is yet another reason for exerting maximal surgical effort on all patients. A second important consideration is that some studies fail to separate these tumors from the more malignant tumors, thus producing better survival figures than are justified. If such studies are advocating conservative treatments, the results can be very misleading. We emphasize that an adequate number of sections of all portions of the tumor and from other specimens must be examined to be sure of the diagnosis.

TABLE 11. PROPORTIONS OF TUMORS CONSIDERED TO BE HISTOLOGICALLY OF "LOW MALIGNANT POTENTIAL" AMONG 990 EPITHELIAL MALIGNANCIES OF THE OVARY

Tumor Type	Low Malignant Potential	Frank Carcinoma
Serous	7.5%	28.6%
Mucinous	8.1%	12.4%
Endometrioid	0.7%	20.8%
Mesonephroid	—	6.2%
Undifferentiated	—	15.7%

(Data from Kolstad P, et al: Obstet Gynecol 37:1, 1971, with permission.)[84]

SURGICAL CONSIDERATIONS: DEFINITIVE SURGERY

The staging, the restaging, and the major mode of treatment of ovarian malignancy is surgical. It is therefore essential that all doctors performing surgery on women with ovarian cancer understand the process of staging, the mode and sites of spread of the disease, and the ways it is treated. The FIGO staging of ovarian carcinoma is shown in Table 12.

A surgeon expecting to find ovarian cancer at surgery is wise to prepare for the most extensive procedure likely. Because of the nature of ovarian cancer, bowel resection or colostomy may be required. The prudent surgeon will therefore prepare the bowel of such patients prior to surgery. In the patient who is nutritionally deficient, total parenteral nutrition for several days preoperatively must be considered.[86] An important practical point is to schedule an adequate amount of time to allow surgery to proceed without concern about other cases, office work, and other routines, because the operation may be tedious and slow. It is obviously an advantage if an experienced gynecologic oncologist, capable of performing all aspects of such surgery, is present or immediately available. We would caution that ignorance about the peculiar features of ovarian cancer can lead to inadequate treatment, and so consultants must be chosen for both their knowledge of this particular disease and their surgical skill.

TABLE 12. CLINICAL STAGING OF CARCINOMA OF THE OVARY—BASED ON FINDINGS AT SURGERY

Stage I	Growth limited to the ovaries
Stage I A	Growth limited to one ovary, no ascites No tumor on the external surface; capsule intact Tumor present on the external surface and/or capsule ruptured
Stage I B	Growth limited to both ovaries; no ascites No tumor on the external surface; capsule intact Tumor present on the external surface and/or capsule(s) ruptured
Stage I C	Tumor either Stage I A or I B but with ascites[a] or positive peritoneal washings
Stage II	Growth involving one or both ovaries with pelvic extension
Stage II A	Extension and/or metastases to the uterus and/or tubes
Stage II B	Extension to other pelvic tissues
Stage II C	Tumor either Stage II A or II B, but with ascites[a] or positive peritoneal washings
Stage III	Growth involving one or both ovaries with intraperitoneal metastases outside the pelvis and/or positive retroperitoneal nodes; or tumor limited to the true pelvis with histologically proved malignant extension to small bowel or omentum
Stage IV	Growth involving one or both ovaries with distant metastases. If pleural effusion is present there must be positive cytology to allot a case to Stage IV. Parenchymal liver metastases equal Stage IV

[a]Special category. Unexplored cases thought to be ovarian carcinoma.

The Three Aims of Surgery in Ovarian Cancer

First, to stage the disease accurately, allowing better choices of adjuvant therapy and a better assessment of prognosis.

Second, to reduce tumor bulk to nodules of less than 1 cm or remove it completely, as well as to perform total hysterectomy, bilateral adnexectomy, and omentectomy. In a few carefully staged and selected patients, conservative therapy may be justifiable, under conditions outlined in a later section.

Third, to relieve or prevent bowel obstruction caused by the tumor.

The Routine of Surgery for Ovarian Tumors

This routine should be followed whenever an ovarian tumor is known or suspected to be present. Only by making this a rule will unpleasant surprises and mistakes be avoided.

1. Surgery should start with a vertical incision. We advocate the use of this incision in all cases where gynecologic malignancy is suspected, and it is especially important to allow adequate exploration of patients with ovarian cancer.
2. Immediately after the peritoneal cavity is opened, and before exploration of the abdominal cavity can shed mesothelial cells to confuse the cytologist, any ascitic fluid is withdrawn and sent for cytology. If no free fluid is present, 300 ml of saline are instilled into the peritoneal cavity. Approximately 100 ml is instilled via a soft rubber catheter between the liver and diaphragm, aspirated, and sent for cytology. We believe that the larger fraction is better able to circulate in the abdominal cavity, and it is easier to withdraw a substantial proportion of it. We aid the circulation of the fluid by placing the patient in a steep Trendelenburg position and then in the reverse Trendelenburg position for aspirating the fluid. If blood is present in the ascites or washings, 1000 units of heparin are added to the specimen for cytologic examination. One can expect peritoneal washings to be positive in approximately 30 percent of patients with disease apparently localized to the ovaries.[87] The finding of positive washings has been shown to indicate a significantly worsened prognosis, and is an indication for adjunctive therapy in early stage lesions.[5,88]
3. Visual and manual exploration of the upper abdomen is the next procedure. This should never be neglected, even in the presence of extensive lower abdominal disease. This part of the examination is essential to accurate staging. It may reveal an upper abdominal source of what had been thought to be primary ovarian disease and allows the accurate documentation of the sites of all metastases. This portion of the examination is commonly inadequate and this fact is documented in the study of Piver and colleagues[67] of 100 consecutive patients referred after surgical diagnosis of ovarian cancer. In 83 percent the incision was considered inadequate to allow upper abdominal explora-

tion, and in 92 percent of patients para-aortic nodes had not been mentioned in the operative reports. In 84 percent the diaphragm was not mentioned, in 76 percent the stomach and pancreas, in 70 percent the colon, and in 59 percent the liver was not mentioned (Fig. 10).

The surface of the liver and the right hemidiaphragm are important places to examine. This is because the removal of particulate matter from the peritoneal cavity is through lymphatics which drain to the inferior surface of the diaphragm before entering mediastinal nodes and the right thoracic trunk.[89] When one remembers that 30 percent of patients with Stage I ovarian cancers have positive peritoneal cytology and that staging at initial surgery is often inadequate, it is hardly surprising to find that when patients referred for therapy of surgical Stage I lesions of the ovary were restaged by repeated surgery within 1 month, 10 percent were found to have diaphragmatic metastases.[87] Visualization of this area depends on a large incision and good light. A sigmoidoscope or fiberoptic light source is useful, but we have not found the laparoscope of great value with the abdomen open.

During the abdominal exploration one must keep in mind the importance of examining the paracolic gutters, stomach, and small and large bowels as well as the mesentery and omentum and all other abdominal organs. The histologic resemblance of some pancreatic cancers to those of the ovary must be kept in mind as well as the fact that alimentary tract cancers frequently metastasize to the ovary.[90,91] Any suspicious lesions should be biopsied, and if possible frozen sections performed. When all peritoneal surfaces and retroperitoneal and intraabdominal organs have been examined, attention is directed to

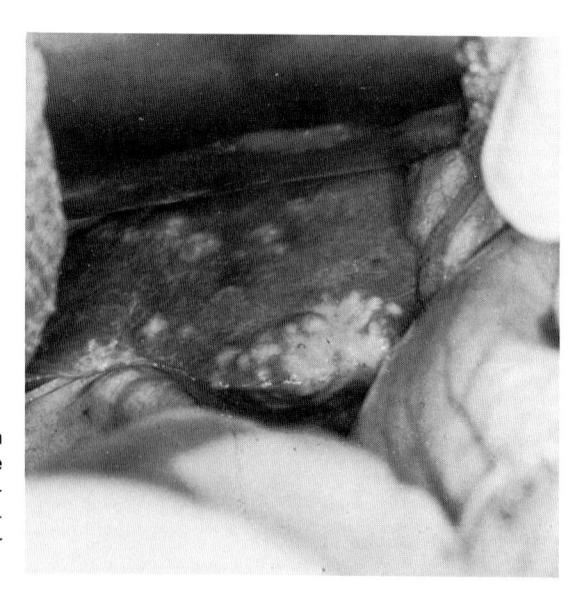

Figure 10. Liver metastases from ovarian carcinoma. These are within the liver parenchyma, indicating a Stage IV tumor. Metastases on the surface of the liver indicate Stage III disease.

the para-aortic nodes. Tumor has been found in these nodes in approximately 10 percent of patients whose disease had otherwise been thought to be confined to the ovaries.[87] This justifies para-aortic dissection especially in women for whom conservative therapy is contemplated. The omentum, "policeman of the peritoneal cavity," has been shown to be the site of microscopic metastases in 3 percent of women with disease otherwise thought to be Stage I.[87] It seems likely that omentectomy performed routinely in all cases of ovarian carcinoma will reveal a higher proportion of microscopic metastases. Infracolic omentectomy is a simple procedure, and performed carefully has minimal morbidity. We believe it should be performed for prognostic reasons, to assure accurate staging if conservative therapy is contemplated, and because it may improve the prognosis[92] though at present no large controlled study has been done.

4. Attention is then turned to the lower abdomen and pelvis. The peritoneum over the bladder and that of the pouch of Douglas and pelvic sidewalls is carefully inspected. The aims of surgery in ovarian cancer are to remove all tumor if possible, together with the uterus, tubes, and ovaries, or if this is not possible, to "debulk" the tumor to make it more amenable to adjunctive therapy. Should there be any doubt about the malignant status of the ovary at this stage, frozen section is invaluable. As DiSaia and Creasman[85] point out, bilateral, partially or wholly solid tumors with extracystic or intracystic papillations, areas of necrosis, and adhesions to bowel and adjacent organs, especially in the presence of ascites, are likely to be malignant (Figs. 11–13). We believe that in the woman who is perimenopausal or postmenopausal and who is explored for possible ovarian carcinoma, the minimal procedure acceptable is the full staging "work-up," omentectomy and total hysterectomy with bilateral salpingo-oophorectomy because the stakes are too high if an error is made.

When More Extensive Disease is Present, How Radical Should One Be?

Griffiths[93] stated that if the largest residual tumor mass was greater than 1.5 cm in diameter, the prognosis was uniformly poor, and that surgery improved survival relative to the reduction of tumor size beyond this point, to a maximal effect when all gross tumor was excised. The same principles have been demonstrated in other studies also.[94,95]

Nelson,[10] although accepting that adequate studies have not and now probably cannot be done, believes that maximal surgery is imperative. He does, however, point out that "a lesion pronounced unresectable by one gynecologist can be resected by another" (Fig. 14).[10] It is our belief that, both to allow the maximal chance for adjuvant surgery to work and to help avoid the unpleasant sequelae of intestinal obstruction, all efforts to resect tumor should be made including bowel resection and colostomy if required. As Piver and colleagues[96] have shown, over the last decade, survival times after surgery

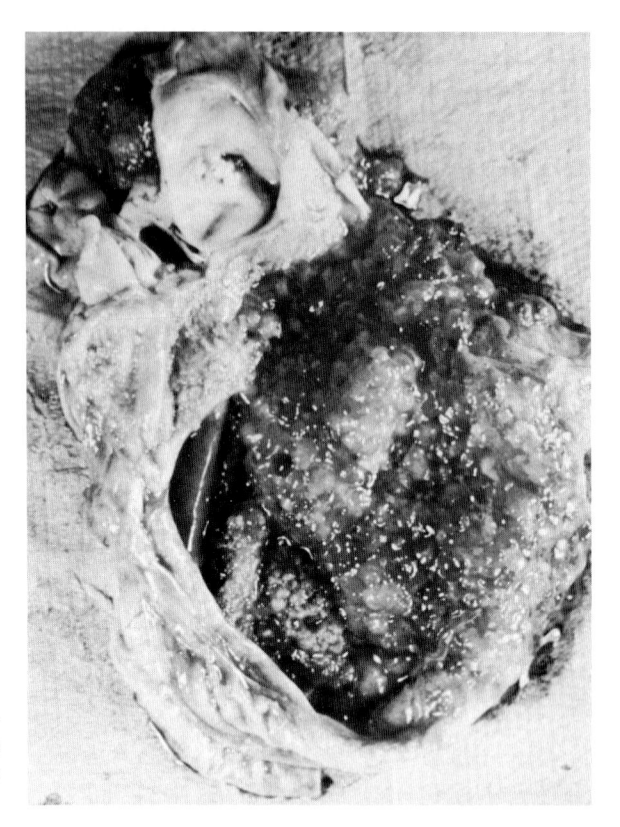

Figure 11A. Typical intracystic papillations of a serous cystadenocarcinoma of the ovary.

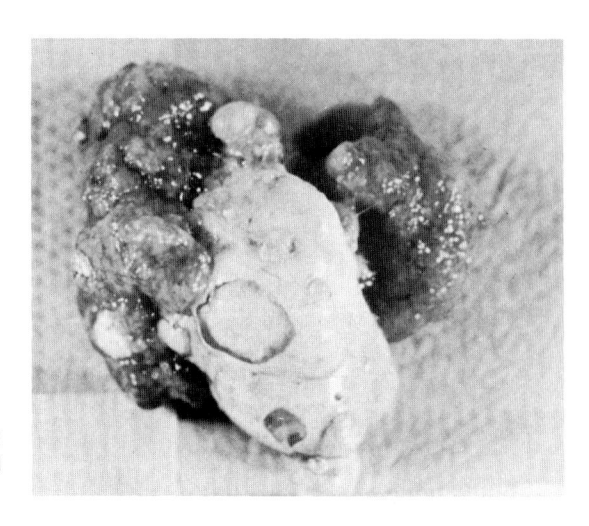

Figure 11B. The contralateral ovary, though smaller in size, had tumor on the ovarian surface.

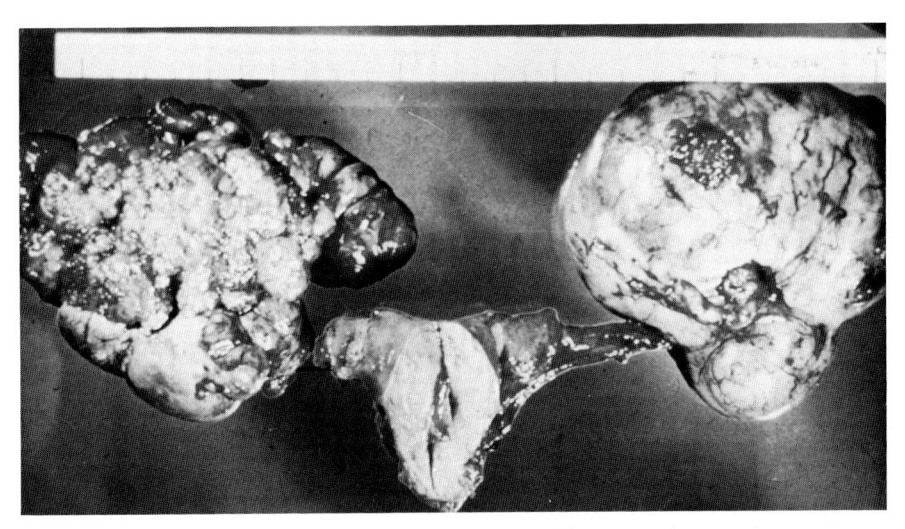

Figure 12. Bilateral serous cystadenocarcinomas with extracystic excrescences. This is a typical finding.

for bowel obstruction caused by ovarian cancer have been relatively short, but the more effective combination chemotherapy now available can be expected to improve these figures. It should also be remembered that bowel obstruction developing in women treated for ovarian cancer may not result from active tumor. Ketcham and associates[97] reported on three patients who died of untreated bowel obstruction on the assumption that it resulted from previously treated cancer who, at postmortem were tumor free. Tunca and coworkers[98] found 12 patients with previously treated ovarian cancer who at surgery for bowel obstruction were tumor free. Remembering that few people

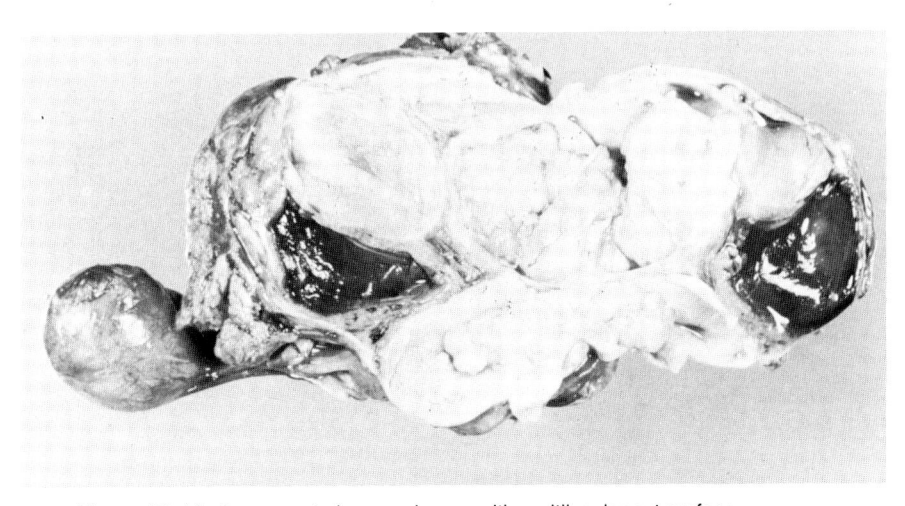

Figure 13. Mucinous cystadenocarcinoma with multilocular cut surface.

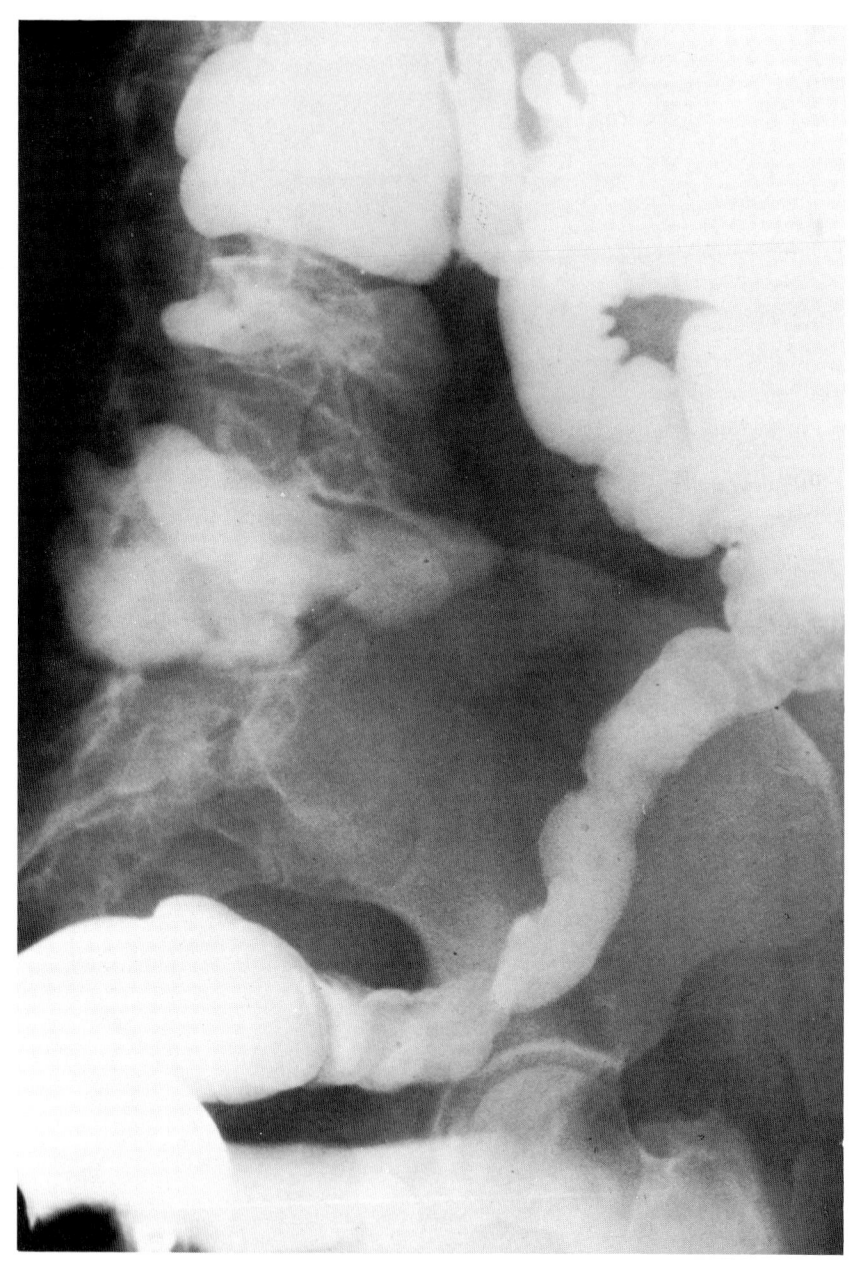

Figure 14A. A barium enema in a patient with ovarian carcinoma shows external compression of the sigmoid colon.

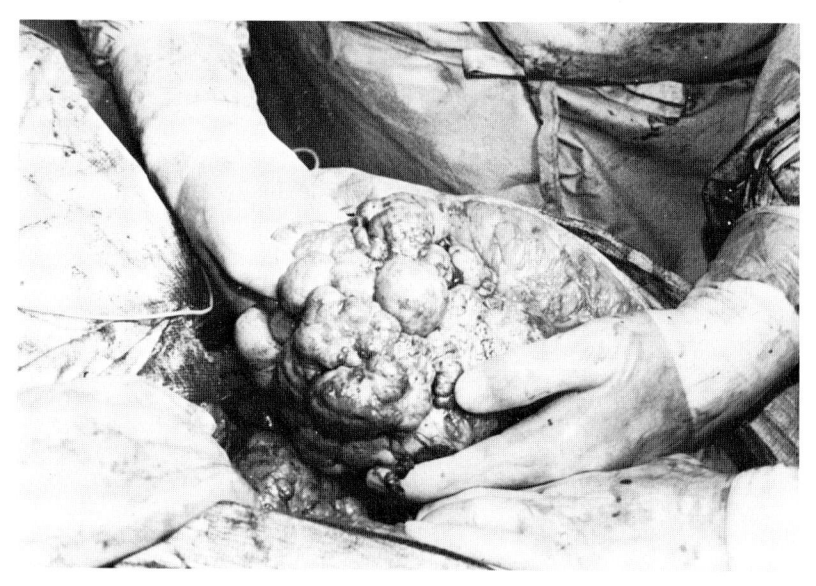

Figure 14B. A solid adenocarcinoma of the left ovary weighing 24 lb was removed, but no bowel resection was required. The patient had 18 liters of ascitic fluid.

die peacefully and in dignity with bowel obstruction, we would not hesitate to divert the bowel even in advanced cases, where obstruction is imminent or probable. As gynecologic oncologists who manage all aspects of our patients' care, we can state confidently that maximal surgical effort, in sensible and experienced hands, is justifiable for the comfort of the patient, even if survival times are not uniformly improved. Other authors have commented on the safety and efficacy of resection of portions of the lower urinary tract involved with tumor, if this is needed to achieve more nearly complete tumor bulk reduction.[99]

The subject of conservative therapy in special circumstances will be discussed later. Here we must state that it is always a calculated risk and one that is totally unacceptable in the postmenopausal woman. Before advising conservative treatment in the young patient, one must consider the fact that recurrence or persistence of tumor is a high price to pay for fertility.

The Unexpected Finding of Ovarian Cancer During Surgery

As has been stated earlier, one would hope that this possibility is always in the mind of every gynecologist, so that such surprises are less likely. But even the most careful of us will occasionally face this situation. If one has chosen a Pfannenstiel incision, exposure is the first problem. This is achieved, albeit not so well as one would like, by extending the skin incision, and dividing the rectus muscles, taking care to secure the inferior epigastric vessels. The management is then as described earlier. If possible, skilled help should be ob-

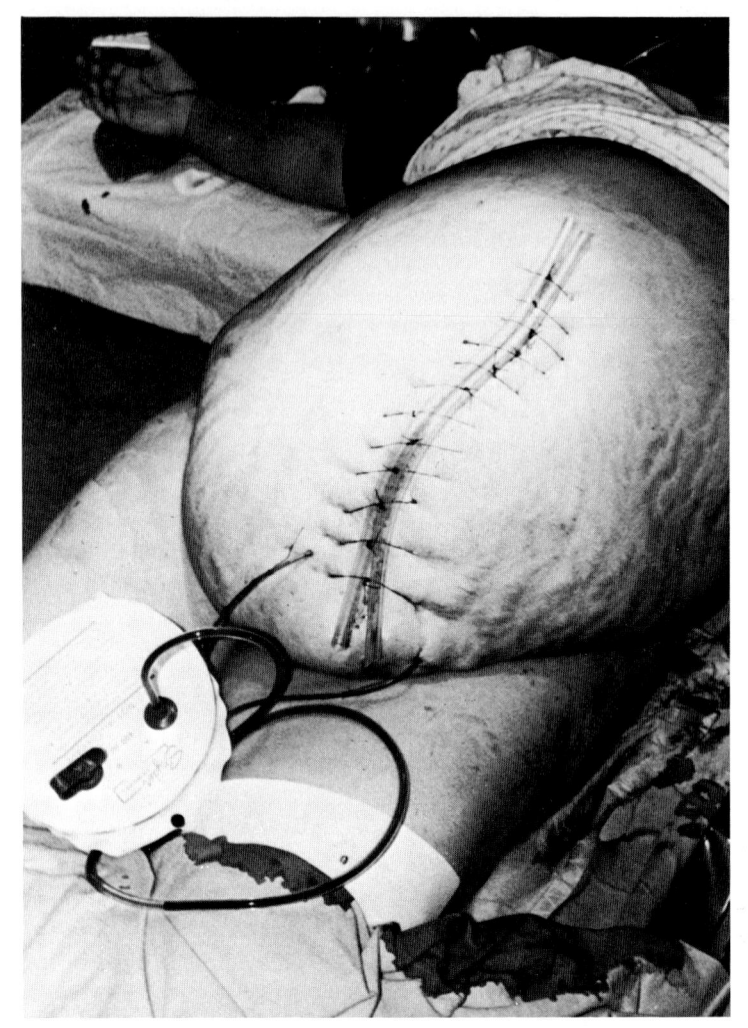

Figure 14C. The abdomen closed after the procedure with bilateral pelvic drains, and retention sutures tied over plastic tubing along each side of the incision.

tained. If you believe that the disease is resectable, but not by you, there may be a case for biopsies, closing, and referral if appropriate aid is not available. However, the first surgical attack is the best opportunity for cure.

The Pathologist Finds Ovarian Malignancy in Specimens Thought to Be Benign

When the pathology report indicating a malignant tumor is received some days after surgery, it is evident that further treatment is required. Free use of frozen sections and careful abdominal exploration in all patients will minimize the chance of such an event. We have discussed the management of this situation in detail elsewhere.[100] Consultation with a gynecologic oncologist should be sought. Reexploration for staging and definitive therapy will usually be required.

ADJUNCTIVE THERAPY

The difficulty of surgically removing all tumor in patients with advanced ovarian cancer, and the poor results even when this was done with early stage lesions, led to the use of a wide range of adjunctive therapies. Historically, radiotherapy, either as intraperitoneal instillation of radiocolloid or as external beam therapy, has been favored. More recently, various forms of chemotherapy and immunotherapy have been utilized. In evaluating the place of any particular therapy, several themes recur. Inadequate staging, poorly defined control groups, variable selection criteria, and the frequent use of a variety of therapeutic agents in many sequences and combinations are the norm for reported studies. The following discussion presents an overview of each adjunctive modality. The current bias is toward the use of combination chemotherapy, which is believed on theoretic and experimental grounds to be the most effective adjunct to adequate surgery.

Intraperitoneal Radiocolloids

These have a great theoretic application for a disease that tends to occur and recur on the peritoneal surfaces of the entire abdominal cavity. Radiocolloid doses to tumor and omental surfaces will be high, while dosage to the liver and kidneys will be low. The dose distribution when 150 millicuries of radioactive gold are instilled into the peritoneal cavity is 4000 rads to the serosa, 6000 rads to the omentum, and 7000 rads to the retroperitoneal and mesenteric lymph nodes, while the liver parenchyma receives only 130 rads and the kidneys 30 rads.[7] Such a distribution would appear to be ideal. ^{198}Au emits 90 percent beta rays and 10 percent gamma rays, and has a relatively short half-life. ^{32}P emits purely beta particles and has a longer half-life. The absence of gamma radiation reduces complications for patients and the prolonged half-life may produce an improved time/dose relationship.[101] The radiocolloids are introduced through catheters placed either at surgery or by paracentesis and 150 millicuries of ^{198}Au or 15 millicuries of ^{32}P are instilled in 1 liter of saline. Side effects include nausea and vomiting in about one-third of patients, fever in 10 to 30 percent, and diarrhea in 5 percent, with small bowel damage and obstruction, occasionally leading to death, occurring in up to 10 percent of patients receiving radioactive gold, especially in association with external beam therapy.[101] These effects are said to be less common with ^{32}P than with ^{198}Au. The consensus appears to be that radioisotope instillation produces improved survival rates in Stages I and II epithelial ovarian cancer.[102-105] Problems of obtaining an even distribution after surgery and the incidence of adhesions and bowel complications tend to weigh against the use of these agents, but in institutions where the procedure is commonly used, the results appear to be good with ^{32}P.

Radiotherapy

External beam radiotherapy has been used for many years to aid in the management of ovarian cancer. Some series have reported the use of radiotherapy to reduce the size of unresectable tumors, allowing resection.[106] Kjorstad and colleagues[107] found that 38 percent of 96 patients with lesions considered resectable at initial surgery could have complete resection after 3000 rads of external therapy over 4 weeks, and 92 percent of 49 patients felt to be unresectable on clinical examination were resected after the radiotherapy. However, the operative mortality was 9 percent and 5-year survival 16 percent, so that one doubts whether anything was gained.

The most common use of radiotherapy has been postoperatively. There are serious problems with radiation as adjunctive therapy. Ovarian cancer tends to have a generalized spread throughout the abdominal cavity, and the incidence of occult extrapelvic metastases is considerable even in apparent Stage I disease. The delivery of cancerocidal doses of radiation to the liver and kidney may lead to irreversible and potentially fatal radiation hepatitis and nephritis. These regions are therefore partially shielded, making "sanctuary areas" of some of the more common metastatic sites.[7] In addition to the severe gastrointestinal side effects associated with total abdominal radiation there are long-term problems such as radiation-induced stenosis, bowel obstruction, and bowel perforation. These problems may be life threatening in themselves and are often extremely difficult to manage.

Some studies have suggested that patients with Stage I ovarian cancer fare worse when given postoperative radiation than when treated by surgery alone. For instance, Munnell[108] reported 5-year survival rates of 78 percent for patients with Stage I A tumors treated by surgery alone, and 53 percent if postoperative radiotherapy was used. In patients with Stage I disease, Clark and associates[109] found 61 and 54 percent 5-year survivals after surgery alone and surgery with radiotherapy, respectively. It seems likely that these results reflect selection bias rather than any cause and effect relationship between radiation and poor prognosis.

It is in Stage II ovarian cancers that radiation has reportedly been of greatest value, with most series showing distinct improvements in survival following adjuvant radiotherapy.[5] In Stage III lesions the results were felt to be equivocal. But many gynecologic oncologists have been skeptical about the benefits of radiation, and considered that, whether given as a whole abdominal bath, or by a moving strip technique, the short-term and long-term side effects outweighed the benefits. Nevertheless, it is the opinion of some authors that "many have prejudged the ultimate value of radiotherapy in the management of ovarian neoplasms, resulting in the development of a polarization in the oncologic community. . . ."[101]

There has been renewed interest in radiation therapy following the publication of work from the Princess Margaret Hospital.[110] This study was a randomized trial comparing pelvic radiation alone, pelvic radiation with chlorambucil, and pelvic and abdominal radiation as adjuncts to surgical treatment for Stages I and II, and selected Stage III patients. With unresectable disease no regimen of treatment was superior. Where optimal tumor reduction was achieved surgically, 5-year survival rates were 81 percent for patients with total abdominal radiation, 55 percent for those receiving pelvic radiation and chlorambucil, and 50 percent for those treated with pelvic radiation alone. In Stage I A lesions adjunctive therapy appeared to be unnecessary. Several comments should be made. First, the technique of radiation used gives a pelvic dose of 4500 rads and a moving strip technique delivers 2250 rads to the abdomen with the liver unshielded. Hence, the "sanctuary area" on the right hemidiaphragm is radiated, in contrast to other techniques. Staging of patients in this study has been questioned and the chemotherapeutic regimen was far from optimal.[111] But as the authors of the paper commented "It is quite clear that no institution has treatment results which are so good that any potentially active therapeutic modality can be disregarded, especially on the very inadequate data which exist in the literature."[110]

Before leaving the subject of radiation for ovarian tumors, we have to mention the one tumor that appears to be uniquely sensitive to radiotherapy, the dysgerminoma. It is unfortunate that the much more common epithelial tumors generally respond poorly to radiotherapy.

Chemotherapy

The poor results of treatment of epithelial ovarian cancers, their propensity for widespread metastasis, and the frequency with which late stage lesions are found have led to an increasing interest in the use of chemotherapy as an adjunct to surgery. In general, chemotherapy is given systemically.

The first group of agents shown to be effective against epithelial carcinomas of the ovary were the alkylating agents and they remain the standard against which all other agents are judged. The most widely used alkylating agent in patients with ovarian cancer is melphalan (Alkeran). The response rates for this drug are between 35 and 65 percent for cases of advanced epithelial cancer, with 20 percent of responders being symptom free for 5 or more years.[112] This response rate is typical of those reported in other series, and with other drugs in the alkylating agent group.[113] Other members of this group of drugs are chlorambucil, thiotepa, cyclophosphamide, and nitrogen mustard and its derivatives. While these drugs produced responses, the rates are much lower among patients relapsing after or resistant to radiotherapy. For example, Beck and Boyes[114] showed 75 percent of patients who had no previous radiation responded to alkylating agents compared with 42 percent where radiation had failed.

But response and cures are very different. Responses are generally based on clinical assessment of tumor regression over a period of 1 to 3 months. The response rate for alkylating agents was encouraging, but the relapse rate was very discouraging. Experience with multiagent chemotherapy in childhood leukemias suggested that this might benefit patients with ovarian cancer. Examples of drugs that are effective as single agents are 5-fluorouracil, which produced a 33 percent response rate; methotrexate, 25 percent; doxorubicin, 25 percent; hexamethylmelamine, 46 percent, and cis-platinum, 24 percent.[115] These drugs had often been used as single agents after the failure of alkylating agents to control the disease, so that there was reason to hope that as first-line drugs the response would be greater. Combination chemotherapy is based on concepts of potentiation whereby a given dose of drug is more effective in the presence of another, the cell cycle specificity of various agents, and the assumption that in combinations smaller doses of toxic agents will be effective.

A prospective randomized trial of a combination of hexamethylmelamine, cyclophosphamide, methotrexate, and 5-fluorouracil (Hexa-CAF) against melphalan alone showed the combination to produce a 76 percent response rate compared with the single agent response of 54 percent: 33 percent exhibited complete response compared with 16 percent with the single agent.[116] The survival time of patients treated with Hexa-CAF was a mean of 29 months compared with 17 months for melphalan. Vogl and colleagues[117] reported initial response rates for the highly toxic combination cyclophosphamide + hexamethylmelamine + adriamycin + cis-platinum (CHAD) of 90 percent. Other studies showed the combination of cyclophosphamide, adriamycin, and cis-platinum (CAP) to produce an initial response rate of 72 percent.[118] It is the latter regimen that we have chosen as our initial chemotherapeutic approach in all cases of ovarian carcinoma where chemotherapy is deemed necessary.

At the University of South Florida we administer CAP chemotherapy on an inpatient basis because we believe this allows better prehydration, more satisfactory control of acute gastrointestinal side effects, and is, in general, more acceptable to patients and their families. Courses are given at 4-week intervals unless toxicity demands a longer recovery period. The drug doses are cyclophosphamide (Cytoxan), 500 mg/m^2; doxorubicin (Adriamycin), 30 mg/m^2; cisplatin (Platinol), 50 mg/m^2. The administration plan is as follows: On the night before chemotherapy is to begin, the patient is admitted to the hospital and an intravenous infusion of 5 percent dextrose in 0.5 normal saline is begun at a rate of 150 ml/hr. Chlorpromazine (100 mg) and promethazine (25 mg) are given by rectal suppositories. The following morning, chemotherapy is begun by giving the calculated dose of cyclophosphamide as an intravenous bolus, followed by the dose of doxorubicin as a bolus. At the same time an infusion of droperidol is begun at the rate of 1 mg per hour for 6 hours. After the cyclophosphamide and doxorubicin have been given, an intravenous infusion containing the calculated dose of cisplatin mixed with 37.5 g of mannitol in 2 liters of 5 percent dextrose with 0.5 percent saline is run at 300 ml/hour. After this the intravenous infusion is usually stopped and the patient returns home, either later in the day or the following morning.

Prior to each treatment cycle, a complete blood count, platelet count, serum creatinine and creatinine clearance, and serum electrolyte assays are obtained. A complete physical examination and pelvic examination are performed and an audiogram obtained. No patient receives more than 550 mg/m^2 of doxorubicin. All patients with hemoglobin concentrations less than 10 mg percent receive packed red blood cells to achieve a minimum hemoglobin concentration of 10 mg percent.

We have treated 47 patients with Stage III or IV ovarian cancer using this regimen, and our actuarial survival rates are 66 percent at 1 year, 39 percent at 2 years, 30 percent at 3 years, and 25 percent at 4 years. The median survival time is 18 months: for patients with Stage III disease it is 26 months, and for those with Stage IV disease, 11 months. Survival rates are better for well-differentiated tumors and after optimal debulking. At the present time, 19 second-look laparotomies have been performed and 10 were negative.

It is worthy of note that combination chemotherapy should be repeated as often as toxicity allows. If the first regimen is not successful, it is unlikely that much response will be obtained with other combinations.

Combination chemotherapy is not without its hazards. Most chemotherapeutic agents produce acute gastrointestinal disturbances, which in some cases have led patients to refuse therapy. In addition, there is myelosuppression, which can be fatal. Adriamycin is cardiotoxic in excessive dosage, cyclophosphamide and doxorubicin produce alopecia, and cisplatin is both nephrotoxic and ototoxic. The management of patients on chemotherapy should only be performed by those with special knowledge of these regimens and their problems and in centers with adequate facilities for the monitoring and care of the immunosuppressed patient. We cannot emphasize strongly enough the importance of careful and regular examinations, including rectovaginal assessment by an experienced gynecologist before each course of chemotherapy.

We believe that after approximately 12 courses of chemotherapy a second-look procedure should be performed to assess response and to resect residual disease. In patients with residual disease at second-look surgery, second-line chemotherapy must be chosen. This is a difficult choice to make. In those free of disease, we give three more cycles of cyclophosphamide alone, orally, because others have reported,[119] and we have anecdotal experience of, rapid recurrence of disease after sudden cessation of chemotherapy.

It must be remembered that as the results of chemotherapy improve and more long-term survivors appear, new complications of therapeutic agents will become obvious. For instance, the strikingly increased risk of leukemia among women treated with alkylating agents may prove to be but one of a series of problems.[120]

Intraperitoneal use of hemisulfur mustard proved ineffective in controlling tumors or ascites, but the idea of intraperitoneal use of some of the newer chemotherapeutic agents has received consideration more recently, in the hope of achieving higher tumor doses and less systemic toxicity. In 1978 Jones and coworkers[121] reported on the use of high volume intraperitoneal chemotherapy as a "belly bath" for ovarian carcinoma. Methotrexate, 5-fluorouracil, and doxorubicin have been used intraperitoneally, and *cis*-platinum would appear to be a very logical choice. The chemotherapeutic agents are administered in two liters of peritoneal dialysate. This "belly bath" technique may have its greatest use in Stage III patients with minimal residual disease or as adjuvant chemotherapy following surgery for Stage I disease.

Immunotherapy

Attempts have been made to enhance the immune response of patients with ovarian carcinoma as an aid to chemotherapy. Injection of live bacillus Calmette-Guérin (BCG) vaccine, or killed suspensions of *Corynebacterium parvum*, the former by scarification and the latter by the intravenous route, both enhance the body's nonspecific immune response.[57] *C. parvum* has produced a range of favorable responses when used alone in a variety of animal models. BCG has been used as an effective adjunct to chemotherapy in leukemias, lymphomas, and some other tumors. Pattillo[122] used BCG in association with other therapy in a small group of patients with recurrent drug-resistant disease and achieved one remission and apparent stabilization in three other patients. The uncertain stage of the disease prevents drawing firm conclusions.

A study by Creasman and colleagues[85] combining *C. parvum* with alkylating agents in treating Stage III ovarian cancer showed an enhanced response rate for patients receiving chemoimmunotherapy, even though cases in this group initially had less favorable prognostic factors present. In another study, BCG was used in conjunction with a combination of doxorubicin and cyclophosphamide.[123] Again, the results suggested that immunotherapy conferred some benefits, but overall results were very poor for either mode of treatment in this study. Nevertheless, this is considered to be an area worthy of further exploration.

Antiestrogen Therapy

The recognition that estrogen and progesterone receptors are present in at least a substantial proportion of ovarian carcinomas[32,33] raises the possibility of utilizing antiestrogens in their treatment, as has been done with breast cancers. Mangioni and colleagues[124] obtained a 15 percent response rate in a group of 33 patients who had progressive disease despite multiagent chemotherapy, when they were treated with high-dose medroxyprogesterone acetate (Depo-Provera). Schwartz and coworkers[125] were able to stabilize disease for substantial periods of time in a small group of patients who had not responded to a variety of other agents, by use of the antiestrogen Tamoxifen. These results are clearly only preliminary, but this area deserves more attention in the future.

"In Vitro" Tumor Sensitivity Studies

Recent advances in the fields of cell culture and pharmacology suggest that it may be possible to develop an accurate tumor culture and sensitivity technique so that anticancer drugs can be selected on the basis of in vitro cultures. In 1980, Alberts and associates[126] reported on an in vitro clonogenic assay for predicting the response of ovarian cancer to chemotherapy. The ovarian cancer cells were grown in a soft agar system and information on 40 patients was published. The predictive accuracy of the assay for complete and partial remissions was 62 percent and the accuracy of the assay for predicting drug resistance was 99 percent. Thus, the assay appears particularly helpful in deciding which drugs will not benefit the patient. Other possible uses of such an assay include:

1. The study of pharmacologic mechanism of drug resistance in human ovarian carcinoma cells.
2. The selection of second-line drugs following failure of an initial drug regimen.
3. The screening of new drugs that might be appropriate for Phase II trials in patients with ovarian carcinoma.

SECOND-LOOK SURGERY

The concept of electively reexploring patients who had surgical removal of intraabdominal malignancies arose over 20 years ago, when Wangensteen[127] eventually cured a woman with colonic cancer after six laparotomies for symptomatic recurrence. He concluded that after resection of all but localized tumors, it would be preferable electively to reexplore patients apparently cancer-free each 6 months to resect residual tumor and perform biopsies. This program was continued until no evidence of disease was detected at routine exploration. The use of this approach for ovarian tumors was reported by Santoro and colleagues in 1961.[127]

Rationale for Second-Look Surgery

Many other authors reported small numbers of patients with resectable residual disease after radiation or chemotherapy, with variable results.[128] Wallach and coworkers in 1975[129] advocated second-look surgery for patients in whom ovaries were left at initial surgery and where complete clinical regression occurred with adjunctive therapy, or for patients where major regressions of tumor made resection possible. They did not advocate exploration of the clinically cured patient.

Improved chemotherapeutic agents have increased the chance of major regressions and even the cure of relatively advanced disease. However, they produce problems of short-term and long-term toxicity and carcinogenesis, making the earliest feasible cessation of therapy desirable. A greater understanding of the mode of spread of the disease made it clear that clinical examination alone was no guarantee that a patient was tumor free nor was it sufficient to justify cessation of chemotherapy. Thus, the concept of planned second-look surgery in patients treated for ovarian cancer arose. Smith and associates in 1976[130] reported on 103 patients with advanced ovarian carcinoma who underwent second-look surgery. These were patients disease free after "sufficient drug," who had completed ten or more courses of chemotherapy, who had regression of tumor to resectable size, who required a change of chemotherapy, or in whom a lesion initially thought to be residual tumor was later thought to be benign.

Currently we advise second-look surgery for virtually all patients who have received treatment for ovarian cancer. The aims of second-look surgery are:

1. To confirm "cure" and allow cessation of chemotherapy.
2. To confirm the presence of residual tumor requiring resection or the modification of treatment regimens.
3. To clarify clinical findings by direct vision.

One should not underestimate the immense value to the morale of a patient who is clinically clear of disease to know that this assumption is supported by gross and microscopic examination.

Use of Laparoscopy

Laparoscopy has been advocated as a method of monitoring patients following chemotherapy of ovarian cancer and saving a proportion from laparotomy.[131,132] In neither of these studies was laparoscopy intended to replace laparotomy. The aim was to perform laparoscopy to confirm whether tumor was actually present in patients where cessation of chemotherapy was being considered. If laparoscopy revealed residual tumor, it was felt that laparotomy was not needed, and chemotherapy was reinstituted. A negative laparoscopy was an indication for a full second-look laparotomy.

There are several problems with this approach. First, it is not always possible to insert the laparoscope in patients with prior abdominal surgery, and in the study of Ozols and colleagues[132] this occurred in 6 percent of the cases. Second, such a procedure is not always safe, though in this study, only 2.5 percent of patients needed medical therapy for complications of laparoscopy. Nevertheless, we would caution that in any patient the insertion of a laparoscope is a potentially dangerous procedure, and occasionally lethal, and that the presence of adhesions from previous major surgery make it more so. A third problem with laparoscopy is that there are strong arguments for resecting as much residual tumor as possible, and it is technically impossible to be sure whether resectable disease is present through a laparoscope. While the idea is attractive we fear that ill-advised use of this technique may lead to unnecessary morbidity and mortality for some patients, and to a return to a situation that existed some years ago where a little information was enough for management. The importance of resecting as much tumor as possible at "second-look" must be kept in mind. The authors of the aforementioned papers emphasized that the findings of "no tumor" at laparoscopy mandated a laparotomy. Ozols and colleagues[132] found that 55 percent of their patients with negative laparoscopies had residual tumor, generally in the pelvis or mesentery.

Procedure for Second-Look Laparotomy

The approach to the second-look laparotomy has been described well by Smith and associates:[130]

> A second-look operation is not a simple laparotomy; it is a well-planned, systematic operation. If cancer is found, an effort should be made to remove all cancer with careful documentation of the residual disease. From these findings the treatment may be modified and subsequent care can be planned. If disease is not found, a complete sampling of the peritoneum of the abdominal cavity, including peritoneal cytology, is done. . . (Fig. 15).[130]

Of particular importance is the biopsy and removal of all adhesions and residual omentum, the biopsy of all old pedicles, and the use of multiple random biopsies. In view of the fact that significant numbers of patients with ovarian cancer have high para-aortic nodal metastases, we advocate biopsy of these nodes also.[87,133] We have found from experience that palpability is not a prerequisite for the presence of tumor, and occasionally, the biopsy of apparently normal nodes yields surprising results. Creasman and coworkers[134] have reported on five patients whose only evidence of residual disease at second-look surgery was in retroperitoneal nodes of the pelvis or para-aortic regions. Failure to sample retroperitoneal nodes can thus lead to the erroneous conclusion that no residual disease is present, and hence to the premature cessation of treatment. The patient is not served by anything but the most thorough of laparotomies when consideration is being given to cessation of therapy.

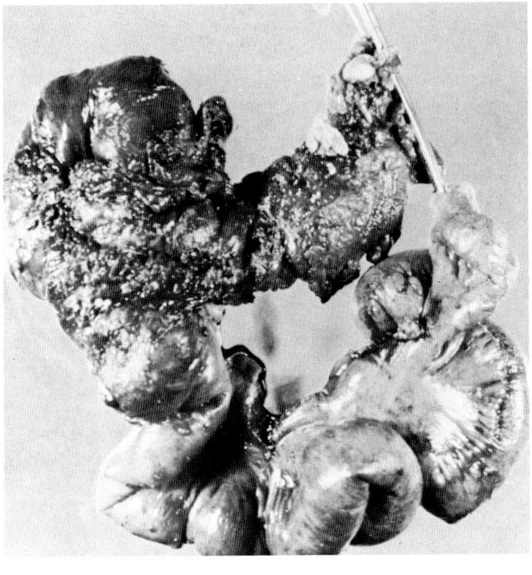

Figure 15. At "second-look" surgery the only remaining bulk tumor encased the terminal ileum and right hemicolon. A right hemicolectomy and primary bowel anastomosis were performed.

Timing of Second-Look Surgery and Subsequent Survival

Second-look laparotomy is an established part of the treatment regimen for ovarian carcinoma.[135]

Two further considerations are important. First, what is the optimal time for the procedure? We presently accept 12 courses of chemotherapy, or roughly 1 year after primary therapy. This is based on studies where chemotherapy was stopped after negative "second-looks" following as few as four courses, with subsequent recurrence.[130] There must be adequate time to allow the optimal drug effect. Second, what is the chance of survival after a negative "second-look" and cessation of chemotherapy? Smith quotes 72 percent 5-year survivals after negative "second-looks," 38 percent when only microscopic disease was present, and 15 percent if macroscopic tumor was present.[2] However, when all residual tumor was resectable, 48 percent of the patients survived 2 years. If resection to less than 2 cm was possible, 38 percent survived 2 years, and if the maximal residual tumors were over 2 cm in diameter, only 9 percent survived 2 years.

Greer and coworkers[4] point out that although early carcinomas of the ovary are not frequently seen, they offer the greatest opportunity for cure, and optimal treatment is essential. This will include "second-look" surgery.

THE YOUNG WOMAN WITH OVARIAN CARCINOMA

Incidence

Fortunately, ovarian malignancies are not common in the reproductive age group. Bennington and associates[61] found 9 percent of 332 ovarian tumors removed from women aged 20 to 44 to be malignant. The malignancy rate of ovarian tumors in varying age groups in an Australian population is shown in Table 13.[136]

The relative rarity is potentially dangerous because it may lead to prolonged observation of patients when, in retrospect, it is obvious that surgery

TABLE 13. MALIGNANCY RATES OF OVARIAN TUMORS AT DIFFERENT AGES

Age	Tumors Sampled	Malignant
Under 20	61	2%
20 to 29	358	3%
30 to 39	343	10%
40 to 49	264	29%
50 to 59	166	52%
60 to 69	130	48%
70 and over	69	48%
Overall	1391	22%

(Data from Beischer NA, et al: Aust NZ J Obstet Gynaecol 11:208, 1970, with permission.)[136]

should have been performed. Failure to consider the possibility of malignancy may lead to a surgeon's finding unexpected malignancy through a small transverse incision. It may be ruptured during attempts to remove it. In this situation neither the surgeon nor the patient is prepared for the performance of optimal surgery. It is essential to remember the vague and nonspecific gastrointestinal symptoms of ovarian cancer, and that all solid tumors, all bilateral tumors, those 10 cm or more in diameter, and adherent or rapidly growing tumors may be malignant in any age group.

Optimal Treatment

We believe that the optimal treatment for all patients with epithelial ovarian cancers is the complete surgery previously detailed: fastidious surgical staging, omentectomy, total hysterectomy and bilateral salpingo-oophorectomy, and maximal tumor bulk reduction. We further believe that all patients with tumors other than Stage I A, of low malignant potential, or grade I, should receive adjunctive chemotherapy postoperatively, and a later second-look procedure. Any treatment less than this, in our opinion, must be recognized as a calculated risk.

There is a small group of patients in the reproductive years where conservative surgery has been considered satisfactory. To qualify for consideration of conservative surgery, the patient must be young, of low parity, desiring further children, and without apparent cause for infertility. Both the doctor and the patient must understand the risks involved. The importance of adequate staging cannot be overemphasized and the frequency of unrecognized metastasis to other sites in apparent Stage I A lesions, as discussed earlier, must be borne in mind. The exact nature of tumors of nonepithelial origin must be absolutely certain, and in epithelial tumors the histologic grading equally certain. Furthermore, the importance of some gross findings at surgery, which may be easily ignored, must be kept in mind (Table 14).[137] The significance of extracystic excrescences is apparent to most surgeons, but even filmy adhesions may be significant, and should be excised for study rather than simply lysed. The significance of cyst rupture draws attention again to the need for an adequate incision.

TABLE 14. FIVE-YEAR SURVIVAL RATES IN PATIENTS WITH STAGE I EPITHELIAL CANCER OF THE OVARY, ACCORDING TO GROSS CHARACTERISTICS AT SURGERY

Gross Characteristics	5-Year Survival
Intracystic lesion	90%
Extracystic excresences	68%
Ruptured at surgery	56%
Adherent cysts	51%

(Data from Webb MT, et al: Am J Obstet Gynecol 116:222, 1973, with permission.)[137]

Criteria for Conservative Therapy
The conditions in which a patient may be considered for conservative surgery for ovarian cancer are as follows:

1. Patient young, of low parity, desiring further children.
2. Tumor carefully staged: Stage I A.
3. Tumor encapsulated, free of adhesions, and removed intact with no spill.
4. Peritoneal washings show no malignant cells.
5. Omentum removed and microscopically free of tumor.
6. Histologic type and grade:
    (a) Epithelial tumor of low malignant potential or grade 1.
    (b) Dysgerminoma.
    (c) Granulosa cell tumor.
    (d) Sertoli-Leydig tumor.
7. No microscopic evidence of invasion of capsule, vessels, lymphatics, or mesovarium.
8. Other ovary carefully bivalved and free of tumor microscopically.

It is apparent that, depending on the circumstances, certain of these requirements will be known to have been met only after pathology reports are available, possibly several days later. We unequivocally advise reexploration and complete surgery in any patient who has had conservative surgery and is subsequently found to have any feature precluding this in the above list. Similarly, we would strongly advise that any woman treated conservatively, in whom there is any doubt about the adequacy of staging, should have a repeat staging laparotomy performed by an experienced gynecologic oncologist, in circumstances where immediate frozen sections are available.[100] Inadequate staging would include exploration through a low transverse incision. As Barber has said "transverse is perverse."[7]

Results of Conservative Therapy
A proper assessment of the risks of conservative therapy is not possible, because of known deficiencies in staging of ovarian cancers in the past. Munnell[138] showed no significant difference in survival rate for patients with Stage I A ovarian cancer treated by either conservative or complete surgery. However, the relative 5-year survival rates overall were only 74 percent for conservative procedures, and 79 percent for complete surgery. His figures are summarized in Table 15.

The poor overall results suggest inadequate staging. The fact that mucinous tumors had a better outcome support this, because stage for stage their outcome has been shown to be the same as for serous tumors.

For tumors of low malignant potential, the safety of conservative surgery for Stage I A lesions has been demonstrated by Julian and Woodruff.[82] Conservative therapy for selected young women with Stage I A, "borderline," or grade 1 epithelial tumors is supported by Williams.[139]

TABLE 15. RELATIVE 5-YEAR SURVIVAL RATES FOR VARIOUS STAGE I A OVARIAN MALIGNANCIES

Tumor Type	Relative Five-Year Survivals	
	Conservative Surgery	Complete Surgery
Serous: Borderline and grade 1	87%	91%
Serous: Grades 2 and 3	45%	52%
Mucinous	100%	90%
Granulosa cell	67%	100%
Other	67%	89%
Overall	74%	79%

(Data from Munnell EW: Am J Obstet Gynecol 103:641, 1969, with permission.)[138]

A further word of warning seems appropriate in view of the fact that Williams and coworkers[140] reported that 2 patients out of 29 treated by conservative surgery for Stage I A tumors developed recurrence in the opposite ovary 7 and 30 years later. In all women conservatively treated, we advise total hysterectomy and the removal of the remaining tube and ovary as soon as childbearing is completed.

Possible Long-Term Effects of Adjuvant Therapy

In the young woman with ovarian cancer one must bear in mind the possibility that chemotherapy and radiotherapy may have undesirable long-term effects. In this respect the increased incidence of leukemia among patients treated with alkylating agents as reported by Reimer and colleagues[120] is important. Briefly, among 5455 patients treated with alkylating agents for between 3 and 90 months (mean 22 months) there were 13 cases of nonlymphocytic leukemia during follow-up ranging from less than 1 year to 7 years. The overall increase in risk for developing leukemia among patients treated with alkylating agents was between 21 and 36 times that of those not so treated, and for those surviving over 2 years, it was 67 to 170 times. Other studies have shown unexpectedly high rates of hematologic neoplasia in women treated with chlorambucil as adjuvant therapy for breast cancer,[141] and of second neoplasms in patients treated by combination chemotherapy and radiation for Hodgkin's disease.[142,143]

Sieber and Adamson[144] indicate that a latent period of approximately 4 years is to be expected between initiation of drug therapy and development of malignant sequelae. Thus, it will only be possible to assess fully this danger of adjunctive therapy when we have larger numbers of long-term survivors. We must keep in mind the fact that we are using toxic drugs to treat a lethal disease. Such drugs should be used for the shortest time compatible with optimal results. Hence, the extreme importance of second-look surgery in the young woman apparently cured of tumor.

The Adnexal Mass in the Pregnant Patient

When an ovarian tumor is found in pregnancy, the chance of malignancy is relatively low. In 1964, Tawa[145] reviewed 9 published series, and added 62 patients of his own to ascertain that approximately 6 percent of 348 reported cases of ovarian tumors in pregnancy were malignant. Later Beischer and coworkers[136] reported 2.4 percent of 164 patients explored for ovarian tumors in pregnancy had ovarian malignancy. If tumors over 15 cm were considered separately the malignancy rate was 5 percent. These rates were one-tenth those seen in nonpregnant women over the same time span. This probably reflects the early age of the patients, and the fact that most pregnant women will seek antenatal care, thus allowing detection of more benign tumors. On the other hand, older, nonpregnant women may only have tumors discovered when they become symptomatic of malignancy.

But a 3 to 5 percent malignancy rate is no grounds for complacency. We therefore advise that any ovarian mass over 5 cm in diameter that does not regress by the end of the first trimester should be investigated by laparotomy. This is best done early in the second trimester because at that time spontaneous abortion is less likely, and emesis has usually stopped, making the postoperative course smoother. Placental function is established so the removal of the corpus luteum is not a problem, and uterine size does not hamper surgery. Any patient with an ovarian tumor that is producing symptoms or is suspicious of malignancy must have an immediate laparotomy regardless of the stage of pregnancy. Asymptomatic and nonsuspicious masses discovered close to term may be followed expectantly until after delivery.

It is worth emphasizing that all women having cesarean section must have their ovaries inspected during the procedure.

Management of Ovarian Cancer in Pregnancy

Munnell[146] has estimated the incidence is only about 1 in every 18,000 pregnancies. The management of ovarian cancer in a pregnant woman is essentially the same as in the nonpregnant patient. If the tumor is low grade and confined to one ovary, unilateral oophorectomy and bisection of the opposite ovary is the immediate treatment of choice, with the pregnancy being allowed to go to term. However, if the ovarian cancer has extended beyond the ovary, then total abdominal hysterectomy, bilateral salpingo-oophorectomy, omentectomy, and appendectomy are carried out. Debulking procedures are performed as in the nonpregnant patient. The 5-year survival rate for pregnant women is in the region of 75 percent. However, these results are a reflection of the generally favorable type of tumor and stage of disease encountered in these young women.

PROPHYLACTIC OOPHORECTOMY

It would be a bold surgeon indeed who advocated elective oophorectomy for all women 40 or older, even though such a move would save 1 percent of these women from developing ovarian carcinoma, and reduce the incidence of the disease by over 80 percent. Every surgeon performing a hysterectomy or pelvic laparotomy for benign disease must consider the advisability of oophorectomy at that time. The problem is to balance the dangers of ovarian disease, principally cancer, in the retained ovaries against the complications of castration. When reproductive function is no longer required, the only function of the ovary is steroid synthesis. Estrogen production normally ceases at the menopause, but androgen production continues postmenopausally, and these androgens may be converted to estrogen by peripheral nonglandular conversion.[147] Loss of ovarian estrogen production leads to menopausal symptoms, possibly an increase in cardiovascular disease, and certainly an increase in osteoporosis, which may, through predisposing to hip fractures, lead to fatal complications. The value of the androgen secretion of the postmenopausal ovary is less certain.

Gibbs[148] suggests that removal of the ovaries in all women having a pelvic operation beyond the age of 35 would prevent 20 percent of all ovarian cancer seen. This estimate is based on his own studies and a review of the available literature.

Terz and colleagues[149] reviewed 624 cases of ovarian carcinoma and found 55 of the patients had a history of previous pelvic laparotomy, over one-third of them within the 5 years prior to diagnosis. The 5-year survival of the 55 women was 18 percent. These figures are in broad agreement with figures from many sources:

> . . . the sad commentary on ovarian carcinoma is the fact that approximately five to eight percent of these tumors occur in women following previous hysterectomy at which time the ovaries were retained.[150]

Ovaries may become too old to function, but not to form cancer. It is our belief that in every woman over 35 years undergoing abdominal hysterectomy, consideration should be given to oophorectomy, and the situation discussed with the patient. Any woman electing conservation of the ovaries at hysterectomy must understand the extreme importance of regular pelvic examinations by a competent gynecologist. *We are strongly opposed to ovarian conservation at abdominal hysterectomy in perimenopausal and postmenopausal women.* Removal of the ovaries at vaginal hysterectomy is technically more difficult, so it is reasonable to advise ovarian conservation at the time of vaginal hysterectomy.

REFERENCES

1. Chamberlain G: Aetiology of gynaecological cancer. Roy Soc Med 74:246, 1981
2. Smith WG: Surgical treatment of epithelial ovarian carcinoma. Clin Obstet Gynecol 22:939, 1979
3. American Cancer Society: Cancer Facts and Figures, New York, 1982

4. Greer BE, Rutledge FN, Gallager HS: Staging or restaging laparotomy in early-stage epithelial cancer of the ovary. Clin Obstet Gynecol 23:294, 1980
5. Tobias JS, Griffiths CT: Management of ovarian carcinoma. Current concepts and future prospects. N Engl J Med 294:877, 1976
6. Smith JP, Day TG: Review of ovarian cancer at the University of Texas Systems Cancer Center, M.D. Anderson Hospital and Tumor Institute. Am J Obstet Gynecol 135:984, 1979
7. Barber HRK: Ovarian carcinoma. Etiology, Diagnosis and Treatment. New York: Masson, 1978
8. Woodruff JD: The pathogenesis of ovarian neoplasia. Johns Hopkins Med J 144:117, 1979
9. Wijnen JA, Rosenshein NB: Surgery in ovarian cancer. Arch Surg 115:863, 1980
10. Nelson JM: Importance of maximum procedure in ovarian cancer. Natl Cancer Inst Mongr 42:109, 1975
11. Morris JM: Invited editorial comment on the paper of Wijnen and Rosenshein, "Surgery in ovarian cancer." Arch Surg 115:868, 1980
12. Schenker JG, Polishuk WZ, Steiner R: An epidemiologic study of carcinoma of the ovary in Israel. Israel J Med Sci 4:820, 1968
13. King H, Maenszel W: Cancer mortality among foreign and native born Chinese in the United States. J Chron Dis 26:623, 1973
14. Buell P, Dunn JE: Cancer mortality among Japanese Issei and Nissei of California. Cancer 18:656, 1965
15. Menck MR, Henderson BE: Cancer incidence rates in the Pacific Basin. Natl Cancer Inst Monogr 53:119, 1979
16. Beral V, Fraser P, Chilvers C: Does pregnancy protect against ovarian cancer? Lancet 1:1083, 1978
17. Fraumeni JF, Lloyd JW, Smith EM, Wagoner JK: Cancer mortality among nuns: Role of marital status in etiology of neoplastic disease in women. J Natl Cancer Inst 42:455, 1969
18. McGowan L, Parent L, Lednar W, Norris MJ: The woman at risk for developing ovarian cancer. Gynecol Oncol 7:325, 1979
19. Fathalla MF: Incessant ovulation—a factor in ovarian neoplasia. Lancet 2:163, 1971
20. De Boer CH: Transport of particulate matter through the human female genital tract. J Reprod Fertil 28:295, 1972
21. Henderson WJ, Joslin CAF, Turnbull AC, Griffiths K: Talc and carcinoma of the ovary and cervix. J Obstet Gynecol Br Cwlth 78:266, 1971
22. Keal G: Asbestosis and abdominal neoplasms. Lancet 2:1211, 1960
23. Newhouse M, Pearson R, Fullerton J, et al: A case control study of carcinoma of the ovary. Brit J Prev Med 31:148, 1977
24. Casagrande JT, Pike MC, Ross RK, et al: "Incessant ovulation" and "ovarian cancer." Lancet 2:170, 1979
25. Joly DJ, Lilienfeld AM, Diamond EL, Bross IDJ: An epidemiologic study of the relationship of reproductive experience to cancer of the ovary. Am J Epidemiol 99:190, 1974
26. Willett WC, Bain C, Hennekens CH, et al: Oral contraceptives and risk of ovarian cancer. Cancer 48:1684, 1981
27. Wynder EL, Hyams L, Shigamatsu T: Correlation of international cancer death rates, an epidemiological exercise. Cancer 20:113, 1967

28. Fox M, Langley FA: Tumors of the Ovary. London: Heinemann, 1976
29. Guthrie MJ: Tumorigenesis in intrasplenic ovaries in mice. Cancer 10:190, 1957
30. Bielschowsky F, Hall WH: Carcinogenesis in parabiotic rats: Tumors of ovary induced by acetyle-aminofluorescence in intact females joined to gonadectomized litter mates. Br J Cancer 5:331, 1951
31. Gondos B: Surface epithelium of the developing ovary: Possible correlation with ovarian neoplasia. Am J Pathol 81:303, 1975
32. Creasman WT, Sasso RA, Weed JC, McCarty KS: Ovarian carcinoma: Histologic and clinical correlation of cytoplasmic estrogen and progesterone binding. Gynecol Oncol 12:319, 1981
33. Schwartz PE, LiVolsi VA, Hildreth N, et al: Estrogen receptors in ovarian epithelial carcinoma. Obstet Gynecol 59:229, 1982
34. Lauchlan SC: The secondary Müllerian system. Obstet Gynecol Surg 27:133, 1972
35. Hsu YK, Parmely TH, Rosenshein NB, et al: Neoplastic and nonneoplastic mesothelial proliferations in pelvic lymph nodes. Obstet Gynecol 55:83, 1980
36. Radiasauljevic SV: The pathogenesis of ovarian inclusion cysts and cystomas. Obstet Gynecol 49:424, 1979
37. Ridley JH, Edwards IK: Experimental endometriosis in the human. Am J Obstet Gynecol 76:783, 1958
38. Merrill JA: Endometrial induction of endometriosis across a millipore filter. Am J Obstet Gynecol 94:780, 1966
39. Novak ER: Pathology of endometriosis. Clin Obstet Gynecol 3:413, 1960
40. Parkley TH, Woodruff JD: The ovarian mesothelioma. Am J Obstet Gynecol 120:234, 1974
41. West RO: Epidemiologic study of malignancies of the ovaries. Cancer 19:1001, 1966
42. Wynder EL, Dodo H, Barber HRK: Epidemiology of cancer of the ovary. Cancer 23:352, 1969
43. Osbourne RH, DiGeorge FV: The ABO blood groups in neoplastic disease of the ovary. Am J Hum Genet 15:380, 1963
44. Liber AF: Ovarian cancer in a mother and five daughters. Arch Pathol 49:280, 1950
45. Li FP, Rappaport AH, Fraumeni JF, Jensen RD: Familial ovarian cancer. JAMA 214:1559, 1970
46. McCrann DJ, Marchant DJ, Bardwil WA: Ovarian carcinoma in three teen-age siblings. Obstet Gynecol 43:132, 1974
47. Fraumeni JF, Grundy GW, Creagan EJ, Everson RB: Six families prone to ovarian cancer. Cancer 36:364, 1975
48. Franceschi A, LaVecchia C, Mangioni C: Familial ovarian cancer: Eight more families. Gynecol Oncol 13:31, 1982
49. Szamborski J, Czerwinski W, Gadomska H, et al: Case control study of high risk factors in ovarian carcinoma. Gynecol Oncol 11:8, 1981
50. Cutler SJ, Myers MH, White PL: Who are we missing and why? Cancer 37:421, 1976
51. Rutledge F, Boronow RC, Wharton JT: Gynecologic Oncology. New York: Wiley, 1976
52. Barber HRK: Ovarian cancer. Part I, American Cancer Society, Ca—A Cancer Journal for Clinicians 29:341, 1979
53. Stone ML, Weingold AB, Sall S, Sonnenblick B: Factors affecting survival of patients with ovarian carcinoma. Surg Gynecol Obstet 116:351, 1963

54. Parker RJ, Parker CM, Willbanks GD: Cancer of the ovary: Survival studies based upon operative therapy, chemotherapy and radiotherapy. Am J Obstet Gynecol 108:878, 1970
55. Johnson GM: Pelvic mass and diagnosis of cancer of the ovary. Clin Obstet Gynecol 22:903, 1979
56. McGowan L: Gynecologic Oncology. New York: Appleton-Century-Crofts, 1978
57. Ballon SC: Immunotherapy and immune diagnosis of ovarian cancer. Clin Obstet Gynecol 22:993, 1979
58. Barlow JJ: Summary of discussion groups: Early diagnosis and staging of ovarian cancer. Natl Cancer Inst Monogr 42:186, 1975
59. Barber HRK, Graber EA: The PMPO syndrome (postmenopausal ovary syndrome). Obstet Gynecol 38:921, 1971
60. Graber EA: Early diagnosis of ovarian cancer. Clin Obstet Gynecol 12:958, 1969
61. Bennington JL, Ferguson BR, Haber SL: Incidence and relative frequency of benign and malignant ovarian neoplasms. Obstet Gynecol 32:627, 1968
62. Spanos WJ: Preoperative hormonal therapy for cystic adnexal masses. Am J Obstet Gynecol 116:551, 1973
63. Lawson TL, Albarelli JN: Diagnosis of gynecologic pelvic masses by Gray Scale ultrasonography: Analysis of specificity and accuracy. Am J Roentgenol 128:1003, 1977
64. Levi S, Delval R: Value of ultrasonic diagnosis of gynecologic tumors in 370 surgical cases. Obstet Gynecol Scand 55:261, 1976
65. Donald I: Ultrasound in the diagnosis of ovarian neoplasia. In DeWatterville M (ed): Diagnosis and Treatment of Ovarian Neoplastic Alterations. New York: Elsevier, 1975
66. Stern J, Buscema J, Rosenshein N, Siegelman S: Can computed tomography substitute for second-look operation in ovarian carcinoma? Gynecol Oncol 11:82, 1981
67. Piver MG, Lele S, Barlow JJ: Preoperative and intraoperative evaluation in ovarian malignancy. Obstet Gynecol 48:312, 1976
68. Severini A, Petrillo R, Kenda R, De Palo G: The value of double contrast enema in the assessment of ovarian carcinoma's diffusion. Gynecol Oncol 11:17, 1981
69. Serov SF, Scully RE, Sobin LH: Histologic typing of ovarian tumors. International Histologic Classification of Tumors, No. 9. Geneva, World Health Organization, 1974
70. Ozols RF, Garvin AJ, Costa J, et al: Histologic grade in advanced ovarian cancer. Cancer Treat Rep 63:255, 1979
71. Decker DG, Malkasian GD, Taylor WF: Prognostic importance of histologic grading in ovarian carcinoma. Natl Cancer Inst Monogr 42:9, 1975
72. Gallager HS: Prognostic importance of histologic type in ovarian carcinoma. Natl Cancer Inst Monogr 42:13, 1975
73. Johansson H: Clinical aspects of metastatic ovarian cancer of extragenital origin. Acta Obstet Gynecol Scand 39:681, 1960
74. Israel SL, Helsel EV, Hausman DM: The challenge of metastatic ovarian carcinoma. Am J Obstet Gynecol 93:1094, 1965
75. Rubin P: Understanding the problem of understaging in ovarian cancer. Semin Oncol 2:235, 1975
76. Broders AC: Carcinoma: Grading and practical application. Arch Pathol 2:376, 1926

77. Ewing J: Neoplastic Diseases. Philadelphia: Saunders, in press.
78. Dyson JL, Beilby JDW, Steele SJ: Factors influencing survival in carcinoma of the ovary. Br J Cancer 25:237, 1971
79. Day TG, Gallager HS, Rutledge RN: Epithelial carcinoma of the ovary: Prognostic importance of histologic grade. Natl Cancer Inst Monogr 42:15, 1975
80. Barber HRK, Sommers SC, Snyder R, Kwon TH: Histologic and nuclear grading and stromal reactions as indices for prognosis in ovarian cancer. Am J Obstet Gynecol 121:795, 1975
81. Nalick RH, DiSaia PJ: Rea TH, Morrow CP: Immunocompetence and prognosis in patients with gynecologic cancer. Gynecol Oncol 2:81, 1974
82. Julian CG, Woodruff JD: The biologic behavior of low grade papillary serous carcinoma of the ovary. Obstet Gynecol 40:860, 1972
83. Hart WR, Norris JH: Borderline and malignant mucinous tumors of the ovary: Histologic criteria and clinical behavior. Cancer 31:1031, 1973
84. Kolstad P, Aure JC, Hoeg K: Clinical and histologic studies of ovarian carcinoma. Long-term follow-up of 990 cases. Obstet Gynecol 37:1, 1971
85. Creasman WT, Gall SA, Blessing JA, et al: Chemoimmunotherapy in the management of primary stage III ovarian cancer; a Gynecologic Oncology Group Study, Cancer Treat Rep 63:319, 1979
86. Griffiths CT, Fuller AF: Intensive surgical and hemotherapeutic management of advanced ovarian cancer. Surg Clin North Am 58:131, 1978
87. Piver MS, Barlow JJ, Lele SB: Incidence of subclinical metastasis in Stage I and II ovarian carcinoma. Obstet Gynecol 52:100, 1978
88. Creasman WT, Rutledge F: The prognostic value of peritoneal cytology in gynecologic malignant disease. Am J Obstet Gynecol 110:773, 1971
89. Feldman GB, Knapp RC: Lymphatic drainage of the peritoneal cavity and its significance in ovarian cancer. Am J Obstet Gynecol 119:991, 1974
90. Wheelock MC, Puting P: Ovarian metastases from adenocarcinomas of the colon and rectum. Obstet Gynecol 14:291, 1959
91. Karsh J: Secondary malignant disease of the ovaries. Am J Obstet Gynecol 61:154, 1951
92. Parker RT, Parker CM, Wilbanks GD: Cancer of the ovary. Am J Obstet Gynecol 108:878, 1970
93. Griffiths CT: Surgical resection of tumor bulk in the primary treatment of ovarian carcinoma. Natl Cancer Inst Mongr 42:101, 1975
94. Declos L, Quinlan EJ: Malignant tumors of the ovary managed with postoperative megavoltage irradiation. Radiology 93:659, 1969
95. Day TG, Smith JP: Diagnosis and staging of ovarian carcinoma. Semin Oncol 2:217, 1975
96. Piver MS, Barlow JJ, Lele SB, Frank A: Survival after ovarian cancer induced intestinal obstruction. Gynecol Oncol 13:44, 1982
97. Ketcham A, Hoye R, Pilch Y, Morton D: Delayed intestinal obstruction following treatment for cancer. Cancer 2:406, 1970
98. Tunca JC, Buchlet DA, Mack CA, et al: The management of ovarian cancer-caused bowel obstruction. Gynecol Oncol 12:186, 1981
99. Berek JS, Hacker NF, Lagasse LD, Leuchter RS: Lower urinary tract resection as part of cytoreductive surgery for ovarian cancer. Gynecol Oncol 13:87, 1982
100. Cavanagh D, Marsden DE: Unexpected carcinoma of the ovary reported by pathology 5 days following unilateral salpingo-oophorectomy for presumed endo-

metrial cyst. In Nichols DH (ed): Clinical Problems in Gynecologic Surgery. Baltimore: Williams & Wilkins, 1983
101. Eltringham JR: Radiation therapy for ovarian carcinoma. Clin Obstet Gynecol 22:967, 1979
102. Piver MS: Radioactive colloids in the treatment of Stage IA ovarian cancer. Obstet Gynecol 40:42, 1972
103. Clark DGC, Hilaris BS, Ochoae M: Treatment of cancer of the ovary. Clin Obstet Gynecol 3:159, 1976
104. Decker DG, Webb MJ: Prophylactic therapy for Stage I ovarian cancer. Gynecol Oncol 1:203, 1973
105. Buchsbaum HJ, Keettel WC, Latourette MB: The use of radioisotopes as adjunct therapy of localized ovarian cancer. Semin Oncol 2:247, 1975
106. Perez CA, Walz BJ, Jacobson PL: Radiation therapy in the management of carcinoma of the ovary. Natl Cancer Inst Monogr 42:119, 1975
107. Kjorstad KE, Welander C, Kolstad P: Preoperative irradiation in Stage III carcinoma of the ovary. Acta Obstet Gynaecol Scand 56:449, 1977
108. Munnell EW: The changing prognosis and treatment in cancer of the ovary: A report of 235 patients with primary ovarian carcinoma—1952–1961. Am J Obstet Gynecol 100:790, 1968
109. Clark DGC, Hilaris B, Rousis C: The role of radiation therapy (including isotopes) in the treatment of cancer of the ovary: Results of 614 patients treated at Memorial Hospital, New York. Prog Clin Cancer 5:227, 1973
110. Dembo AJ, Bush RS, Beale FA, et al: The Princess Margaret Hospital Study of Ovarian Cancer: Stages I, II and asymptomatic III presentations. Cancer Treat Rep 63:249, 1979
111. Willson HKV, Ozols RF, Lewis BJ, Young RC: Current status of therapeutic nodalities for treatment of gynecologic malignancies with emphasis on chemotherapy. Am J Obstet Gynecol 141:81, 1981
112. Smith JP, Rutledge F: Chemotherapy in the treatment of cancer of the ovary. Am J Obstet Gynecol 107:691, 1970
113. Young RC: Chemotherapy of ovarian cancer: Past and present. Semin Oncol 2:267, 1975
114. Beck RE, Boyes DA: Treatment of 126 cases of advanced ovarian cancer with cyclophosphamide. Can Med Assoc J 98:539, 1968
115. Eyre JH: Chemotherapy of ovarian cancer. Clin Obstet Gynecol 22:957, 1979
116. Young RC, Chabner BA, Hubbard SP, et al: Advanced ovarian carcinoma: Prospective clinical trial of melphalan (L-PAM) versus combination chemotherapy. N Engl J Med 229:1261, 1978
117. Vogl SE, Berenzweig M, Kaplan BH, et al: The CHAC and HAD regimens in advanced ovarian cancer: Combination chemotherapy including cyclophosphamide, hexamethylmelamine, Adriamycin and *cis*-dichlorodiamine platinum. Cancer Treat Rep 63:311, 1979
118. Bruckner HW, Ratneil LH, Cohen CJ, et al: Combination chemotherapy for ovarian carcinoma with cyclophosphamide, Adriamycin and *cis*-dichlorodiamine platinum after failure of initial chemotherapy. Cancer Treat Rep 62:1021, 1978
119. Barr W, Cowell MA, Chatfield WR: The management of ovarian carcinoma—A review of 420 cases. Scot Med J 15:250, 1970
120. Reimer RR, Hoover R, Fraumeni JF, Young RC: Acute leukemia after alkylating agent therapy of ovarian cancer. N Engl J Med 297:177, 1977

121. Jones RB, Myers CE, Guarina AM, et al: High volume intraperitoneal chemotherapy ("belly bath") for ovarian cancer. Pharmacologic basis and early results. Cancer Chemother Pharmacol 1:161, 1978
122. Pattillo RA: Immunotherapy and chemotherapy of gynecologic cancers. Am J Obstet Gynecol 124:808, 1976
123. Alberts DS, Moon TE, Stephens RA, et al: Randomized study of chemoimmunotherapy for advanced ovarian cancer: A preliminary report of a southwest oncology group study. Cancer Treat Rep 63:325, 1979
124. Mangioni C, Francesci S, LaVecchia C, D'Incalci M: High dose medroxy progesterone acetate (MPA) in advanced epithelial ovarian cancer resistant to first- or second-line chemotherapy. Gynecol Oncol 12:314, 1981
125. Schwartz PE, Keating G, MacLuskey N, Gisenfeld A: Tamoxifen (T) therapy for advanced ovarian cancer. Proc Am Assoc Cancer Res Am Soc Clin Oncol 21:430, 1980
126. Alberts DS, Salmon SE, Chen HSG, et al: In vitro clonogenic assay for predicting response of ovarian cancer to chemotherapy. Lancet 2:340, 1980
127. Santoro BT, Griffen WO, Wangensteen OM: The second-look procedure in the management of ovarian malignancies and pseudomyxoma peritoneal. Surgery 50:354, 1961
128. Tepper E, Sanfillippo LJ, Gray J, Romney SL: Second-look surgery after radiation therapy for advanced stages of cancer of the ovary. Am J Roentgenol Radium Ther Nucl Med 112:755, 1971
129. Wallach RC, Kabakow B, Blinick G: Current status of the second-look operation in ovarian carcinoma. Natl Cancer Inst Monogr 42:105, 1975
130. Smith JP, Delgado G, Rutledge F: Second-look operation in ovarian carcinoma postchemotherapy. Cancer 38:1438, 1976
131. Smith WG, Day TG, Smith JP: The use of laparoscopy to determine the results of chemotherapy for ovarian cancer. J Reproductive Med 18:257, 1977
132. Ozols RF, Fisher RI, Anderson T, et al: Peritoneoscopy in the management of ovarian cancer. Am J Obstet Gynecol 140:611, 1981
133. Delgado G, Chow BK, Caglar H, Bepko F: Paraaortic lymphadenectomy in gynecologic malignancies confined to the pelvis. Obstet Gynecol 50:418, 1977
134. Creasman WT, Abu-Ghazaleh S, Schmidt HJ: Retroperitoneal metastatic spread of ovarian cancer. Gynecol Oncol 6:447, 1978
135. Curry SL, Zembo MM, Nahhas WA, et al: Second-look laparotomy for ovarian cancer. Gynecol Oncol 11:114, 1981
136. Beischer NA, Buttery BW, Fortune DW, Macafee CAJ: Growth and malignancy of ovarian tumors in pregnancy. Aust NZ J Obstet Gynaecol 11:208, 1971
137. Webb MJ, Decker DG, Mussey E, Williams TJ: Factors influencing survival in Stage I ovarian cancer. Am J Obstet Gynecol 116:222, 1973
138. Munnell EW: Is conservative therapy ever justified in Stage I (IA) cancer of the ovary? Am J Obstet Gynecol 103:641, 1969
139. Williams TJ: Management of ovarian carcinoma in young women. Clin Obstet Gynecol 19:673, 1976
140. Williams TJ, Symmonds RE, Litwak O: Management of unilateral and encapsulated ovarian cancer in young women. Gynec Oncol 1:143, 1973
141. Lerner H: Second malignancies diagnosed in breast cancer patients while receiving adjuvant chemotherapy at the Pennsylvania Hospital. Proc Am Assoc Cancer Res 18:340, 1977

142. Canellos GP: Second malignancies complicating Hodgkin disease in remission. Lancet 1:1294, 1975
143. Williams CJ, Coleman CN, Glatstein EJ, et al: Hematologic malignancies in remission of Hodgkin's disease (HD). Proc Am Assoc Cancer Res 18:288, 1977
144. Sieber SM, Adamson RH: Toxicity of antineoplastic agents in man: Chromosomal aberrations, antifertility effects, congenital malformations and carcinogenic potential. Adv Cancer Res. 22:57, 1975
145. Tawa K: Ovarian tumors in pregnancy. Am J Obstet Gynecol 90:511, 1964
146. Munnell EW: Primary ovarian cancer associated with pregnancy. Clin Obstet Gynecol 6:983, 1963
147. Speroff L, Glass RH, Kase NG: Clinical Gynecologic Endocrinology and Infertility, 2nd ed. Baltimore: Williams & Wilkins, 1978
148. Gibbs EK: Suggested prophylaxis for ovarian cancer. Am J Obstet Gynecol 111:756, 1971
149. Terz JJ, Barber HRK, Brunschwig A: Incidence of carcinoma in the retained ovary. Am J Surg 113:511, 1967
150. Mattingly RF: TeLind's Operative Gynecology. Philadelphia: Lippincott, 1977

CHAPTER 8
Primary Nonepithelial Ovarian Cancer

Discussions of ovarian cancer generally center around the so-called "common epithelial tumors" which occur with far greater frequency than the malignant ovarian tumors of nonepithelial origin. It is only in girls under the age of 15 that the incidence of nonepithelial malignant tumors exceeds that of the epithelial tumors (Fig. 1). The nonepithelial tumors of the ovary form a heterologous group which demonstrate the true pluripotentiality of ovarian cell lines. One sees tumors containing one or more cell types which may recreate any stage of embryonal or extraembryonal development, tumors in which stromal elements produce structures analogous to those seen in immature or mature testes, and tumors that produce estrogens, androgens, and various oncofetal antigens. Furthermore, it is not uncommon to find combinations of several nonepithelial tumor elements combined in a single neoplasm.

The classification of nonepithelial tumors of the ovary (Table 1) looks formidable, but many of the tumors are extremely rare, so that those that are of importance from the clinical point of view form a much smaller group (Table 2). Uncommon though these tumors are, they are of particular interest for several reasons. First, they are the most common ovarian malignancies in children, though a glance at Figure 1 shows that the designation "tumors of young women" is inappropriate, as the actual incidence of germ cell tumors remains relatively constant throughout life, while the incidence of sex cord stromal tumors increases gradually with age.[1] Second, within this group are some of the most rapidly growing malignant tumors known, which until the advent of combination chemotherapy were invariably fatal. Also of considera-

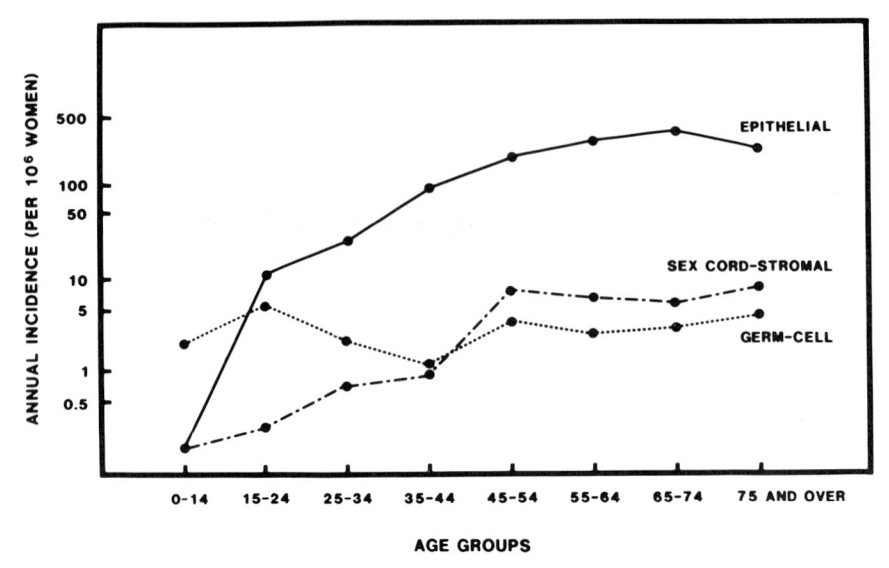

Figure 1. The relative incidence of epithelial and nonepithelial ovarian tumors by age group. Note that the scale is logarithmic. (*Modified from Weiss, et al: Gynecol Oncol 5:161, 1977, with permission.*)[1]

ble interest is the histogenesis of the various tumors, a subject that has exercised scholars since the turn of the century. Other unusual features of tumors within this grouping are the presence of some which are exquisitely sensitive to radiotherapy, others which are prone to very late recurrences after apparent cure, and the ability of chemotherapy to "convert" malignant metastases of certain tumors to benign lesions.

GRANULOSA CELL TUMORS

Granulosa cell tumors, "though by no means common, are not excessively rare."[2] One was described in 1859, but the term "granulosa cell tumor" was first used in 1914 when von Werdt reported six cases of "granulosazell tumoren des ovariums."[3]

Histogenesis. Meyer[4] proposed as an origin "rests" of primitive granulosa cells unused in folliculogenesis, but in 1930 Robinson[5] stated that "this type of ovarian cancer takes its origin from the follicles and not from hypothetical embryonal rests."

In 1936, Furth and Butterworth[6] showed that a sterilizing dose of radiation to the ovaries of mice could produce granulosa cell tumors, which were often associated with uteromegaly, endometrial hyperplasia, and breast malignancy. Geist and colleagues[7] believed that these radiation-induced tumors originated in undifferentiated ovarian parenchymal cells.

TABLE 1. CLASSIFICATION OF PRIMARY NONEPITHELIAL OVARIAN TUMORS (FIGO)

1. *Sex Cord Stromal Tumors*
   A. Granulosa-stromal cell tumors
      1. Granulosa cell tumors
      2. Tumors of the thecoma fibroma group
         i. Thecoma
         ii. Fibroma
         iii. Unclassified
   B. Androblastomas: Sertoli-Leydig cell tumors
      1. Well-differentiated
         i. Tubular androblastoma (Sertoli cell tumor)
         ii. Tubular androblastoma with lipid storage
         iii. Tubular adenoma with Leydig cells (Sertoli-Leydig cell tumor)
         iv. Hilus cell tumor (Leydig cell tumor)
      2. Intermediate differentiation
      3. Poorly differentiated (sarcomatoid)
      4. With heterologous elements
   C. Gynandroblastoma
   D. Unclassified
2. *Lipid (Lipoid) Cell Tumors*
3. *Germ Cell Tumors*
   A. Dysgerminoma
   B. Endodermal sinus tumor
   C. Embryonal carcinoma
   D. Polyembryoma
   E. Choriocarcinoma
   F. Teratomas
      1. Immature
      2. Mature
         i. Solid
         ii. Cystic
            a. Dermoid cyst (benign cystic teratoma)
            b. Dermoid cyst with malignant change
      3. Monodermal teratomas
         i. Struma ovarii
         ii. Carcinoid
         iii. Struma ovarii with carcinoid
         iv. Others
   G. Mixed forms
4. *Gonadoblastoma*
   A. Pure
   B. Mixed with dysgerminoma or other germ cell tumor
5. *Soft Tissue Tumors Not Specific to Ovary*
6. *Unclassified Tumors*
7. *Tumor-like Conditions*

In 1944, Biskind and Biskind[8] produced granulosa cell tumors in rats by transplanting their ovaries into the spleen. Estrogen traveled directly to the liver and was metabolized without entering the systemic circulation. Gonadotropin levels subsequently rose. In 36 rats where the transplant was in place for 317 days or longer, luteomas developed and granulosa cell tumors were

TABLE 2. APPROXIMATE FREQUENCY OF DIAGNOSIS OF VARIOUS FORMS OF NONEPITHELIAL MALIGNANCIES OF THE OVARY WITHIN EACH OF THE MAJOR SUBGROUPS[a]

Malignant germ cell tumors
    Dysgerminoma
    Endodermal sinus tumor
    Immature teratoma
    Choriocarcinoma
    Embryonal carcinoma
    Polyembryoma
    Mixed germ cell tumor
Sex-cord stromal tumors
    Granulosa cell tumor
    Thecoma
    Androblastoma

[a]It must be appreciated that the exact incidences are difficult to determine accurately.

later found in 24 of these.[9] Some produced sufficient estrogen to cornify the vagina and produce uteromegaly despite the passage of the hormone directly into the portal circulation. Only isolated case reports[10,11] link radiation with the genesis of granulosa cell tumors in humans, but McKay and associates[11] noted that both ovarian transplantation and radiation led to the degeneration of ova and atresia of follicles before granulosa cell tumors developed. They believed the tumors arose from granulosa cells persisting after follicular atresia, a process which in humans begins in fetal life and continues to the menopause. This is still the most plausible hypothesis, but the nature of the stimulus that causes their uncontrolled replication is not known. Radiation is unlikely, and although falling estrogen and rising gonadotropin levels in the postmenopausal years might appear to parallel ovarian transplantation in animals, it fails to explain tumors in the reproductive years or in prepubertal girls.

Incidence. Granulosa cell tumors account for less than 10 percent of malignant ovarian neoplasms. They have been reported in a stillborn infant[12] and a 14-week-old baby,[13] but less than 5 percent occur before the menarche. In a recent series from Sweden, the mean age was 53 years.[14] Over 70 percent of the patients were postmenopausal, a finding comparable to the 60 percent reported in other recent studies from Israel[15] and the Mayo Clinic.[16]

Presentation. Isosexual precocious pseudopuberty is the most common presentation in children, although less than 10 percent of cases of precocious puberty are due to estrogenic tumors.[17] Among 75 women of reproductive age with granulosa cell tumors, Bjorkholme and Pettersson[14] found that 64 percent had menometrorrhagia and 16 percent had secondary amenorrhea. Of

188 postmenopausal patients, 71 percent complained of uterine bleeding. The majority of hormonally active granulosa cell tumors are estrogenic but some are androgenic.

Up to 30 percent of patients complain of abdominal pain, distention, or the feeling of a mass.[14,18] Acute abdominal pain secondary to torsion of the tumor was noted in 10 percent of the cases reported by Sjostedt and Wahlen.[19]

Diddle[20] reviewed almost 1000 cases reported in the literature and found that 75 percent of patients had symptoms less than 1 year with a median duration of 9 months. Bjorkholme and Petersson[14] found that in half their patients the symptoms had been present for less than 6 months.

Some women with granulosa cell tumors are infertile or suffer frequent abortions because of the abnormal hormonal milieu. Diddle[20] found reports of 13 previously infertile women, 8 others who had suffered at least 1 spontaneous abortion, and 1 with habitual abortion, who had successful pregnancies after the removal of a granulosa cell tumor. In 16 cases the tumor was diagnosed during pregnancy. Such an association is potentially hazardous. Gillibrand[21] found details of the outcome of pregnancy in 23 of the 27 cases of granulosa cell tumors associated with pregnancy reported in the literature. Of 14 patients in whom the diagnosis was made in the third trimester, 6 had premature labor, 3 had cesarean sections because the tumor obstructed labor, and in another 4 the tumor ruptured. One rupture occurred before labor and the mother survived, but three patients died when the rupture was discovered immediately after delivery.

Gross Pathology. Granulosa cell tumors are unilateral in over 97 percent of cases,[12,14,16] and approximately 90 percent are Stage I.[14,16] The size varies from microscopic lesions in apparently normal ovaries[10] to tumors weighing over 10 kg.[22] In one series, over half were between 8 and 11 cm in diameter.[14]

In the cases studied by Fox and colleagues,[23] 41 percent of the tumors were completely solid, 50 percent had cystic areas, and the remainder were totally cystic. The cystic areas may contain serous, serosanguinous, or gelatinous material. Hemorrhagic and necrotic areas may be seen. The cut surface, often said to be characteristically yellow or orange, may in fact be white, brown, pink, or gray (Fig. 2).

Histology. The typical cell type of a granulosa cell tumor is small, round, polygonal, or less commonly spindle-shaped, with a small amount of eosinophilic cytoplasm and ill-defined boundaries. The nuclei are large, round or oval in shape, often with longitudinal grooving, and may contain a single nucleolus. These cells are arranged in a variety of patterns within a matrix of spindle-shaped stromal cells. Although one pattern generally dominates, most tumors contain areas with a variety of different patterns. Some granulosa cell tumors are luteinized, containing large polyhedral lipid-laden cells.

In the trabecular pattern (Fig. 3), granulosa cells are arranged in cords

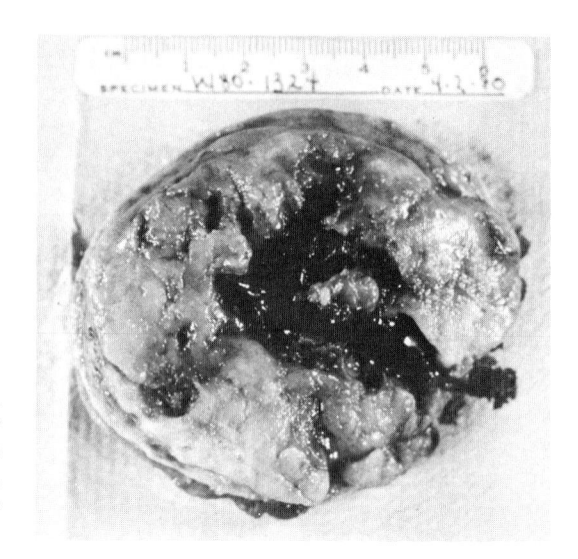

Figure 2. Granulosa cell tumor. This is an extremely soft, cellular tumor, with little connective tissue stroma. As seen in this specimen, hemorrhage, necrosis, and eventually cystic change may occur.

one or more cells wide within the stroma. The stromal cells immediately adjacent to the granulosa cells may be arranged with their axis at right angles to the cords. Where long, narrow, ribbons of tumor cells are set in a scanty stroma a "moire silk" pattern results, while a trabecular arrangement with relatively larger amounts of hyalinized stromal tissue produces a "cylindromatous" pattern. The "insular" pattern (Fig. 4) contains small islands of granulosa

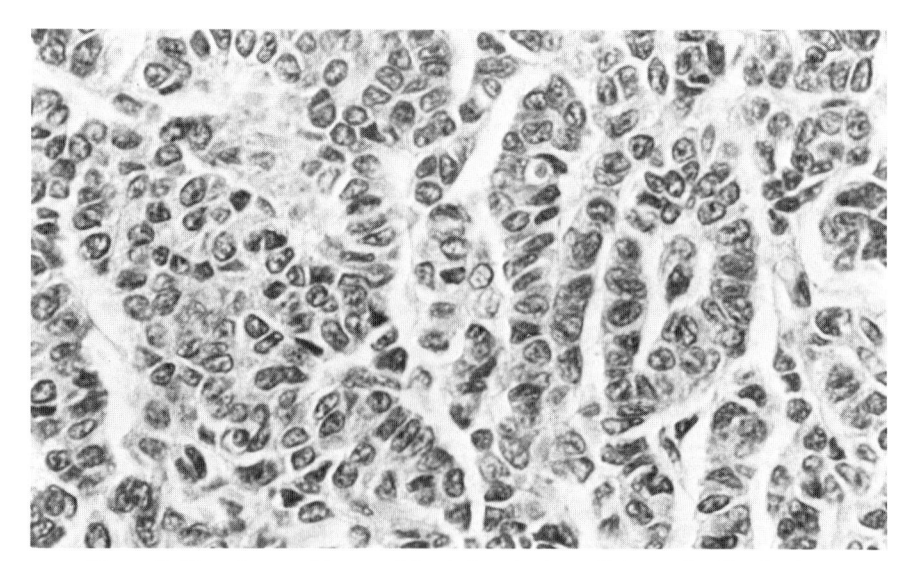

Figure 3. Granulosa cell tumor of the trabecular type. Pale, oval, rather benign looking nuclei, set in a sparse amount of cytoplasm.

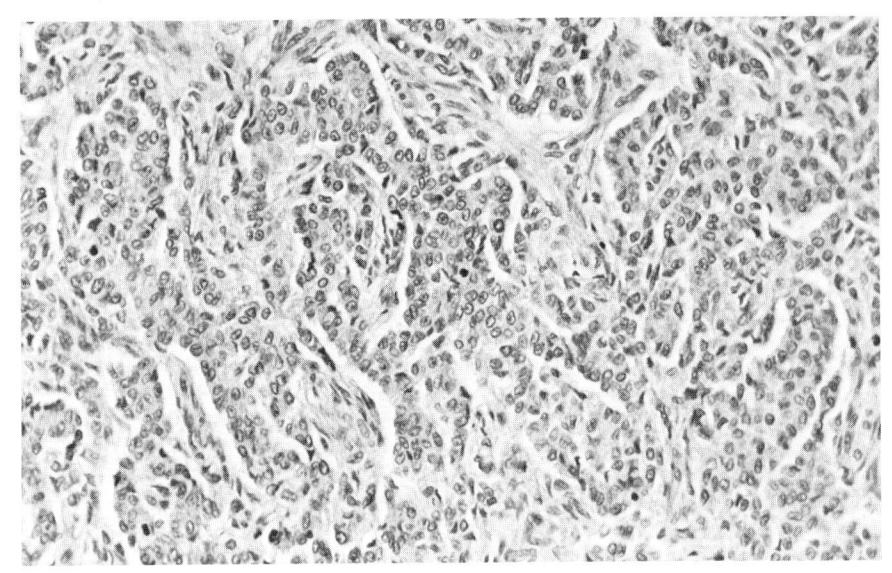

Figure 4. Granulosa cell tumor of the insular pattern. Here the cells are forming distinct islands within a background of spindle-shaped fibrothecal cells.

cells within the stroma. Although the majority of cells in the islands are randomly arranged, the outermost row may show radial symmetry. The "sarcomatoid" pattern consists of closely packed oval or spindle-shaped cells arranged in sheets.

Call-Exner bodies, though pathognomic, are seen in less than half of granulosa cell tumors. They consist of microfollicles of randomly arranged granulosa cells surrounding a small space containing dense eosinophilic material or nuclear fragments. Other forms of cystic pattern occur, with larger follicles containing mucoid material or less commonly granulosa cells arranged radially around an empty space in a manner resembling the Graafian follicle of a newborn, but without the ovum.

Scully[24] has drawn attention to a "juvenile type" of granulosa cell tumor, most often seen in the first two decades of life, which are usually of either the diffuse or macrofollicular type, and may be extensively luteinized. The overall appearance may "give the tumor a more malignant appearance than is supported by its clinical behaviour."

Associated Abnormalities. The precise incidence of coexistent endometrial hyperplasia and carcinoma are uncertain. Novak and colleagues[25] found 23 percent of endometrial specimens from women with feminizing tumors showed carcinoma and 65 percent hyperplasia. However endometrial specimens were only available for 79 of the 307 patients represented in their registry, and registry figures are biased by the referral of "interesting" cases. In no study was the endometrium from all women with granulosa cell tumors studied (Table 3). Emge[26] estimated the true incidence of endometrial cancer in women with feminizing tumors to be about 2 percent, and claimed the much higher figures often quoted were the results of small samples and selected populations. Fox and associates[23] believe that 5 percent of women with granulosa cell tumors will have or later develop endometrial carcinoma. Bjorkholme and Pettersson[14] estimate that Swedish women with feminizing tumors are ten times as likely to develop endometrial carcinoma as the general population.

The studies of Ohel and colleagues[15] and of Evans and associates[16] both showed that approximately 6 percent of women with feminizing tumors developed breast cancer, though the former group found most breast tumors after the treatment of the ovarian lesion, while the latter group found the diagnosis of breast cancer to have been made on the average 4.5 years before the ovarian tumor was found.

Clinical Course and Prognosis. Diddle[20] commented that "a five year survival rate does not necessarily indicate a cure in patients with these tumors and does not carry the same evaluation as it does in some other types of cancer." Norris and Taylor[12] reported corrected 5-year survival rates for granulosa cell tumors of 97 percent at 5 years and 93 percent at 10 years, stating that the figures in other studies resulted from the use of "crude survival, an archaic method that does not distinguish deaths from tumor from deaths from unrelated conditions." Fox and associates[23] disagree, commenting that "if no patient died from any other disease, it would be expected that nearly 50 percent of women with granulosa cell tumors would be dead within 20 years as a result of this neoplasm." Sjostedt and Wahlen[19] calculated the corrected survival figures shown in Table 4. Evans and colleagues[16] compared the survival rates of patients with granulosa cell tumors with survival data for women in the same area of the United States. The relative survival rates for women with granulosa cell tumors were 88 percent at 5 years, 83 percent at 10 years, 75 percent at 20 years, and 56 percent at 30 years. The crude survival rate for

TABLE 3. INCIDENCE OF ENDOMETRIAL HYPERPLASIA AND CARCINOMA ASSOCIATED WITH GRANULOSA CELL TUMORS (GCT)[a]

Authors	Total GCT	Endometrium Studied	Proportion Studied with (%) Hyperplasia	Cancer
Norris and Taylor (1968)[18]	97	38	65	11
Fox et al. (1975)[23]	92	58	50	10
Bjorkholme and Pettersson (1980)[14]	263	"over half"	45	—
Evans et al. (1980)[16]	118	76	55	13
Ohel et al. (1983)[15]	172	63	59	11

[a]Pure thecomas are excluded.

TABLE 4. LONG-TERM SURVIVAL RATES FOR PATIENTS WITH GRANULOSA CELL TUMORS

Interval from Treatment	Number of Patients	Crude Survival (%)	Corrected Survival (%)
5 years	157	84	87
10 years	104	75	83
15 years	51	63	71
20 years	24	58	67

(From Sjostedt S, Wahlen T: Acta Obstet Gynecol Scand 40[suppl]6:1, 1961, with permission.)[19]

172 cases of granulosa cell tumors diagnosed in Israel after 1960 was only 55 percent at 5 years.[15]

In the Mayo Clinic study,[16] only 8 percent of patients with an intact, encapsulated, unilateral granulosa cell tumor (Stage I Ai) died of their tumor, compared to 67 percent of those with Stage III disease. Furthermore, only 9 percent of Stage I Ai tumors recurred, compared to 30 percent for all other stages combined. Seventy percent of patients with recurrences died of their tumor. Bjorkholme and Pettersson[14] report 5- and 10-year survivals of 91 and 81 percent respectively for Stage I A tumors, compared to 50 and 32 percent respectively for Stage II B disease. The 5-year survival in the study from Israel[15] was 72 percent for Stage I disease, as compared to 11 percent for Stages III and IV.

The majority of granulosa cell tumors are Stage I, but within this group there are a number of prognostic factors. Some authors have found that women over 40 have a poorer prognosis,[18,19] though a detailed study of prognostic factors in 198 cases failed to substantiate this relationship.[20] Patients presenting with abdominal pain or a palpable mass have a poorer outlook than those with abnormal uterine bleeding.[15,18,19] The prognosis appears to be worse for patients with a short duration of symptoms,[19] a finding that may relate to the presence of specific symptoms such as pain, tumor rupture, or a rapidly growing abdominal mass. Bjorkholm and Silfversward[27] found that only 4 percent of women with tumors less than 5 cm in diameter died of their disease, compared to 20 percent with larger tumors. Tumor-related deaths occurred in 8 percent of patients with intact tumors, compared with 38 percent where the tumor ruptured. The histologic pattern is probably not significant,[12,18] but nuclear atypia and a high mitotic count are indicators of a poorer prognosis, at least in the more advanced stages.[23,27]

Treatment. A fastidious staging laparotomy must be performed through a generous vertical incision. Ascitic fluid, or in its absence, peritoneal washings, are sent for cytology. Possible metastases and enlarged or suspicious lymph nodes are biopsied. If conservative therapy is being considered, frozen section is invaluable.

The optimal treatment for Stage I granulosa cell tumors is total abdominal hysterectomy and bilateral salpingo-oophorectomy. We do not agree with Fox and colleagues[23] that "there is no convincing evidence that surgery radically alters the ultimate fate of the patients." As Evans and associates[16] demonstrated, "the young woman with a Stage I Ai granulosa cell tumor incurs a 7.5 percent risk of dying from the tumor, and only an 8.9 percent risk of developing recurrences. . . . unfortunately one-third of recurrences were in the reproductive tract, which would have been removed by initial total abdominal hysterectomy and bilateral salpingo-oophorectomy." In their study 25 percent of women who had conservative surgery developed recurrences, compared to 6 percent of those who had the "complete" surgery. Diddle[20] commented that "women who initially had only one ovary involved not uncommonly proved later to have a similar tumor in the other ovary."

We do not condemn conservative surgery for young women with Stage I Ai tumors who desire to maintain their fertility. Prerequisites include careful and accurate staging, wedge biopsy of the contralateral ovary, a tumor less than 10 cm in diameter without adhesions, extracystic excrescences or leakage, in a patient desirous and capable of childbearing, who understands the need for careful follow-up. In view of the incidence of associated endometrial abnormalities, it is prudent to perform endometrial curettage in patients treated conservatively. Tumor recurrence is fatal in 75 percent of cases[16] so we advise total hysterectomy and removal of the other adnexa when the family is complete.

The basic approach to advanced or recurrent granulosa cell tumors is the surgical "debulking" of the tumor together with a total hysterectomy, bilateral salpingo-oophorectomy, and omentectomy. The slow growth of these tumors may justify repeated surgical debulking in some cases.

Stenwig and colleagues[28] could demonstrate no benefit from adjuvant pelvic radiotherapy following surgery for Stage I granulosa cell tumors, though they concede that where there is a high mitotic count and marked cellular atypia it might be worthwhile. Following surgery, Schwartz and Smith[29] advise adjunctive radiotherapy for patients with ruptured tumors or for Stage I B to Stage III disease, provided residual tumor masses are all less than 2 cm in diameter. Where residual masses are larger, or for Stage IV disease, they advise combination chemotherapy with actinomycin D, 5-fluorouracil, and cyclophosphamide monthly for 12 courses followed by a second-look laparotomy. Kolstadt[30] recommends adjuvant pelvic radiotherapy for patients with Stage I tumors with high mitotic counts or marked anaplasia. Where there is extrapelvic spread he advises abdominopelvic radiation, unless there is tumor that could not be encompassed within radiation fields, when he suggests combination chemotherapy with vincristine, actinomycin D, and cyclophosphamide.

It is our opinion that adjuvant chemotherapy should be used for all tumors over 10 cm in diameter, especially in the presence of high mitotic counts or marked anaplasia, in all cases of tumor rupture and all Stages II, III, and IV tumors. The regimen we prefer is a combination of vincristine, adriamycin, and cyclophosphamide. A second-look procedure should be performed after approximately 1 year of chemotherapy. Radiotherapy is reserved for patients with minimal persistent or recurrent tumor after 12 cycles of such chemotherapy.

For premenarchial girls with Stage I tumors, unilateral oophorectomy is probably satisfactory treatment, and even in the presence of tumor spill the prognosis appears favorable.[31]

THECOMAS

Thecomas occur approximately one-fifth as frequently as granulosa cell tumors and are almost exclusively benign. They are most frequently seen in postmenopausal women. The tumors commonly produce estrogen and are often associated with abnormal uterine bleeding, endometrial hyperplasia, and occasionally with endometrial carcinoma.

Gross Pathology. Theca cell tumors are usually unilateral and between 5 and 10 cm in diameter, though they are reported in all sizes from microscopic to huge (Fig. 5). They are firm and rubbery in consistency and are demarcated

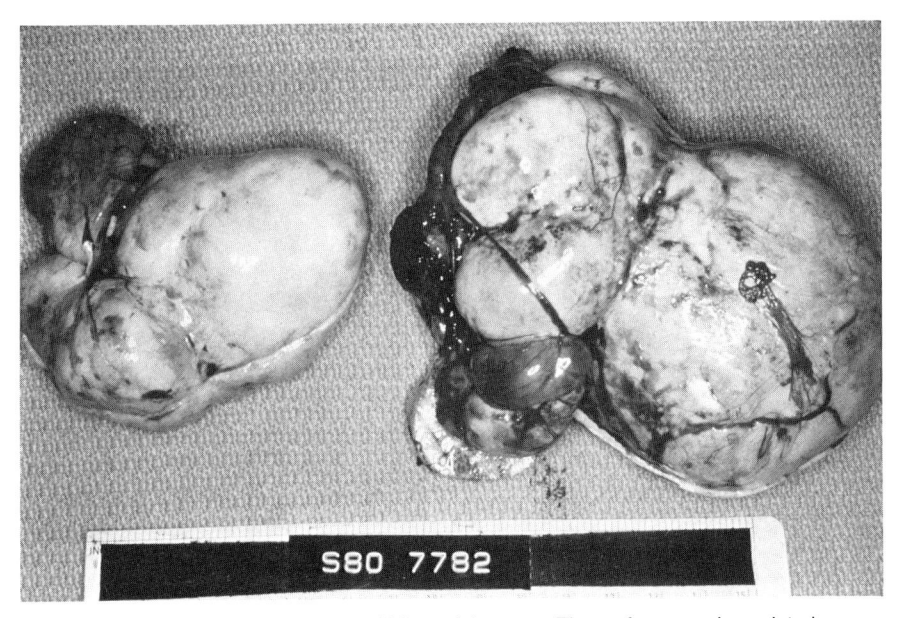

Figure 5. An unusual instance of bilateral thecoma. The surfaces are bosselated, smooth, and glistening. The tumor is extremely firm to touch. On sectioning, the surfaces vary from grey to yellow. One should always suspect a Krukenberg tumor whenever bilateral, solid, ovarian tumors are encountered.

from the normal ovarian tissue by a pseudocapsule. The cut surface is usually solid, though varying degrees of cyst formation are sometimes seen as are focal areas of hemorrhage. The most common pattern is of islands of yellow tissue separated by grey fibrous septa.

Microscopic Pathology. Thecomas consist of plump, pale-staining spindle cells of "epithelioid" appearance set in bundles or trabeculae separated by bands of fibrous tissue (Fig. 6). The cellular elements represent lipid-laden stromal or mesenchymal cells which resemble thecal cells. The proportions of epithelioid and connective tissue elements varies throughout the tumor. In less cellular areas the cells tend to be more spindle-shaped, while in the more cellular areas they tend to be plumper, with more abundant cytoplasm, poorly defined borders, and small ovoid nuclei. Both the cells and the intercellular spaces contain fat. Reticulin fibers are often present and may surround individual cells.

Management. The fact that most, if not all, thecomas are benign makes the conservation of reproductive function in younger women acceptable. Less than 20 malignant thecomas have been reported.[2] In older women and especially in the perimenopausal and postmenopausal age groups, total hysterectomy and bilateral salpingo-oophorectomy is the treatment of choice. Regard-

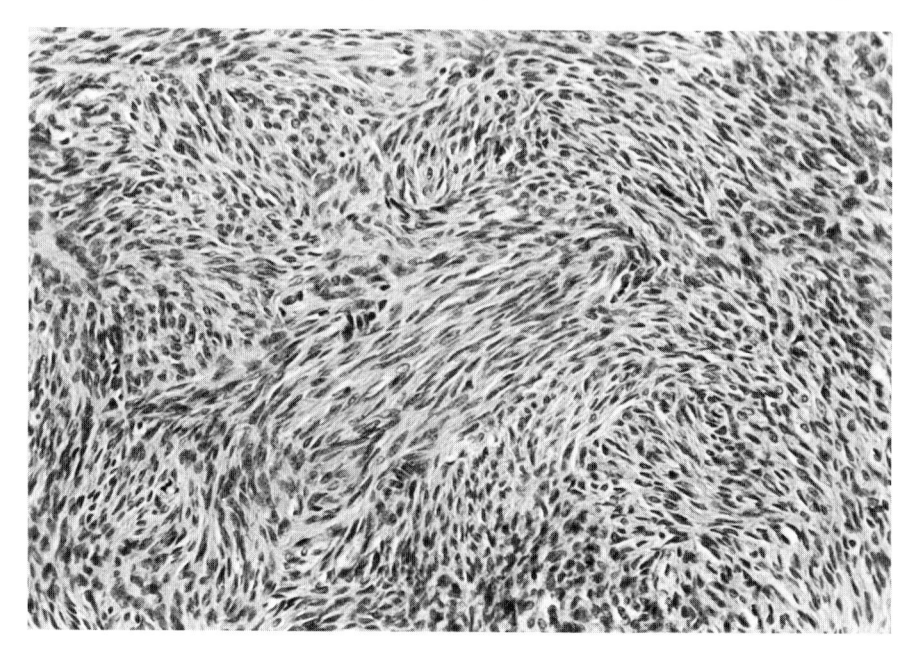

Figure 6. Thecoma. Interlacing bundles of benign spindle cells are seen. In the grossly yellow areas the cells are plump or epithelioid, and fat stains will demonstrate the steroid containing lipid. Mitotic figures or other evidence of malignancy are rare.

less of the suspected nature of any ovarian tumor, it is essential that the surgeon thoroughly explore the entire abdominal cavity prior to deciding on the appropriate therapy. Consideration must be given to the possibility of endometrial carcinoma being coexistent with the tumor and, if the uterus is to be preserved, curettage should be performed.

ANDROBLASTOMAS

Androblastomas account for 0.5 percent of ovarian tumors.[32] They are composed of Sertoli cells, Leydig cells, or their precursors. Scully[24] states that the designation androblastoma "emphasizes the fact that the more primitive tumors in this category may recapitulate, albeit imperfectly, the development of the testis" and the term Sertoli-Leydig tumor "focuses on the direction of differentiation of the neoplastic cells, even though such differentiation is realized only focally or to a minimal degree in some cases." Arrhenoblastoma, the term formerly used for this group of tumors, implies virilization which is not always present.

"The origin of these tumors is even more obscure than that of granulosa-theca cell tumors."[24] Among the origins proposed are from an ovotestis, from "male directed" cell rests in the hilum of the ovary, from granulosa cells, and from teratomas.[33] Teilum[34] recognized the homology of granulosa and Sertoli cells, and of Leydig and theca cells. His "blastemic" theory postulates that an unknown stimulus causes pluripotent ovarian cells to differentiate along one of several pathways. Other authors claim that up to 5 percent of androblastomas are derived from teratomas.[2]

WELL-DIFFERENTIATED ANDROBLASTOMAS

Among 240 androblastomas reported up to 1960, Pedowitz and O'Brien[35] found 24 percent to be well-differentiated, as were 28 percent of 111 cases in the Emil Novak Ovarian Tumor Registry.[36]

Tubular Androblastoma (Sertoli Cell Tumor)

This tumor is extremely rare and Fox and Langley[2] could find only 24 adequately documented cases in the literature up to 1976. Many tumors reported in the past as "Sertoli cell tumors" were in fact Sertoli-Leydig tumors, granulosa cell tumors, or testicular tumors in patients with congenital androgen insensitivity (testicular feminization). Tubular androblastomas are homologs of Sertoli cell tumors of the testis.[37] Their origin from cells of the undifferentiated gonadal mesenchyme is widely accepted (the "blastemic" theory of Teilum[37]) although some may be hamartomas rather than true neoplasms.[2]

Clinical Features. They are seen at any age. About 70 percent produce estrogen, 20 percent androgens, and the remainder are inactive. The most common presenting complaints are dysfunctional uterine bleeding, postmenopausal bleeding, or isosexual precocious pseudopuberty with estrogenic tumors and defeminization, hirsutism, virilization, or oligomenorrhea with androgenic tumors. Infertility may be present with either type.

Gross Pathology. These tumors are usually unilateral. Few exceed 10 cm in diameter and most are less than 5 cm. The cut surface usually reveals an encapsulated, lobular tumor which is solid and yellow in color.

Microscopic Pathology. Well-differentiated tubules are set in a connective tissue stroma which may, on occasion, contain a considerable amount of collagen, causing a superficial resemblance to a Brenner tumor. The tubules are lined by a layer of radially arranged columnar cells with basal nuclei and a clear cytoplasm. Droplets or vacuoles of lipid are often present in the stromal cells.

Management. Pure Sertoli cell tumors are almost always benign and oophorectomy will cure the patient and cause regression of the hormonal effects. In younger women pregnancy may follow.[38] Perimenopausal or postmenopausal women should have a total abdominal hysterectomy and bilateral salpingo-oophorectomy. Although most pure Sertoli cell tumors are benign, some highly malignant forms are seen. The possibility of congenital androgen insensitivity (testicular feminization) must be considered.

Tubular Adenoma with Leydig Cells

This tumor, otherwise known as a well-differentiated Sertoli-Leydig cell tumor, is uncommon. Only 34 cases had been reported by 1976.[2]

Clinical Features. Over half the reported cases have been in women between 20 and 35 years of age.[2] Androgenic effects are present in about 60 percent, being manifested as defeminization, virilization, amenorrhea, or infertility. Symptoms are often mild, and present for many years. Abdominal pain is the presenting complaint in about 10 percent of cases.

Gross Pathology. Very large tumors have been reported, but the majority are in the vicinity of 5 cm in diameter. Almost all are unilateral and well encapsulated.

Microscopic Pathology. Well-differentiated Sertoli-Leydig tumors consist of tubules lined by Sertoli cells, separated by a stroma containing varying numbers of regular, polyhedral Leydig cells. These have large basophilic nuclei centrally placed in a finely granular cytoplasm. The cells may contain fat. About half of the Leydig cells contain Reinke's crystalloids, slender rod-shaped crystals approximately 10 to 20 microns in length.

Management. These tumors are benign and in young women may be managed with conservative surgery. Total hysterectomy and bilateral salpingo-oophorectomy is the appropriate treatment for older women. The tumor may develop in association with congenital androgen insensitivity (testicular feminization).

Hilus Cell Tumor (Leydig Cell Tumor)
Like the other well-differentiated androblastomas, the hilus cell tumor is rare. Some may be incorrectly diagnosed as lipid cell tumors or as the hilar cell rests commonly seen in the normal ovary. It is not clear whether the tumor arises from these hilus cells or whether it is derived from the ovarian stroma.

Clinical Features. Approximately 80 hilus cell tumors have been reported,[2] and in over 80 percent the patient presented with defeminization and virilization. Some tumors are estrogenic and a few patients have presented with postmenopausal bleeding and associated mild virilization.[2] The majority occur between 50 and 70 years of age.

An interesting but poorly understood clinical correlation is the high incidence of hypertension in women with these tumors. The blood pressure may return to normal after removal of the tumor and it has been postulated that in these cases the tumor produces catecholamines as well as sex hormones.[39]

Gross Pathology. Hilus cell tumors are generally unilateral and less than 5 cm in diameter, often originating in the hilus of the ovary and expanding into the mesovarium. The cut surface is brownish-yellow and fleshy.

Microscopic Pathology. These tumors consist of tightly packed polyhedral cells with acidophilic cytoplasm and a large basophilic central nucleus. The cytoplasm may contain lipid. Reinke's crystalloids, slender rod-shaped crystals 10 to 20 microns in length, are seen in about half of the cells. These crystals are pathognomic of Leydig cells, but may be absent or irregularly distributed within the tumor. Morphologically the cells are identical to testicular Leydig cells.[37,40]

Management. Although these tumors are generally benign, occasional cases with metastasis have been reported.[41,42] Thus, although conservative treatment is reasonable in young women desiring further pregnancy, "complete" surgery is prudent in older women.

Androblastomas (Sertoli-Leydig) Tumors of Intermediate and Poor Differentiation
Most androblastomas fall into this grouping, but even so they are not common. Much of our information is gained from case reports and reviews of the literature. Pedowitz and O'Brien[35] found 238 cases in the literature to 1960, and added 2 of their own, while Novak and Long[36] reported 111 cases from

the Emil Novak Ovarian Tumor Registry. In 1962, O'Hern and Neubecker[43] described their experience with 31 cases and Roth and associates[32] recently reported 34 cases. All series contained some well-differentiated androblastomas, but over 80 percent were of intermediate or poor differentiation.

Clinical Features. Cases have been reported in patients as young as 2 years[36] and as old as 84,[32] but over 75 percent of patients are under 40[35,36] with a median age of 25 to 30.[32,43] The median age of patients with well-differentiated tumors was 41 years, compared to 23 and 19 years respectively for tumors of intermediate and poor differentiation.[32]

The tumors are usually androgenic and symptoms were generally present for at least a year before diagnosis, presumably because of their insidious onset.[35] Amenorrhea, sterility, and breast atrophy precede virilization, manifested by hirsutism, clitoromegaly, and deepening of the voice. These symptoms are present in approximately 75 percent of patients.[32] Others have postmenopausal bleeding, abdominal pain, a palpable mass, or have an asymptomatic tumor found on routine examination.

Pedowitz and O'Brien[35] found reports of ten Sertoli-Leydig tumors in pregnancy. In eight cases where the outcome of pregnancy was known there were two spontaneous abortions and six live births. One child was a "female pseudohermaphrodite" and another had clitoral hypertrophy.

Gross Pathology. Most are unilateral and confined to the ovary. Over 50 percent are less than 10 cm in diameter.[35] The cut surface is fleshy and grey to yellow in color. Hemorrhage and cystic change are not uncommon in larger tumors.

Microscopic Pathology. Better differentiated tumors have immature Sertoli cells arranged in tubules, cords, or trabeculae in an abundant mesenchymal stroma. Leydig cells are scattered through the stroma either as isolated cells or in clusters or sheets. Reinke's crystalloids are uncommon. Less differentiated tumors are made up of sheets of spindle-shaped cells resembling the stroma of the undifferentiated gonad. Occasional poorly formed tubules or cords of Sertoli cells are present, together with groups or clusters of Leydig cells. In the very poorly differentiated or "sarcomatoid" form, the diagnosis may only be made by the recognition of occasional Leydig cells.

Prognosis. Pedowitz and O'Brien[35] report an overall malignancy rate of over 20 percent with the least differentiated tumors being malignant in over 40 percent of cases. O'Hern and Neubacker[43] found only 3 percent to be malignant, and Roth and associates[32] agree. Of 90 patients in the Ovarian Tumor Registry followed at least 5 years, 34 percent died.[36]

Extraovarian spread of the diffuse intraperitoneal type is common at the time of diagnosis.[35] In other tumors, malignancy becomes obvious when they recur, generally within 2 years. The 5-year survival for malignant Sertoli-Leydig tumors was 14 percent. Recurrence may be heralded by the return of defeminization and virilization.

Management. Conservative surgery is generally advised for young women who want children. Such treatment carries an element of risk, especially with large, poorly differentiated tumors. For older women total hysterectomy and bilateral salpingo-oophorectomy is appropriate. Where the tumor is more advanced than Stage I A, total hysterectomy, bilateral salpingo-oophorectomy, omentectomy, and tumor bulk reduction are employed.

Schwartz and Smith[29] advise adjuvant whole abdominal radiation for ruptured tumors and for advanced disease where residual tumor masses are less than 2 cm in diameter and can be encompassed in the radiation fields. For bulky residual disease, or Stage IV tumors, they recommend cyclic chemotherapy with vincristine, actinomycin D, and cyclophosphamide, followed by a second-look procedure after approximately 24 cycles. We use adjuvant chemotherapy with the same regimen for patients with ruptured tumors or disease beyond Stage I A, and reserve radiation for patients with minimal residual disease at second-look surgery, which we perform after 12 cycles of chemotherapy.

MALIGNANT GERM CELL TUMORS

Dysgerminoma

In 1931, Meyer[4] gave the name "disgerminoma" to a group of tumors first described in 1906 as "seminoma ovarii." He believed they arose "from an undifferentiated form of germinal cells which had lost their facility for becoming either masculine or feminine in type" within disgenetic gonads. "Dysgerminoma" implies an origin from primitive germ cells that have migrated to the germinal ridge from the yolk sac. This explains the occurrence of dysgerminomas in the testis and along the route of migration of the primitive germ cells, and the frequent association of dysgerminoma with other tumors such as endodermal sinus tumor, malignant teratomas, and choriocarcinoma. Primitive germ cells do not contain Barr bodies. Asadourian and Taylor[44] failed to demonstrate Barr bodies in dysgerminoma cells. They showed that resting tumor cells contained twice the DNA of lymphocytes, which is consistent with the fact that primary oocytes are arrested in prophase, with twice the DNA of diploid cells.

Incidence. In Western countries, dysgerminomas account for about 5 percent of primary malignant ovarian tumors,[45] although in Japan they account for approximately 13 percent of ovarian tumors.[46] The difference may be due to the rarity of epithelial ovarian tumors. The high incidence rates in India[47] are similarly explained.

The youngest patient reported was aged 7 months[48] and the oldest 76 years.[45] Over 90 percent are diagnosed before the age of 30 and the median age is in the early 20s.[44,49,50] Half the cases in the Emil Novak Ovarian Tumor Registry were in patients under 20 years of age.[49] Approximately 25 percent of malignant ovarian tumors in children under 17 years of age are dysgerminomas.[48]

Clinical Features. Half of the patients complain of nonspecific symptoms such as vague abdominal pain, dyspepsia, pelvic pressure, or abdominal distention.[44,49,50] From 10[44] to 30 percent[50] of patients are asymptomatic and their tumors are found on routine examination. Up to 15 percent are diagnosed during pregnancy or immediately postpartum.[44,49] Dysgerminomas only are slightly less common than the epithelial tumors in pregnancy.[51]

Human chorionic gonadotropin (hCG) assays are sometimes positive in the presence of dysgerminomas, and a false diagnosis of pregnancy has occasionally been made.[44] This raises the possibility of choriocarcinoma within the tumor but a small proportion of dysgerminomas may produce hCG.[52] Menstrual abnormalities such as amenorrhea or menorrhagia have been reported in some series[44] and there have been case reports of virilization[53] and precocious puberty.[54]

The duration of symptoms prior to diagnosis is less than 6 months in over half the cases.[44,50] A small proportion of patients present with an acute abdomen, usually due to torsion of the tumor.[45,50]

Approximately 80 percent tumors are Stage I and 10 percent Stage II.[49] Bilaterality rates of 10 to 15 percent have been reported[44,50] but the disease in the contralateral ovary may be microscopic.

Gross Pathology. Dysgerminomas range in size from microscopic to massive, with a median diameter of 15 cm.[44] They tend to compress and destroy surrounding tissues and a pseudocapsule is visible around smaller tumors. The shape is usually round, oval, or lobulated. They are solid, with a firm rubbery texture and a pink or yellow cut surface. Hemorrhage or necrosis occur in larger tumors, but these findings or the presence of calcification or cystic change may be indicative of a mixed germ cell tumor. Some studies have found dysgerminoma to be more common in the right ovary than the left[44] and although this has been explained in terms of the slower embryologic development of the right gonad[55] the relationship appears tenuous.

Microscopic Pathology. The histologic appearance of dysgerminoma is distinctive (Fig. 7). Islands or strands of large uniform cells resembling primordial germ cells are set in a delicate connective tissue stroma which is often infiltrated with lymphocytes. The cells are round or polygonal, 15 to 20 microns in diameter, with clear or granular cytoplasm and a prominent vesicular nucleus containing one or more nucleoli. Mitotic activity varies from one area of the tumor to another. Giant tumor cells with a single nucleus and collections of syncytial cells may be present, but the absence of cytotrophoblast excludes choriocarcinoma.

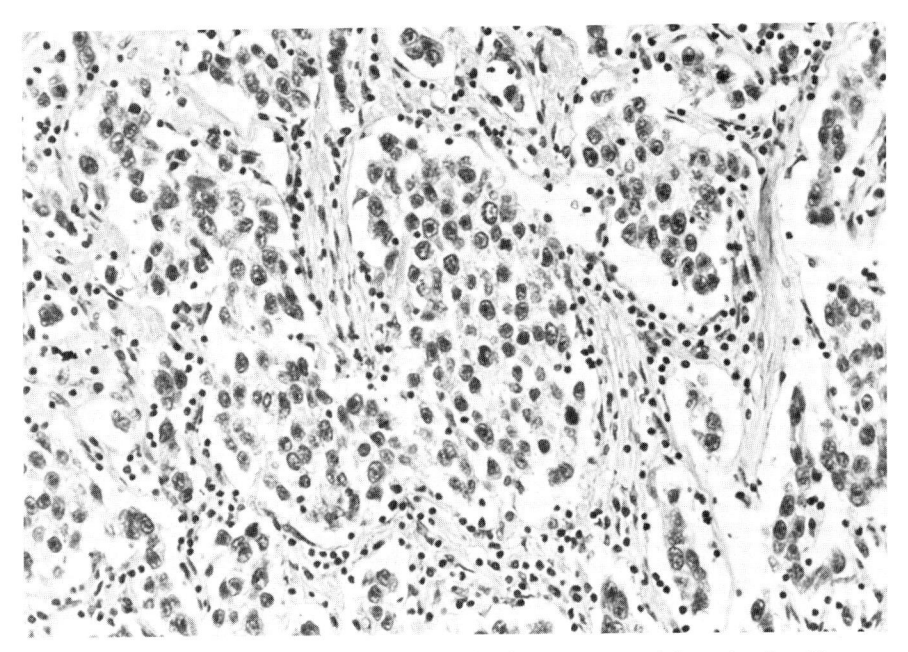

Figure 7. Dysgerminoma. This is the classic pattern, consisting of cells with abundant cytoplasm containing large vesicular nuclei with prominent nucleoli, compartmentalized by fibrous septa within which is a variable degree of lymphocytic infiltrate.

About 15 percent of dysgerminomas contain other germ cell elements,[44,49] most commonly gonadoblastoma, endodermal sinus tumor, and teratoma. Finding the admixed germ cell tumor may require an exhaustive search. Abell and colleagues[56] reported a case where 19 tissue blocks from a pelvic tumor showed only dysgerminoma, but metastatic deposits in the inguinal nodes contained endodermal sinus tumor, choriocarcinoma, and teratoma.

Pattern of Spread. Eighty percent of dysgerminomas are Stage I at diagnosis, and 10 to 15 percent have involvement of both ovaries. Extraovarian spread occurs by either the lymphatic route, or in the manner of the epithelial ovarian tumors.[52,55] Hematogenous spread may occur in advanced disease. The liver, lungs, and kidneys are the most common sites of metastasis.[52,55]

Prognostic Factors. Some reports have indicated a 5-year survival of less than 30 percent[45,57] but it is generally believed that those figures are unduly pessimistic, probably because of the inclusion of mixed germ cell tumors. Asadourian and Taylor[44] have reported 5- and 10-year actuarial survival rates of 90 and 84 percent respectively, while the equivalent figures from Gordon and colleagues[49] are 83 and 74 percent.

Clinical Features. The short duration of symptoms is the most striking feature of these tumors. Kurman and Norris[65] found that symptoms had been present for less than 2 weeks in 66 percent of cases and less than 1 week in 45 percent. In 10 percent of patients the symptoms had been present for less than 24 hours. In the M.D. Anderson series,[66] the duration of symptoms ranged from 2 days to 6 months, with a median of 4 weeks. There are many well-documented cases where large endodermal sinus tumors developed within weeks of a normal pelvic examination.

Abdominal pain is reported by 80 percent of patients[65,66] and about 75 percent complain of an abdominal mass.[65,66] A mass was the sole reason for presentation in 20 percent of cases in one series.[67] Nonspecific abdominal distention occurs in about 30 percent. Many patients are febrile at diagnosis.[66] Torsion, hemorrhage, or rupture may occur. The combination of an "acute abdomen" with fever has led to the erroneous diagnosis of acute or ruptured appendicitis.[65]

Gross Pathology. Among 41 endodermal sinus tumors in the Emil Novak Ovarian Tumor Registry, 80 percent exceeded 15 cm in diameter, and the weights were generally between 2 and 10 pounds.[67] In the AFIP series the median diameter was 15 cm[65] while in the M.D. Anderson series it was 17 cm.[66] Between 50[65] and 70 percent[66,67] were Stage I, the contralateral ovary was generally only involved if there was spread to other pelvic or abdominal organs. It is very rare to find occult endodermal sinus tumor in a macroscopically normal contralateral ovary.

The tumor spreads by diffuse metastases to all peritoneal surfaces and the omentum. In the AFIP series, 13 percent ruptured before and 14 percent during surgery[65] while in the M.D. Anderson series the figures were 7 and 29 percent respectively.[66] Ascites is present in about one-quarter of cases.[66] It is seen in about 15 percent of patients with Stage I disease and 45 percent of patients with more advanced disease.[65]

Endodermal sinus tumors are generally encapsulated, round or globular and may adhere to and invade contiguous structures. The cut surface is generally solid although gelatinous cysts or areas of hemorrhage are not uncommon.

Microscopic Pathology. There are several histologic patterns seen in endodermal sinus tumors. The "festoon" pattern containing Schiller-Duvall bodies is pathognomic (Fig. 8). Perivascular structures consisting of a central capillary surrounded by mesenchyme, covered with cuboidal or columnar epithelium, project into sinusoidal spaces to form a pattern resembling mesonephric glomeruli. Intracellular and extracellular periodic acid Schiff (PAS)-positive hyaline droplets containing alpha-fetoprotein are usually present. Though pathognomic, this pattern is not the most common, nor is it present in all tumors. The "reticular" pattern is most common and is characterized by a meshwork of empty vacuoles lined by flattened cells. Other patterns described are a "polyvesicular viteline" type, an "alveolar glandular" type, and a

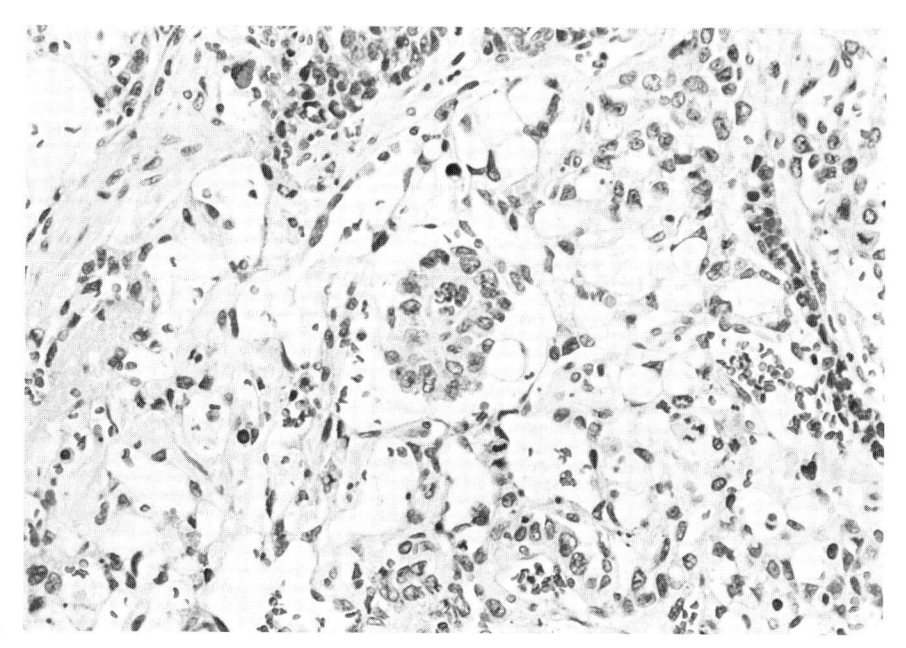

Figure 8. Endodermal sinus tumor. A Schiller-Duvall body is seen in the center of the field. There is a capillary surrounded by a mantle of cells, set within a space resembling a renal glomerulus. Colloid bodies are also present, and these stain positive for alpha-fetoprotein with immunoperoxidase stains. The delicate reticular network surrounding the Schiller-Duvall body is also characteristic.

"solid" type. In all types mitotic activity is brisk. The heterogeneity of histologic patterns within a given tumor may make diagnosis difficult without an exhaustive pathologic examination of many sections of the tumor.

Endodermal sinus tumors frequently occur in combination with other germ cell tumors, including benign cystic teratoma, dysgerminoma, embryonal carcinoma, and less frequently choriocarcinoma.

Prognostic Factors. Until recently the outlook for patients with this tumor was dismal, regardless of the stage of disease, its histologic pattern, the extent of surgical resection, or the use of postoperative radiation or single agent chemotherapy.[65,68,69] Multiagent combination chemotherapy has dramatically changed the prognosis. As Gershenson and colleagues[66] comment: "Earlier reports describing the extremely poor prognosis and almost uniformly fatal outcome need no longer apply. With adequate surgery, aggressive combination chemotherapy, and meticulous monitoring, most patients should survive." Furthermore, patients can have normal pregnancies following treatment for endodermal sinus tumor.

Treatment. The initial management is surgical. A generous vertical incision is used, to allow accurate staging and increase the chance of removing the tumor intact. The affected ovary is removed. In Stage I or more advanced stages without macroscopic tumor on the uterus or contralateral ovary, these structures may be preserved to retain fertility. Biopsy of an apparently normal contralateral ovary is not justified for endodermal sinus tumors, but should be done if the diagnosis is in doubt. Tumor masses should be debulked to the maximum possible extent.

All patients should receive adjuvant chemotherapy postoperatively. The most commonly used regimen involves monthly cycles of a combination of vincristine, actinomycin D, and cyclophosphamide. In the M.D. Anderson series, this regimen resulted in 16 survivals among 22 patients, with the mean survival not reached at 162 months.[66] Alternatively a combination of vinblastine, bleomycin, and *cis*-platinum may be given monthly. This regimen was first used by Einhorn and Donohue[70] for disseminated testicular cancer, and has been effective as first-line adjuvant treatment for endodermal sinus tumors, and following failure of other chemotherapy.[71-73]

We favor the use of vincristine, actinomycin D, and cyclophosphamide for the treatment of patients with minimal residual disease after surgery. The regimen has a good response rate and low toxicity. Second-look surgery is performed after approximately 12 cycles. For patients with a large residual tumor burden or with persistent or recurrent disease after other chemotherapy, we favor the use of the *cis*-platinum, vinblastine, bleomycin regimen. If this combination of drugs is used, second-look surgery may be performed after six to nine cycles.

Endodermal sinus tumors produce alpha-fetoprotein, and it is possible to assay this hormone to monitor regression and detect recurrence.[74,75] While we advocate the serial assay of this tumor marker throughout treatment, and monthly for at least 1 year after apparent "cure," and would consider either repeat surgery or a change of chemotherapy regimen in the face of rising levels, we do not believe the test obviates the need for second-look surgery at the present time. In one case a patient developed massive disseminated disease which was fatal with only a minimal rise in alpha-fetoprotein levels.[76]

Embryonal Carcinoma of the Ovary

This rare tumor is analogous with embryonal carcinoma of the testis. Previously the term has been used in a less specific manner and often included endodermal sinus tumors. In 1976, Kurman and Norris[77] reported 14 cases erroneously classified as other tumor types, most frequently endodermal sinus tumor, in the files of the Armed Forces Institute of Pathology.

Over half the patients were children and most presented with precocious puberty. Older women presented with dysfunctional bleeding or amenorrhea. The duration of symptoms was usually short. Embryonal carcinoma normally produces both alpha-fetoprotein and hCG and this, together with the symptoms of endocrine disturbance, set it apart clinically from endodermal sinus tumors.

Approximately 60 percent of cases are Stage I. They are macroscopically similar to endodermal sinus tumors. Microscopically they consist of sheets or nests of large cells or sheets of primitive pleomorphic cells. Gland-like clefts and papillary processes may be present in the solid areas. Mitoses are frequent. The tumors contain areas of syncytiotrophoblast but no cytotrophoblast. These areas produce hCG, while large mononuclear cells with hyaline droplets are the source of the alpha-fetoprotein.

The management of these tumors is the same as for endodermal sinus tumor, except that both hCG and alpha-fetoprotein should be monitored. Kurman and Norris[77] found an overall actuarial survival of 39 percent, with a survival of 60 percent for Stage I, but few of their cases had the benefit of combination chemotherapy.

Polyembryoma

This tumor which is seen in both sexes, is extremely rare and less than ten cases have been reported in females.[78] All have been found in association with other germ cell tumors and may represent a partial differentiation of primitive germ cell lines.[79] The striking histologic feature is the presence of "embryoids," structures replicating the features of presomitic embryos. The management is as for the endodermal sinus tumors.

Ovarian Choriocarcinoma

Choriocarcinoma of the ovary may be gestational, arising in an ovarian pregnancy or as metastases from uterine choriocarcinoma, or it may be of the nongestational type which is most commonly one element in a mixed germ cell tumor. Turner and associates[80] estimate the chance of choriocarcinoma developing in the ovary as one in four million. Fox and Langley[2] found only 42 appropriately documented cases in the literature up to 1976. Most were combined with dysgerminoma, endodermal sinus tumor, or malignant teratoma.

Clinical Features. The mean age of reported cases is 13 years,[2] but older women may have been excluded by a reluctance to accept ovarian trophoblastic disease as nongestational when there is any possibility of pregnancy. The most common presenting complaints are abdominal distention and pain. Half of the prepubertal girls presented with precocious puberty,[2,80,81] related to the high levels of hCG. In older women the presence of severe abdominal pain, an adnexal mass, and a positive pregnancy test has occasionally led to the diagnosis of ectopic pregnancy.[82]

Macroscopic Pathology. The tumors are usually large, nodular, and hemorrhagic (Fig. 9). Adhesions to pelvic or extrapelvic structures, ascites, and diffuse intraperitoneal studding are not uncommon. Among eight cases reported by Gerbie and colleagues,[83] half had extrapelvic metastases, and three others had widespread pelvic disease.

On cut section the tumor is usually variegated in appearance, with prominent areas of hemorrhage and necrosis; it is less commonly cystic. The

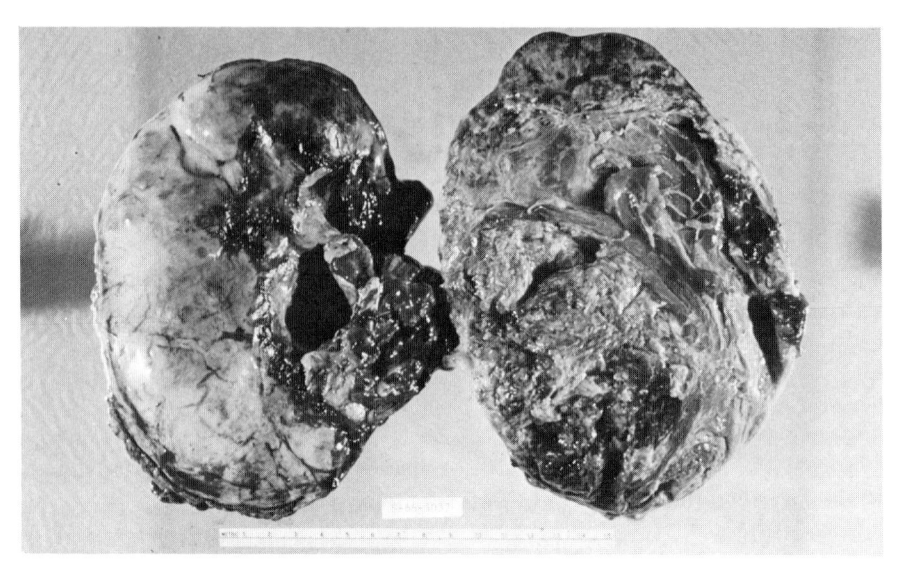

Figure 9. Choriocarcinoma within a mixed germ cell tumor. The child presented because of isosexual precocious pseudopuberty. The tumor was large, friable, partially necrotic, and had areas of hemorrhage.

appearance is generally determined by the characteristics of the admixed germ cell tumor.

Microscopic Pathology. The diagnosis is based on the presence of both cytotrophoblast and syncytiotrophoblast. Generally the cytotrophoblastic cells are surrounded or capped by collections of syncytiotrophoblast. The relative proportions of each is variable. Mitotic activity is common (Fig. 10).

When mixed with other germ cell tumors, choriocarcinoma is often found as scattered nodules within the "host" tumor. Attention may be drawn to these areas by the presence of hemorrhage and necrosis.

Prognosis and Therapy. Methotrexate revolutionized the management of gestational choriocarcinoma, but the nongestational form is much more resistant to treatment. Surgery alone or surgery with radiation or methotrexate produced only rare remissions. In 1969, Wider and colleagues[84] reported sustained remissions in germ cell tumors containing choriocarcinoma utilizing a combination of methotrexate, chlorambucil, and actinomycin D. While multiagent chemotherapy is essential if cures are to be achieved, the optimal regimen is yet to be defined. We favor the use of a combination of *cis*-platinum, vinblastine, and bleomycin on the basis of its known effectiveness against other germ cell tumors and gestational trophoblastic disease.

Immature Teratoma

This term describes a pure teratoma containing immature tissue from one or more of the three germ cell layers.

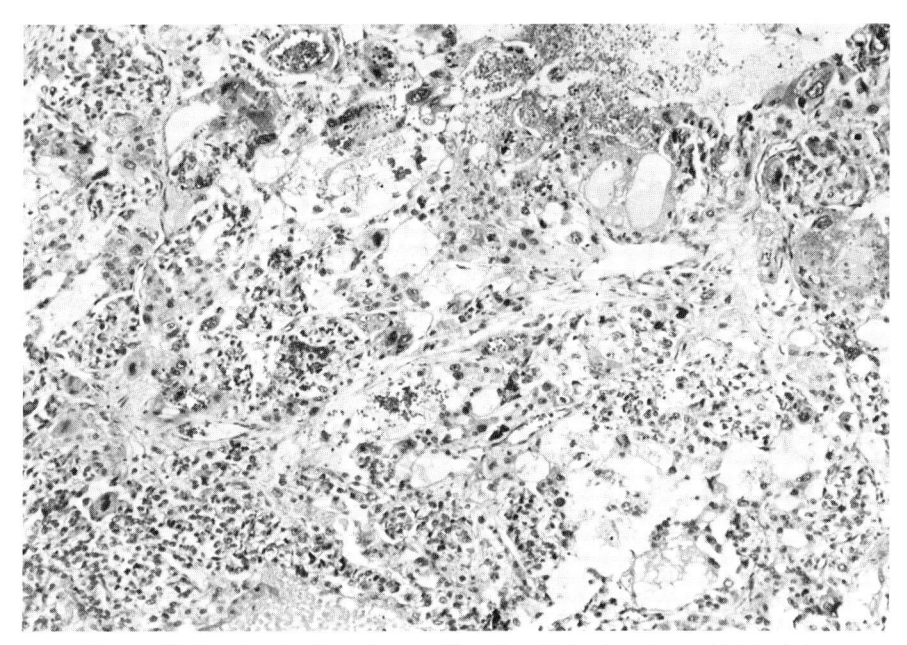

Figure 10. Ovarian choriocarcinoma. There is a biphasic pattern which includes bizarre nuclei within a cytoplasmic syncytium (syncytiotrophoblast) as well as individual cytotrophoblastic cells, set within a hemorrhagic and necrotic background.

Incidence. Immature teratoma is the third most common germ cell malignancy of the ovary[85] and accounted for approximately 20 percent of malignant germ cell tumors seen at the M.D. Anderson Hospital over a 30-year period.[86]

Clinical Features. These tumors have been seen in children as young as 14 months and women as old as 45 but the median age of occurrence is 19 years.[86,87] Symptoms are nonspecific, with abdominal pain, distention, and a palpable mass being the most common. About 25 percent of patients have fever and leukocytosis. Symptoms are often present for less than a month.

Macroscopic Pathology. Stage I disease is present in over half the patients and bilateral ovarian involvement is uncommon, except as part of a pattern of widely disseminated disease.[86,87] Benign cystic teratomas may be present in the other ovary but this should not be mistaken for metastatic disease.

These are large tumors with a mean size of almost 20 cm and ranging from 7 to 35 cm.[87] In one series the mean tumor weight was 2.5 kg.[88] The typical appearance is of a smooth, glistening, encapsulated lesion with a visible cystic component. Hemorrhage and necrosis may be seen. The cut surface shows cysts of various size interspersed with soft fleshy solid areas. Hair, cartilage, bone, and sebaceous material are common. The appearance may be little different from that of a so-called "benign cystic teratoma."

Microscopic Pathology. The tumors are graded according to the amount and type of immature tissue present (Table 5). Neural tissue is the most common and the easiest to grade.[87-89] Norris and associates[87] emphasize that for meaningful grading a minimum of one block for every centimeter of tumor diameter should be examined, together with blocks from all metastatic lesions. Metastases may be more or less differentiated than the primary tumor.

Prognosis. Norris and colleagues[87] found an overall actuarial survival of 63 percent at 5 and 10 years, but for grade 1 tumors the survival was 81 percent, for grade 2, 60 percent, and for grade 3, 30 percent. If metastases were "benign," progression of disease was rare. No patient with grade 3 metastases survived more than 3 years. One problem in assessing the prognosis of patients with these tumors is that the majority of cases were treated before the advent of modern combination chemotherapy.

Treatment. Young women with Stage I disease may be treated with unilateral salpingo-oophorectomy. Where the other ovary is free of disease, but extrapelvic metastasis is present, conservative surgery is still reasonable in younger women, but the metastases should be debulked to the maximum possible extent.

The main question is which patients should receive chemotherapy. Norris and associates[87] advocate surgery alone for patients with grade 1 primary tumor, provided any metastases are "benign." Curry and colleagues[86] are more cautious, pointing out that in their series no patients treated by surgery alone survived, regardless of the stage or grade of the tumor. The combination chemotherapeutic regimen most widely used is vinblastine, actinomycin D, and cyclophosphamide, which in the M.D. Anderson series produced almost 90 percent survivals.

We do not use chemotherapy for patients with adequately sampled grade 1 tumors without metastases, or with "benign" metastases. All others receive combination chemotherapy, usually with vincristine, adriamycin, and cyclophosphamide. For the less well-differentiated tumors, those in whom extensive disease remains, or for those with recurrent or persistent disease, vinblastine, *cis*-platinum, and bleomycin is used.

TABLE 5. GRADING SYSTEM USED FOR MALIGNANT TERATOMAS[a]

Grade 0:	All tissues mature: no mitotic activity.
Grade 1:	Minor foci of abnormally cellular or embryonal tissue mixed with mature elements: slight mitotic activity.
Grade 2:	Moderate quantities of embryonal tissue mixed with mature elements: moderate mitotic activity.
Grade 3:	Large quantities of embryonal tissue present: high mitotic activity.

[a]*Note.* The tumors may not be uniform throughout, so the worst area is graded.
(*From Talerman A: Pathology of the Female Genital Tract*, 2nd ed. New York, Springer-Verlag, 1982, with permission.)[52]

Second-look surgery is advised in all patients 6 to 12 months after initial surgery. It is not uncommon, after combination chemotherapy, to find that previously malignant peritoneal implants have become "benign,"[90] so adequate sampling is essential to avoid the incorrect conclusion that the condition is not improved.

Mixed Germ Cell Tumors

While the foregoing discussion centered on "pure" forms of germ cell tumors, two or more germ cell elements may be combined in the one tumor. Mixed tumors account for about 40 percent of malignant germ cell tumors of the testis, but only 8 percent in the ovary.[91] Dysgerminoma is found in 80 percent of tumors, endodermal sinus tumor in 70 percent, teratoma in 53 percent, choriocarcinoma in 20 percent, and embryonal carcinoma in 16 percent.[91]

The clinical features and presentation of the patients were similar to those with other germ cell malignancies. They tended to be found in children, adolescents, and young women and symptoms were generally of short duration.

The main prognostic factors for Stage I disease were the size of the tumor and its histologic cell types. Where one-third or more of the tumor is endodermal sinus tumor, choriocarcinoma, or poorly differentiated teratoma, the outlook is poor. Tumors with smaller proportions of these elements or with combinations of dysgerminoma, embryonal carcinoma or well-differentiated teratoma

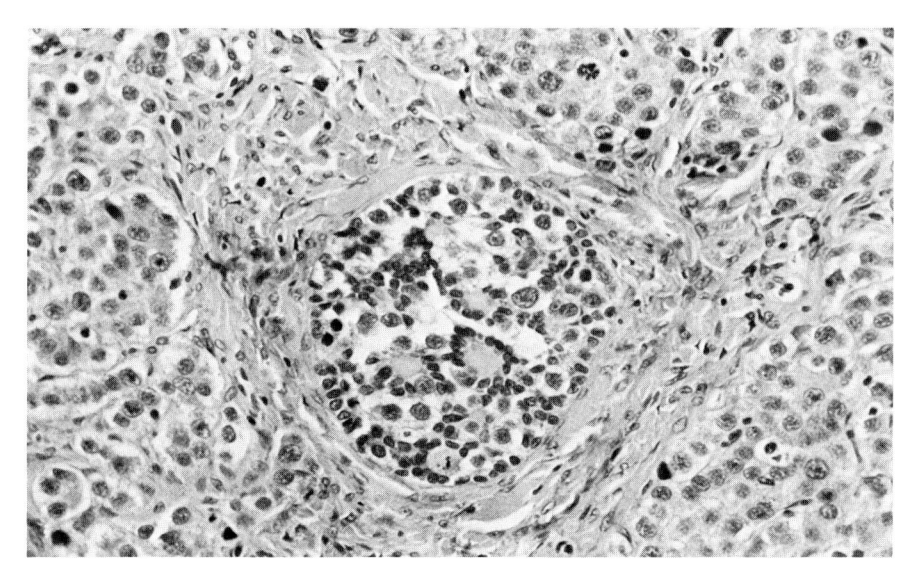

Figure 11. Gonadoblastoma. In the center of the field are small granulosa and germ-like cells surrounding laminated eosinophilic masses which resemble Call-Exner bodies. These may calcify. Surrounding this typical focus of gonadoblastoma is a proliferation of dysgerminoma.

had a good outlook. All patients in one series with tumors less than 10 cm in diameter survived, regardless of the composition of the tumor.[91]

Mixed tumors are treated as appropriate for the germ cell component of the tumor which is present in significant amounts and carries the worst prognosis.

Gonadoblastoma

This tumor arises almost exclusively in dysgenetic gonads, of indeterminate type, although some originate in streak gonads or cryptorchid dysgenetic testes.[92] Most occur before age 40 and are not large. Most contain a mixture of germ cells. Leydig cells may be present (Fig. 11). Half contain dysgerminoma and these are benign, but those with endodermal sinus tumor, embryonal carcinoma, or choriocarcinoma are often lethal.[93]

Treatment is total hysterectomy and bilateral gonadectomy. Radiation or chemotherapy is utilized according to the type of tumor cells present and the stage of the disease.

REFERENCES

1. Weiss NS, Homonchuck T, Young JL: Incidence of the histologic types of ovarian cancer: The US third national cancer survey, 1969–1971. Gynecol Oncol 5:161, 1977
2. Fox H, Langley FA: Tumours of the Ovary. London: Heinemann, 1976
3. von Werdt, quoted by Busby T, Anderson GW: Feminizing mesenchymomas of the ovary. Am J Obstet Gynecol 68:1391, 1954
4. Meyer R: The pathology of some special ovarian tumors and their relation to sex characteristics. Am J Obstet Gynecol 22:697, 1931
5. Robinson MR: Primary and secondary ovarian cancer. Surg Gynecol Obstet 51:321, 1930
6. Furth J, Butterworth JS: Neoplastic diseases occurring among mice subjected to general irradiation with x-rays. Am J Cancer 28:66, 1936
7. Geist SH, Gaines JA, Pollack AD: Experimental biologically active ovarian tumors in mice. Am J Obstet Gynecol 38:786, 1939
8. Biskind MS, Biskind GR: Development of tumors in the rat ovary after transplantation into the spleen. Proc Soc Exper Biol Med 55:176, 1944
9. Biskind GR, Biskind MS: Experimental ovarian tumors in rats. Am J Clin Pathol 19:501, 1949
10. Fathalla MF: The occurrence of granulosa and theca cell tumors in normal ovaries. J Obstet Gynaecol Brit Cwlth 74:279, 1967
11. McKay DG, Hertig AT, Hickey WF: The histogenesis of granulosa and theca cell tumors of the human ovary. Obstet Gynecol 1:125, 1953
12. Norris HJ, Taylor HB: Virilization associated with cystic granulosa tumors. Obstet Gynecol 34:629, 1969
13. Zemke EE, Herrell WE: Bilateral granulosa cell tumors: Successful removal from a child fourteen weeks of age. Am J Obstet Gynecol 41:704, 1941
14. Bjorkholm E, Pettersson F: Granulosa cell and theca cell tumors. Acta Obstet Gynecol Scand 59:361, 1980

15. Ohel G, Kaneti H, Schenker JG: Granulosa cell tumors in Israel: A study of 172 cases. Gynecol Oncol 15:278, 1983
16. Evans AJ, Gaffey TA, Malkasian GD, Annegers JT: Clinicopathologic review of 118 granulosa and 82 theca cell tumors. Obstet Gynecol 55:213, 1980
17. Rayner PHW: Early Puberty. In Brook CGD (ed): Clinical Pediatric Endocrinology. Oxford: Blackwell Scientific Publications, 1981, p 224
18. Norris HJ, Taylor HB: Prognosis of granulosa theca tumors of the ovary. Cancer 21:255, 1968
19. Sjostedt S, Wahlen T: Prognosis of granulosa cell tumors. Acta Obstet Gynecol Scand 40 [suppl] 6:1, 1961
20. Diddle AW: Granulosa and theca cell tumors: Prognosis. Cancer 5:215, 1952
21. Gillibrand PN: Granulosa theca cell tumors of the ovary associated with pregnancy. Am J Obstet Gynecol 94:1108, 1966
22. Dockerty MB, McCarty WC: Granulosa cell tumors, with a report of a 34 pound specimen and a review. Am J Obstet Gynecol 37:425, 1939
23. Fox H, Agrawal K, Langley FA: A clinicopathologic study of 92 cases of granulosa cell tumor of the ovary with special reference to the factors influencing prognosis. Cancer 35:231, 1975
24. Scully RE: Ovarian tumors: A review. Am J Pathol 87:686, 1977
25. Novak ER, Kutchmesgi J, Mupas RS, Woodruff JD: Feminizing gonadal stromal tumors: Analysis of the granulosa theca cell tumors of the ovarian tumor registry. Obstet Gynecol 38:701, 1971
26. Emge LA: Endometrial cancer and feminizing tumors of the ovaries. Significance of their coexistence. Obstet Gynecol 1:511, 1953
27. Bjorkholme E, Silfversward C: Prognostic factors in granulosa cell tumors. Gynecol Oncol 11:261, 1981
28. Stenwig JT, Hazekamp JT, Beecham JB: Granulosa cell tumors of the ovary. A clinicopathological study of 118 cases with long-term follow-up. Gynecol Oncol 7:136, 1979
29. Schwartz PE, Smith JP: Treatment of ovarian stromal tumors. Am J Obstet Gynecol 125:402, 1976
30. Kolstadt P: Malignant tumors of the ovary: Norwegian experience and protocols for management. In Coppleson M (ed): Gynecologic Oncology. Fundamental Principles and Clinical Practice. Edinburgh: Churchill Livingston, 1981, p 721
31. Lack E, Perez-Atayde AR, Murthy ASK, et al: Granulosa theca cell tumors in premenarchial girls. A clinical and pathologic study of ten cases. Cancer 48:1846, 1981
32. Roth LM, Anderson MC, Govan ADT, et al: Sertoli-Leydig cell tumors: A clinicopathologic study of 34 cases. Cancer 48:187, 1981
33. Janouski NA, Paramanandhan TL: Ovarian Tumors. Philadelphia: Saunders, 1973, p 73
34. Teilum G: Special Tumors of the Ovary and Testis, 2nd ed. Philadelphia: Lippincott, 1976
35. Pedowitz P, O'Brien FB: Arrhenoblastoma of the ovary: A review of the literature and report of 2 cases. Obstet Gynecol 16:62, 1960
36. Novak ER, Long JH: Arrhenoblastoma of the ovary. A review of the Ovarian Tumor Registry. Am J Obstet Gynecol 92:1082, 1965
37. Teilum G: Classification of testicular and ovarian androblastoma and Sertoli cell tumors. A survey of comparative studies with consideration of histogenesis, endocrinology and embryological theories. Cancer 11:769, 1958

38. Dougal D: A granulosa cell tumor of tubular or adenomatous type. J Obstet Gynaecol Br Emp 52:370, 1945
39. Costero I, Barroso-Mochel R: Hipertension de origen neoplasico. I. Tumor de cellulas hiliares del ovario. Arch Inst Cardiol Mexico 42:52, 1970
40. Merkow LP, Slifkin M, Aceverdo HF, et al: Ultrastructure of interstitial (hilar) cell tumors of the ovary. Obstet Gynecol 37:845, 1971
41. Stewart RS, Woodward DE: Malignant ovarian hilus cell tumor. Arch Pathol 73:91, 1962
42. Echt CR, Hadd HE: Androgen excretion patterns in a patient with a metastatic hilus cell tumor of the ovary. Am J Obstet Gynecol 100:1055, 1968
43. O'Hern TM, Neubecker RD: Arrhenoblastoma. Obstet Gynecol 19:758, 1962
44. Asadourian LA, Taylor HB: Dysgerminoma. An analysis of 105 cases. Obstet Gynecol 33:370, 1969
45. Mueller CW, Topkins P, Lapp WA: Dysgerminoma of the ovary. An analysis of 427 cases. Am J Obstet Gynecol 60:153, 1950
46. Higuchi K, Kato T: Dysgerminoma of the ovary. J Japan Obstet Gynecol Soc 5:206, 1958
47. Jatoi AF: Dysgerminoma of the ovary. A study of 22 cases. J Postgrad Med 5:22, 1959
48. Breen JL, Neubecker RD: Ovarian malignancy in children with special reference to the germ cell tumors. Ann NY Acad Sci 142:658, 1967
49. Gordon A, Lipton D, Woodruff JD: Dysgerminoma: A review of 158 cases from the Emil Novak Ovarian Tumor Registry. Obstet Gynecol 58:497, 1981
50. De Palo G, Pilotti S, Kenda R, Ratti E, et al: Natural history of dysgerminoma. Am J Obstet Gynecol 143:799, 1982
51. Novak ER, Lambroo CD, Woodruff JD: Ovarian tumors in pregnancy. An ovarian tumor registry review. Obstet Gynecol 46:401, 1975
52. Talerman A: Germ cell tumors of the ovary. In Blaustein A (ed): Pathology of the Female Genital Tract, 2nd ed. New York: Springer–Verlag, 1982, p 602
53. Castleman BC, Scully RE, McNeely BU: Case reports of the Massachusetts General Hospital. Case 11-1972. N Engl J Med 286:594, 1972
54. Hain AM: An unusual case of precocious puberty associated with ovarian dysgerminoma. J Clin Endocrin 9:1349, 1949
55. Santesson L: Clinical and pathologic survey of ovarian tumors treated at the Radiumhemmet. 1. Dysgerminoma. Acta Radiol 28:643, 1947
56. Abell MR, Johnson VJ, Holz F: Ovarian neoplasms in childhood and adolescence. I. Tumors of germ cell origin. Am J Obstet Gynecol 92:1059, 1965
57. Pedowitz P, Felmus LB, Grayzel DM: Dysgerminoma of the ovary. Prognosis and treatment. Am J Obstet Gynecol 70:1284, 1955
58. Brody S: Clinical aspects of dysgerminoma of the ovary. Acta Radiol 56:209, 1961
59. Marshall AHE, Dyan AD: An immune reaction in man against seminomas, dysgerminomas, pinealomas, and the mediastinal tumors of similar appearance. Lancet 2:1102, 1964
60. Freel JH, Cassir JF, Pierce VK, et al: Dysgerminoma of the ovary. Cancer 43:798, 1979
61. Boyes DA, Pankratz E, Galliford BW, et al: Experience with dysgerminoma at the cancer control agency in British Columbia. Gynecol Oncol 6:123, 1978
62. Schiller W: Mesonephroma ovarii. Am J Cancer 35:1, 1939
63. Teilum G: Endodermal sinus tumors of the ovary and testis. Comparative mor-

phology of the so called mesonephroma ovarii (Schiller) and extraembryonic (yolk sac-allantoic) structures of the rat placenta. Cancer 12:1092, 1959
64. Norris HJ, Jensen RD: Relative frequency of ovarian neoplasms in children and adolescents. Cancer 30:713, 1972
65. Kurman RJ, Norris HJ: Endodermal sinus tumor of the ovary. A clinical and pathologic analysis of 71 cases. Cancer 38:2404, 1976
66. Gershenson DM, Del Junco G, Herson J, Rutledge FN: Endodermal sinus tumor of the ovary: The M.D. Anderson experience. Obstet Gynecol 61:194, 1983
67. Jimerson GK, Woodruff JD: Ovarian extraembryonal teratoma. I. Endodermal sinus tumor. Am J Obstet Gynecol 127:73, 1977
68. Smith JP, Rutledge F: Advances in chemotherapy for gynecologic cancer. Cancer 36:669, 1975
69. Forney JP, Disaia PJ, Morrow CP: Endodermal sinus tumor. A report of two sustained remissions treated postoperatively with a combination of actinomycin D, 5-fluorouracil and cyclophosphamide. Obstet Gynecol 45:186, 1975
70. Einhorn LH, Donohue J: Cis-diamminedichloroplatinum, vinblastine and bleomycin combination chemotherapy in disseminated testicular cancer. Ann Intern Med 87:293, 1977
71. Julian CG, Barrett JM, Richardson RL, Greco FA: Bleomycin, vinblastine, and *cis*-platinum in the treatment of advanced endodermal sinus tumor. Obstet Gynecol 56:396, 1980
72. Lokey JL, Baker JJ, Price NA, Winokur SH: Cis-platin, vinblastine and bleomycin for endodermal sinus tumor of the ovary. Ann Intern Med 94:56, 1981
73. Williams S, Slayton R, Silverberg S, et al: Response of malignant ovarian germ cell tumors to *cis*-platinum, vinblastine, and bleomycin (PVB). Proc Am Assoc Cancer Res. Am Soc Clin Oncol 22:463, 1981
74. Talerman A, Haije WG, Baggerman L: Serum alpha-fetoprotein (AFP) in diagnosis and management of endodermal sinus (yolk sac) tumors of the ovary. Cancer, 41:272, 1978
75. Romero R, Schwartz PE: Alpha-fetoprotein determinations in the management of endodermal sinus tumors and mixed germ cell tumors of the ovary. Am J Obstet Gynecol 141:126, 1981
76. Sell A, Soggaard H, Norgard-Pedersen B: Serum alpha-fetoprotein as a marker for the effect of postoperative radiation therapy and/or chemotherapy in eight cases of ovarian endodermal sinus tumor. Int J Cancer 18:574, 1976
77. Kurman RJ, Norris HJ: Embryonal carcinoma of the ovary. A clinicopathologic entity distinct from endodermal sinus tumor, resembling embryonal carcinoma of the adult testis. Cancer 38:2420, 1976
78. Beck JS, Fulmer HF, Lee ST: Solid malignant ovarian teratoma with "embryoid bodies" and trophoblastic differentiation. J Pathol 99:67, 1969
79. Pierce GB, Dixon FJ: Testicular teratomas. I. Demonstration of teratogenesis by metamorphosis of multipotential cells. Cancer 12:573, 1959
80. Turner HB, Douglas WM, Gladding TC: Choriocarcinoma of the ovary. Obstet Gynecol 24:918, 1964
81. De Haan QC: Nongestational choriocarcinoma of the ovary. Report of a case. Obstet Gynecol 26:708, 1965
82. Marrubini G: Primary chorionepithelioma of the ovary. Report of two cases. Acta Obstet Gynaecol Scand 28:251, 1948

83. Gerbie MV, Brewer JI, Tamimi H: Primary choriocarcinoma of the ovary. Obstet Gynecol 46:720, 1975
84. Wider JA, Marshall JR, Bardin CW, et al: Sustained remissions after chemotherapy for primary ovarian cancers containing choriocarcinoma. N Engl J Med 280:1439, 1969
85. Norris HJ, Jensen RD: Relative frequency of ovarian germ cell neoplasms in children and adolescents. Cancer 30:713, 1972
86. Curry SL, Smith JP, Gallagher HS: Malignant teratoma of the ovary. Prognostic factors and treatment. Am J Obstet Gynecol 131:845, 1978
87. Norris HJ, Zirkin HJ, Benson WL: Immature (malignant) teratoma of the ovary. A clinical and pathologic study of 58 cases. Cancer 37:2359, 1976
88. Nogales FF, Favara BE, Major FJ, Silverberg SG: Immature teratoma of the ovary with a neural component ("solid teratoma"). Hum Pathol 7:625, 1976
89. Breen JL, Neubecker RD: Malignant teratomas of the ovary. Obstet Gynecol 21:669, 1963
90. Disaia PJ, Salz A, Kagan AR, Morrow CP: Chemotherapeutic retroconversion of immature teratoma of the ovary. Obstet Gynecol 49:346, 1977
91. Kurman RJ, Norris HJ: Malignant mixed germ cell tumors of the ovary. A clinical and pathologic analysis of 30 cases. Obstet Gynecol 48:579, 1976
92. Scully RE: Gonadoblastoma. A review of 74 cases. Cancer 25:1340, 1970
93. Talerman A: Gonadoblastoma associated with embryonal carcinoma. Obstet Gynecol 43:138, 1974

CHAPTER 9
Gestational Trophoblastic Neoplasia

Chorionic tissue behaves in a pseudomalignant fashion even under normal circumstances. It invades the uterine wall but ordinarily stops at the decidual-myometrial junction. Embolization occurs, but the deposits do not behave in a malignant fashion.[1] The tissue itself may show bizarre histologic patterns, which vary through all stages of anaplasia and degrees of proliferation. They may be seen in any specimen of chorionic tissue. In 1894, Gottschalk[2] described the neoplasm as arising from the chorion and called it choriocarcinoma. In 1895, Marchand[3] presented further evidence that the chorion was the source of the tumor and termed it chorioepithelioma. In 1910, Ewing[4] observed that this was a very unpredictable type of malignancy and described three forms of the neoplasm: hydatidiform mole, chorioadenoma destruens, and choriocarcinoma.

It is now well recognized that histopathologic features do not completely predict malignant potential and that this classification is inadequate. The difference between the relatively benign and very malignant forms are more accurately expressed in terms of biologic function, that is, production and excretion of human chorionic gonadotropin (hCG). Furthermore, the amount of hCG produced is related to the amount of trophoblastic tissue present.[5] Thus, variation from the excretion pattern for normal pregnancies suggests abnormal growth. Similarly, the reappearance of hCG in body fluids suggests renewed growth of trophoblast whether in utero or elsewhere. Incidence of gestational trophoblastic neoplasia (GTN) shows highest rates among the poor in the developing countries with the frequency of hydatidiform mole being greatest in the

Far East.[6] There, the incidence is seven to eight times higher than it is in the United States. Molar pregnancy occurs in about 1 in 1200 pregnancies in the United States compared with 1 in 82 pregnancies in Taiwan, which has the highest reported rate of hydatidiform mole in the world.[7] Approximately 3000 hydatidiform moles occur each year in the United States.[8] Data from the United Kingdom and Italy indicate that pregnancy in women under 20 and over 40 years of age is more likely to result in molar neoplasia and persistent trophoblastic disease.[9-11] Low socioeconomic status and malnutrition are commonly seen in patients with the highest rates of hydatidiform mole.[12,13] It has also been noted that in areas indigenous for hydatidiform mole the common foods are rice, beans, and corn which are cooked by prolonged boiling.

A molar incidence of 1 in 600 for therapeutic abortions has been reported.[14,15] It seems likely, however, that this is an overreading based upon gross appearance, with molar degeneration (transitional mole) being interpreted as hydatidiform mole, because most abortion clinics do not send specimens for histopathologic examination.

While GTN is certainly not common, a busy obstetrician-gynecologist will see approximately one case of molar pregnancy each year. Approximately 15 percent of patients with hydatidiform mole will develop malignant gestational trophoblastic neoplasia. Chorioadenoma destruens (invasive mole) occurs in 1 of every 15,000 pregnancies. Choriocarcinoma occurs in 1 of every 40,000 pregnancies with approximately 50 percent of these being after hydatidiform mole, approximately 25 percent after an abortion, 22 percent after term pregnancy, and approximately 3 percent after ectopic pregnancy.

NATURAL HISTORY OF GTN

Most of our information on the natural history of GTN comes from the prechemotherapy era. The data available have been summarized by Surwit and Hammond[16] as shown in Table 1. In a more recent report, Lurain and associates[17] analyzed 738 patients with hydatidiform mole who were referred to the John I. Brewer Trophoblastic Disease Center of Northwestern University for follow-up and human chorionic gonadotropin (hCG) testing after evacuation. There was spontaneous regression of trophoblastic disease in 596 (80.8 percent) of the 738 patients. Of these 596 patients, regression occurred in 11 (1.8 percent) by day 10 after evacuation, in 124 (20.8 percent) between days 11 and 30, in 255 (42.8 percent) between days 31 and 60, and in 206 (34.6 percent) between days 61 and 170. Treatment with chemotherapeutic agents was required in 142 (19.2 percent) of the 738 patients; 125 (16.9 percent) of these had invasive mole (107 nonmetastatic and 18 metastatic) and 17 (2.3 percent) had choriocarcinoma (13 nonmetastatic and 4 metastatic). All 596 patients whose hCG titers declined spontaneously to normal levels have remained well and free of disease. All 142 treated patients experienced permanent remission. Thus, all 738 patients are well and free of disease 4 to 18

TABLE 1. GESTATIONAL TROPHOBLASTIC NEOPLASIA—NATURAL HISTORY

	Incidence	Morbidity	Mortality	Outcome
Hydatidiform mole	1/1200 pregnancies	Moderate, (sepsis, hemorrhage, toxemia)	Low	80+% spontaneous remission after evacuation; 15+% progression to malignancy requiring therapy
Chorioadenoma destruens (invasive mole)	1/15,000 pregnancies, anteceded by hydatidiform mole	Major (sepsis, hemorrhage, uterine perforation, loss of reproductive capacity)	15% (prechemotherapy) even with hysterectomy	
Choriocarcinoma	1/40,000 pregnancies, 50% after hydatidiform mole, 25% after term pregnancy 25% after abortion, or ectopic pregnancy	Major	Nonmetastatic—60% (prechemotherapy); Metastatic—98% with surgery and loss of reproductivity (prechemotherapy)	

(From Surwit EA, Hammond CB: Yearbook of Obstetrics and Gynecology—1980. Chicago, Year Book, 1980, with permission.)[16]

years after evacuation of the hydatidiform mole. The follow-up regimen described in this report furnishes information on natural history of molar pregnancies after evacuation and provides an excellent means by which all patients can be safely managed following termination of a hydatidiform mole.

THE HUMAN GONADOTROPIN ASSAY

Human chorionic gonadotropin (hCG) is elaborated by both normal and neoplastic human trophoblast. It is seen in virtually all patients with GTN.[8,17] The titer of hCG produced is proportional to the number of trophoblastic cells present.[18] Thus, hCG determinations, together with histopathologic studies, permit early diagnosis and afford a method of monitoring the effects of treatment. Human chorionic gonadotropin is a glycoprotein composed of alpha and beta subunits. The range of techniques for assaying for hCG together with their degree of sensitivity have been summarized by Surwit and Hammond[16] and are shown in Table 2.

Most pregnancy tests are positive when the hCG level is over 50 IU per liter of urine. It is important to know that they extend down to the normal range of pituitary LH and up to the lower levels of detectability for hCG

TABLE 2. ASSAY TECHNIQUES FOR hCG DETERMINATIONS

Test	hCG Sensitivity
Immunologic commercial pregnancy test (latex agglutination and inhibition)	>700–5000 IU/L
Biologic assay (mouse uterine weight)	0.5–10 IU/L (5 muu/L)
Radioimmunologic[a] LH-hCG whole molecule	<5mIU/ml
Beta subunit hCG	<5 mIU/ml

[a]Note that only the beta subunit radioimmunoassay is hCG specific.
(From Surwit EA, Hammond CB: Yearbook of Obstetrics and Gynecology—1980, Chicago, Year Book, 1980 with permission.)[16]

patients with trophoblastic neoplasia.[8,17,19] Thus, pregnancy tests may be helpful if positive but are worthless if negative. Human chorionic gonadotropin can now be measured in serum as well as urine, and the serum estimations are more accurate. Early radioimmunoassay studies cross-related hCG and pituitary LH.[20] In 1972, however, Vaitukaitis and colleagues[21] reported on a radioimmunoassay technique utilizing an antibody specific for the beta subunit of hCG, and this has allowed the separation of hCG from LH. The sensitivity of this test is adequate to detect hCG at very low levels (less than 5 mIU/ml) and has become very useful for the diagnosis, treatment, and follow-up of patients with GTN. It has been shown that normal trophoblastic cells have higher secretory rates of hCG than choriocarcinoma cells. A single choriocarcinoma cell in tissue culture produces about 10^{-5} IU of hCG in 24 hours. At this rate 10^5 tumor cells are required to produce approximately 1.0 mIU/ml which is the limit of detectability by the most sensitive radioimmunoassay. Thus, it follows that the patient whose serum beta subunit of hCG has just become undetectable may still have a tumor burden of just under 10^5 viable cells present.[22] This fact is taken into account in the treatment of persistent trophoblastic disease. Thus, chemotherapy is continued beyond the point at which the beta subunit of hCG is undetectable. Indeed at least three negative tests should be obtained before chemotherapy is discontinued so that cell killing of trophoblastic tissue may continue to the theoretic last cell. It is vital that a gynecologist taking care of a patient with trophoblastic disease understands the assay results being reported. It should be kept in mind that serum value of 40,000 mIU/ml is equivalent to a 24-hour urine value of 100,000 IU.[16] It must also be understood that even with three negative tests, choriocarcinoma may still be present and clinical acumen should not be abandoned.[23] The effect of methotrexate on the growth and hCG secretion of human choriocarcinoma cell lines in vitro is being studied, and from these studies a better understanding of mechanisms of resistance is to be expected.

CLASSIFICATION

Technical Bulletin No. 59 of the ACOG[14] gives a simple classification on the basis of which therapy can be individualized (Table 3). GTN is primary hydatidiform mole. Malignant GTN may be nonmetastatic or metastatic, with the latter group being further divided into good prognosis and poor prognosis categories. With clinical observation and adequate use of serum beta subunit hCG assays, the treatment applied can result in very high cure rates for patients with GTN. This monitoring system is based on the article by Hammond and associates published in 1973.[24]

BENIGN GTN (PRIMARY HYDATIDIFORM MOLE)

Benign gestational trophoblastic neoplasia takes one of three forms: hydatidiform mole, molar degeneration (transitional mole), and hydropic degeneration of villi in a blighted ovum. Hydatidiform mole is the most easily recognized of these, and so we will confine our remarks in this section to the treatment of primary hydatidiform mole. Benign hydatidiform mole is an abnormal gestation characterized by hydropic degeneration of villi, decreased vasculature, and trophoblastic proliferation. These changes usually occur in the absence of an intact fetus.

TABLE 3. GESTATIONAL TROPHOBLASTIC NEOPLASIA (GTN)[a]

I. Benign GTN
   A. Hydatidiform mole
   B. ? Molar degeneration (transitional mole)
   C. ? Hydropic villi in blighted ovum
II. Malignant GTN
   A. Nonmetastatic
      1. Persistent hydatidiform mole
      2. Invasive mole (chorioadenoma destruens)
      3. Choriocarcinoma
   B. Metastatic GTN
      1. Good prognosis, low-risk
         a. Initial urinary hCG titer <100,000 IU/24 hr or serum hCG titer <40,000 mIU/ml
         b. Duration of symptoms <4 months
         c. No liver or brain metastasis
         d. No previous chemotherapy
      2. Poor prognosis, high-risk
         a. Initial urinary hCG titer >100,000 IU/24 hr or serum hCG titer >40,000 mIU/ml
         b. Duration of symptoms >4 months
         c. Liver or brain metastasis
         d. Previous chemotherapy
         e. Disease following term pregnancy

[a]Classification of GTN used as a basis for treatment.
(From ACOG Tech Bull No. 59, Dec. 1980, with permission.)[14]

Pathogenesis of Hydatidiform Mole

Hertig and Edmonds[25] suggest that trophoblastic neoplasia results from a defective (blighted) ovum which fails to abort spontaneously and gives rise to vascular insufficiency of the placental tissue. Functioning trophoblastic tissues take up fluid from the maternal blood flowing in the intervillous space. This fluid collects in the villous stroma because the pathologic ovum fails to develop fetal circulation to the trophoblasts. The result is progressive fluid accumulation within the chorionic villi and hydropic degeneration. An alternative view has been suggested by Park.[26] He states that the primary defect lies in the trophoblastic tissue, which in its abnormal state does not support the growth of a potentially normal ovum, so that the embryo either aborts or becomes blighted in the first 3 to 5 weeks of development with the formation of characteristic hydropic villi of hydatidiform mole.

More recent morphologic and cytogenetic studies of molar specimens have shown that at least two distinct categories of mole exist.[27,28] These are the partial (incomplete) mole, and the classic (complete) mole. These two variants of benign GTN have differences in their gross morphology, histopathology, and karyotype.

Partial moles have normal villi intermingled with swollen hydropic villi, a fetus, a cord, and/or amnionic membrane associated with them. Microscopic examination of partial moles shows scant or absent trophoblastic hyperplasia and anaplasia. Some villi contain a fetal circulation. Chromosomal analysis of partial moles reveals a polyploid karyotype, which is most frequently triploid.[28]

Complete moles have hydropic swelling of all villi on gross examination with absence of a fetus, cord, and amniotic membrane. Complete moles exhibit marked hyperplasia and anaplasia of the trophoblasts. The villi show no evidence of a fetal circulation. The karyotype of complete moles is uniformly 46×x.[29,30] Kajii and Ohama[29] studied molar chromosomes by fluorescence-banding techniques, and found that the chromosomal material of complete hydatidiform moles is totally inherited from the paternal contribution. GTN has been observed in homozygous twins and this suggests that patients who develop trophoblastic disease have a genetic factor which interferes with meiosis and favors the production of ova with absent or inactivated nuclei.[31]

The clinical usefulness of distinguishing between partial and complete moles lies in the fact that malignant trophoblastic sequelae (chorioadenoma destruens or choriocarcinoma) in a patient who has a partial mole, by these morphologic or karyotypic criteria, are very unlikely.[28,30] One patient with a partial mole that required chemotherapy to achieve remission has been reported. In contrast, clinical follow-up of patients with complete hydatidiform moles confirms that they are at risk for development of malignant gestational trophoblastic neoplasms especially, but not exclusively, with a 46×× karyotype.[28,32] Thus, cases of partial mole rarely need to be regarded as potentially malignant. However, this point needs to be confirmed by additional studies with adequate clinical follow-up. At present, all patients with documented partial moles should have the same careful surveillance as patients with complete moles.[33]

Pathology of Primary Hydatidiform Mole

Grossly, hydatidiform mole is characterized by a mass of vesicles which replace the normal placental architecture. The vesicles may resemble grapes and are individual villi that have become edematous (hydropic degeneration). The hydropic villi may vary in size from 3 mm to 3 cm in diameter, depending on the gestational age of the mole. In a typical specimen the diagnosis is obvious (Fig. 1). However, it may be difficult if the amount of tissue is small, or if it has been mechanically distorted with rupture of the characteristic vesicles by suction curettage. Microscopically there are three major features of hydatidiform mole: (1) edematous swelling of chorionic villi, (2) absence of fetal blood vessels in the villi, and (3) proliferation of trophoblast (Fig. 2). Trophoblastic proliferation is variable in its degree and involves one or both layers which surround the villi, the inner cytotrophoblastic layer and the outer syncytiotrophoblast.

Histologic Grading Linked to Prognosis. Hertig and Sheldon[34] extensively reviewed the histopathology of molar tissue in an attempt to correlate tissue appearance with subsequent biologic behavior. They studied 200 cases of hydatidiform mole and initially reported 6 groups ranging from benign to malignant based on the amount and appearance of the trophoblast. There is

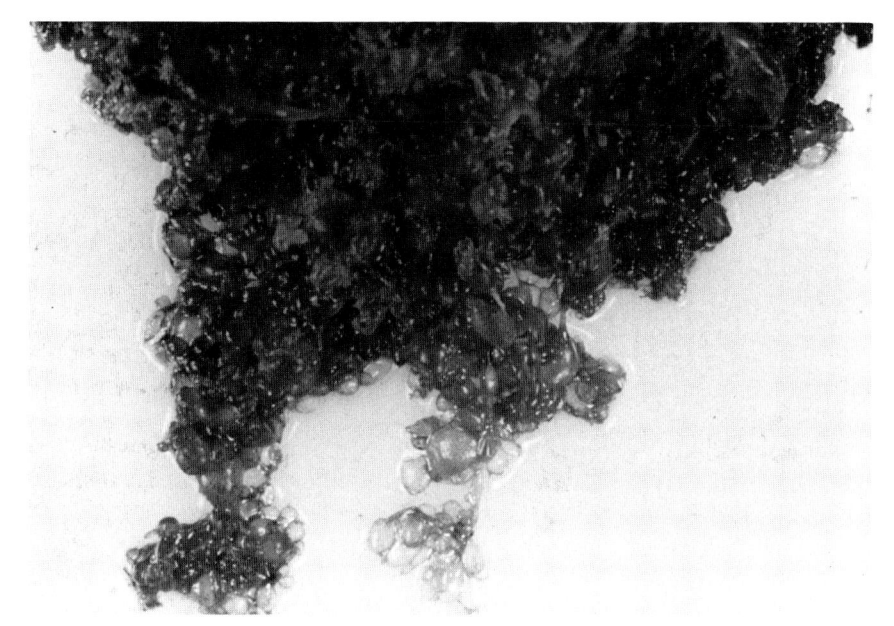

Figure 1. Hydatidiform mole. Individual villi are edematous, cystic, enlarged and appear as translucent clusters of grapes.

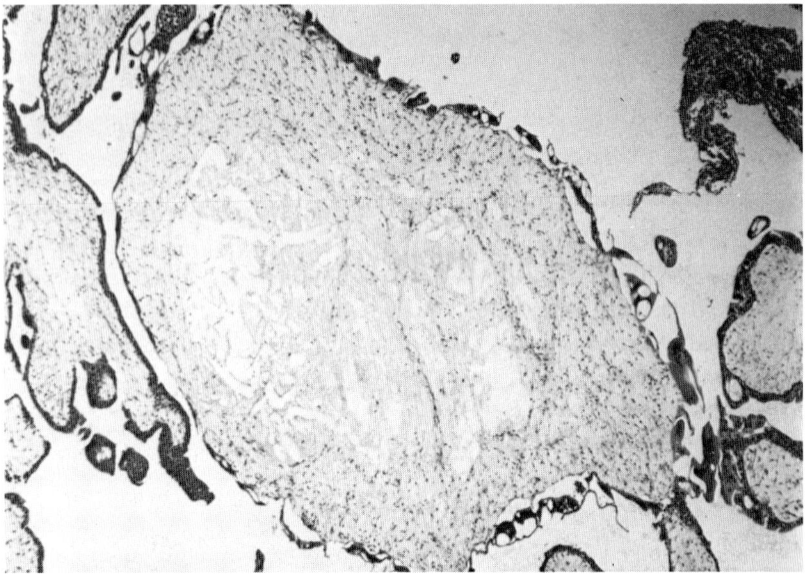

A

B

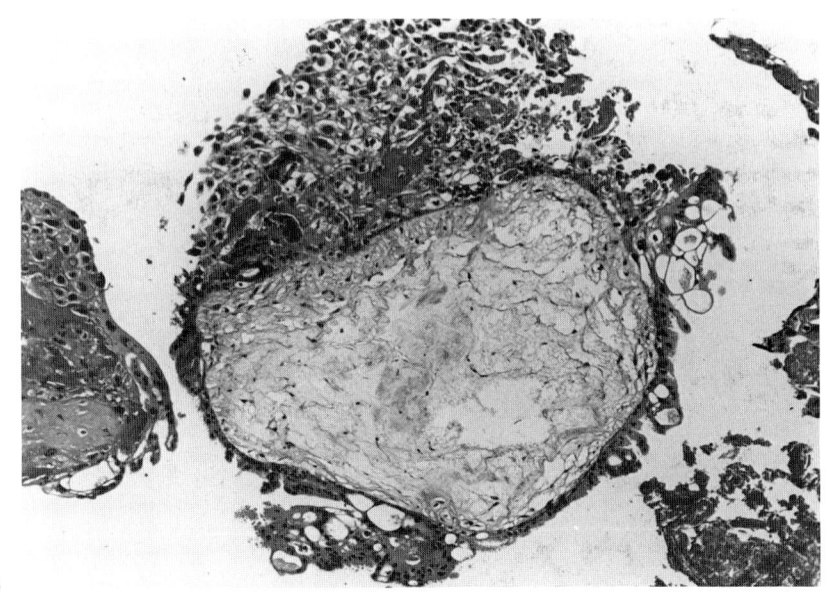

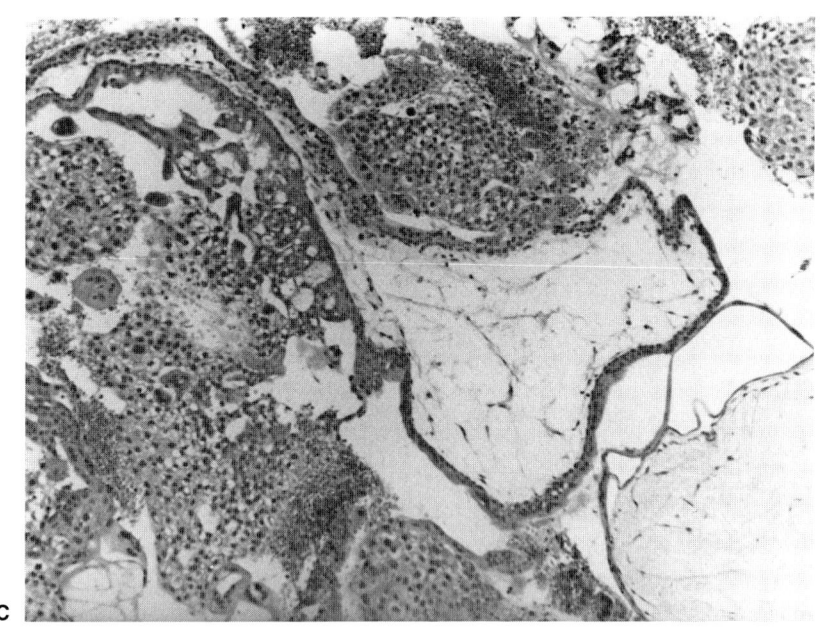

Figure 2. Microscopic findings in hydatidiform mole include edematous enlargement with eventual cyst formation within the individual villus, avascularity, various degrees of trophoblastic proliferation; minimal in (**A**), moderate in (**B**) and marked in (**C**).

variation in the degree of trophoblastic proliferation within a single mole which makes it necessary to sample multiple areas. The villi that are attached to the uterine wall are considered more reliable for microscopic evaluation so that a dilation and curettage is often done to sample this tissue after a mole has aborted spontaneously. Hertig and Mansell[35] simplified the microscopic classification to three grades, varying from "apparently benign" to "apparently malignant." They concluded that there is a general, but not an absolute, correlation between the histopathologic grade of trophoblast and the clinical course. Using the criteria of Hertig and Sheldon to classify 70 patients with hydatidiform mole, Elston and Bagshawe[36] concluded that grading of hydatidiform moles is of no predictive value and may lead to delayed diagnosis of choriocarcinoma. They emphasize that biologic parameters are more important as prognostic indicators.

Clinical Picture

Hydatidiform mole is diagnosed for the first time in 50 percent of patients only when vesicles are passed. Patients usually abort at about 16 weeks' gestation. Vaginal bleeding is present in almost 100 percent of cases. Protracted nausea and vomiting are often features and hyperemesis gravidarum has been described. Hypertension, edema, and proteinuria before 24 weeks of gestation is seen in about 12 percent of patients with molar gestation (Table 4).

Physical examination will reveal disproportionate uterine size in most patients, being increased in 50 percent and decreased in 25 percent. Fetal parts and fetal heart tones are absent in almost every case, although the incidence of molar gestation with a coexistent fetus is reported as from .005 to .01 percent of all pregnancies.[37-40] Less than 20 living children have been born of these pregnancies, and the majority of these are probably cases in which a molar change occurred in only 1 of a pair of twins.[41] Bilateral ovarian masses (theca lutein cysts) are a response to the exceedingly elevated levels of hCG and are found in approximately 30 percent of patients with primary hydatidiform mole. Anemia is often present due to blood loss, and evidence of hyperthyroidism is present in about 3 percent of patients with hydatidiform mole.[42] Supraventricular tachycardia, palpable goiter, increased sweating, heat intolerance, and elevated levels of the free thyroid hormone triiodothyronine (T3) and thyroxin (T4) complete the picture. This is explained by the similarity of hCG and thyroid stimulating hormone (TSH) on a molecular basis, with almost identical alpha subunits and a relative lack of specificity at TSH receptor sites. With elevated levels of hCG there is binding of the hCG molecule by the TSH receptor sites with resultant hyperfunction of the thyroid gland.[43] Acute pulmonary complications of molar pregnancy occur in approximately 10 percent of patients.[44]

Diagnostic Methods

In the absence of passage of vesicles, the diagnosis of hydatidiform mole may be difficult to make at early stage. The following are the most important diagnostic steps:

1. Ultrasonography has virtually replaced all other means of preoperative diagnosis of hydatidiform mole. With a skilled ultrasonographer, diagnostic accuracy is very high. Serial ultrasonography of patients with suspected missed abortion, or threatened abortion, will further tend to exclude hydatidiform mole as a cause of bleeding.
2. Failure to hear fetal heart tones with a Doppler instrument after the fourteenth week of pregnancy should suggest GTN.
3. When a radiograph of the abdomen in the latter part of the midtrimester fails to visualize the fetal skeleton, this should arouse suspicion of GTN.
4. Quantitative urinary hCG value in excess of 100,000 IU per 24 hours, or a serum beta subunit radioimmunoassay value of over 40,000 mIU/ml, increases suspicion that GTN is present. However, such values are occasionally seen with normal pregnancy and are quite consistent with multiple gestation. The hCG assay confirms the presence of pregnancy but is of less importance in the early diagnosis of GTN.

TABLE 4. CLINICAL PICTURE IN BENIGN GTN

Symptoms	Patients[a]	%
Bleeding	309	89
Nausea, vomiting	50	14
Preeclampsia	41	12
Pain	33	10
Hyperthyroidism	2	2

Total Patients[a]

[a]Several patients had more than one symptom complex.
(From Curry SL, et al: Obstet Gynecol 45:1, 1975, with permission.)[19]

Management

This was well outlined by Curry and colleagues in 1975.[19] As soon as the diagnosis of hydatidiform mole has been made, hospitalization, investigation, and evacuation should be promptly performed. Initial management includes diagnosis and treatment of associated medical problems which often coexist with a hydatidiform mole. These include anemia, infection, hyperthyroidism, toxemia, or occasionally disseminated intravascular coagulation. Included in the initial investigation should be a complete blood count, including platelet count, coagulation profile, blood chemistry studies to include liver function tests (SMA complete), renal function tests, blood type and cross-match, chest x-ray, preoperative serum for beta subunit of hCG, thyroid function studies, and pelvic ultrasonography.

After appropriate treatment of any medical complications present, management is based upon (1) the need to evacuate the mole and (2) the need to follow the patient subsequently in order to detect malignant change in any remaining trophoblastic tissue. These steps apply in all cases, no matter what the histologic appearance of the tissue obtained, because approximately 10 percent of patients with hydatidiform moles will require treatment for malignant GTN.[16]

Hemorrhage, sepsis, and possible uterine perforation pose the immediate problems associated with evacuation. Postevacuation, the urinary output, and hemoglobin should be monitored carefully. Hemorrhagic shock must be treated if present on admission or after evacuation of the mole depending upon when it is diagnosed. The condition of the cervix, the amount of bleeding, the size of the uterus, and whether the patient is in the process of aborting the mole or not must all be taken into account in formulating a plan of management.

Surgical Treatment. The essence of this is removal of the mole, and the method used for evacuation will depend upon the circumstances.

1. *Small uterus* (less than 12 weeks). Blood should be available. A laminaria tent is usually unnecessary for dilation as an 8 mm suction catheter is usually sufficient for evacuation. If necessary, an oxytocin infusion (10 units in 1000 ml of 5 percent dextrose in water) should be maintained at a slow drip throughout the procedure. Prostaglandins have been used but present no obvious advantage. General anesthesia is preferable, but no uterine relaxing agents, such as halothane, should be used. After the bulk of the tumor has been evacuated, gentle but thorough, sharp curettage should be carried out. The oxytocin infusion is continued as necessary until the uterus is well retracted, bleeding has stopped, and the patient has recovered from the procedure. Methylergonovine (Methergine) 0.2 mg is given intramuscularly every 8 hours for three doses, unless the patient is hypertensive.
2. *Large uterus*. The larger the mole the more likely a patient is to have persistent trophoblastic disease.[45] Severe hemorrhage may occur either spontaneously or during evacuation. If the patient is not already aborting, an oxytocin infusion may be used to initiate the process. The solution used is 1000 ml of 5 percent dextrose in water with 10 to 20 units of oxytocin. The drip rate is adjusted to effect uterine contractions. If more than one infusion is necessary, the oxytocin may be increased by 10 units, and the vehicle changed to saline or lactated Ringer's solution. It must be remembered that excessive oxytocin (greater than 40 mIU/ml) and large volumes of hypotonic solutions may induce water intoxication with water retention, hyponatremia, and convulsions. Once the abortive process is initiated, evacuation may be aided by the finger. Nitrous oxide (40 percent) with oxygen (60 percent) analgesia may be adequate. Bleeding will usually be heavy and transfusions may be necessary. If the mole is evacuated without the use of suction curettage the uterus should be allowed to involute, if possible, for several days before a repeat sharp curettage is attempted. Extreme care must be taken not to perforate the uterus, nor should the myometrium be damaged by too deep curettage, for fear of producing a subsequent Ascherman's syndrome.
3. *Hysterotomy* is rarely necessary today. Suction curettage has become the recommended approach, and even a molar pregnancy over 30 weeks in size can be emptied within 2 to 3 minutes. In partial moles, a hysterotomy may be necessary because of the large size of the coexisting fetus and excessive maternal hemorrhage.
4. *Hysterectomy*. In women over 35, or in those who have completed their childbearing, hysterectomy should be considered because of the relative frequency with which choriocarcinoma develops in older women.[46]
5. *Ovarian enlargement*. Significant enlargement (greater than 8 cm) of the ovaries, due to the presence of the multiple theca lutein cysts, occurs in 10 to 15 percent of patients (Fig. 3). These should generally

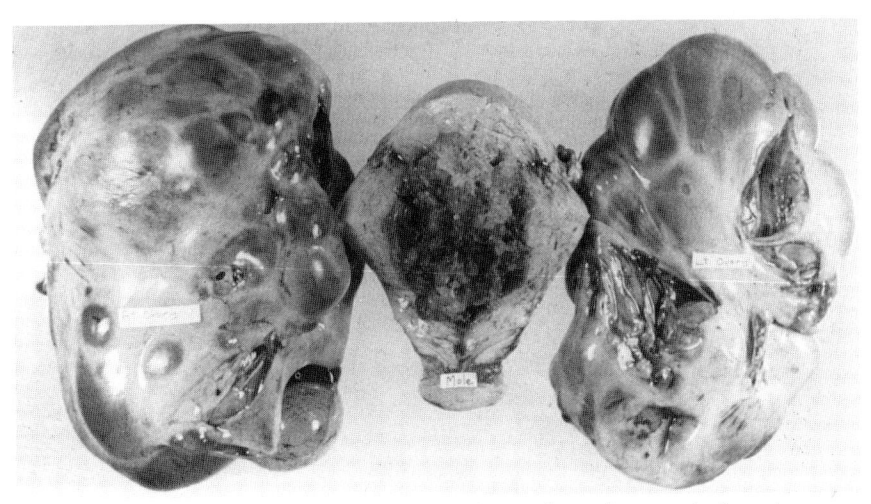

Figure 3. Intrauterine hydatidiform mole with massive enlargement of ovaries caused by theca lutein cysts. These ovaries are prone to torsion, infarction, rupture, and hemorrhage.

be left alone, although it should be kept in mind that persistent trophoblastic disease is more common when theca lutein cysts are present.[47] Occasionally, torsion or hemorrhage into the ovary may create acute abdominal pain with evidence of peritoneal inflammation, and the involved adnexa must be removed. Enlargement, especially in association with a large-for-date uterus, may portend a greater risk of malignant sequelae. Patients over the age of 35 should be advised to have their ovaries removed if a hysterectomy is being performed. Following initial evacuation of a mole, approximately 90 percent of patients are cured. Malignant GTN will develop in the other 10 percent.

Follow-up Management

Regardless of the method of evacuation of the uterus there are two essential points in follow-up management: (1) adequate contraception and (2) adequate serial hCG determinations.

1. *Adequate contraception.* This must be used, as most authorities suggest, at least 1 year without intervening pregnancy. Oral contraceptives provide the best protection against pregnancy, and some earlier fears of increasing the incidence of persistent mole with the use of contraceptives have not yet been supported. Stone and associates[10,48] in England reported a 75 percent increase in the need for chemotherapy among patients given oral contraception during the follow-up period, compared with patients who did not receive oral contraceptives. Goldstein and Berkowitz,[49] Hammond and Surwit,[50] and Eddy and co-

workers[51] have found no significant problems with the use of oral contraceptives, so continue to advise their use. In addition to providing excellent contraception, oral contraceptives suppress production of pituitary LH which, unless specific assays are done, may be confused with hCG. If any other method of contraception is used it must be followed fastidiously. An intrauterine device should not be used for contraception, at least until well after the time of evacuation of the mole and the documentation of remission.

2. *Serial hCG determinations.* These should be performed in a good laboratory using the radioimmunoassay for the beta subunit of hCG in serum. The same laboratory should be used for all of the determinations and the blood should be drawn at approximately the same time each day. Under no circumstances should routine pregnancy tests be utilized to follow patients suspected of having GTN. Following evacuation, hCG determinations should be performed every week until negative (less than 5 mIU/ml), and repeated in 1 month to ensure a negative value. Additional titers are done every 2 to 3 weeks until 1 year has elapsed from the time of the first negative titer. At this point pregnancy is an acceptable risk and hCG monitoring may be discontinued. Interval examinations and chest x-rays are needed to follow the involution of the pelvic structures and aid in the early detection of metastases. Malignant gestational trophoblastic disease which requires treatment is detected in the follow-up period by the finding of serum hCG determinations with "plateaus" for 3 consecutive weeks. A rise in the serum hCG titer at any time after a previous value is an indication for treatment. In the United States about 80 percent of benign GTN will completely resolve after evacuation, but the remainder will develop malignant GTN, with about 15 percent having chorioadenoma destruens and 3 to 5 percent having choriocarcinoma.[52-54] After an initial molar gestation the risk for a second mole is increased four to five times. Repeated episodes of gestational trophoblastic disease have been observed in 0.8 to 3 percent of cases in different series.[19,55-58] Federschneider and associates[55] reported seven patients from the New England Trophoblastic Disease Center. All seven of these patients had spontaneous resolution of their disease after their initial episode of benign GTN, but five of the seven patients required chemotherapy to achieve complete remission of the repeat episode of molar gestation. At the present time it appears that repeat molar gestations have a higher incidence of neoplastic trophoblastic sequelae, and patients with more than one episode of trophoblastic neoplasia have few subsequent normal pregnancies. Patients with repeat GTN probably have some predisposing factor, which makes them more susceptible to GTN, and to poor pregnancy outcome. A follow-up of patients after a single hydatidiform mole with spontaneous resolution after evacuation shows that their fertility and reproductive function is normal. They

have no increase in stillbirth, prematurity, spontaneous abortion, or congenital anomaly rates.[19,59,60] Patients treated with chemotherapy for malignant GTN show a slightly increased incidence of spontaneous abortions[61] and placenta accreta[62] but their pregnancies are otherwise normal. Even in patients with two consecutive moles (1.5 percent) successful pregnancy outcomes have been reported.[63,64]

The Place of Prophylactic Chemotherapy
Some authors[65] have suggested that patients with primary hydatidiform moles be given chemotherapy at the time of evacuation of the mole. Although this has been demonstrated to reduce the number of patients with malignant GTN, it does not prevent it in all patients. Thus, the prevailing opinion at the present time is that, because no more than 10 to 15 percent of patients will eventually require chemotherapy, it is not justified to give the other 85 to 90 percent of patients dangerous drugs. It is not recommended to start prophylactic chemotherapy before 100 days after molar evacuation.[66]

MALIGNANT GTN

Malignant GTN includes invasive mole and choriocarcinoma. At least 50 percent of malignant GTN follows hydatidiform mole but it may follow any type of pregnancy including spontaneous and therapeutic abortion (25 percent), ectopic gestation (3 percent), and term pregnancy (22 percent). High-risk GTN is especially likely after a term pregnancy.[67,68] Indeed, choriocarcinoma can arise during a normal pregnancy.[69]

Chorioadenoma Destruens (Invasive Mole)
The term chorioadenoma destruens was first applied by Ewing[4] because he found that it produced greater enlargement and deformity of the uterus than a hydatidiform mole, with these changes resulting from invasion of the myometrium. This neoplasm may invade the pelvic blood vessels. It metastasizes to the vagina and occasionally to the lungs.[70] Perforation of the uterus with massive intraperitoneal hemorrhage may occur (Fig. 4). Prior to the discovery of chemotherapy, Green[71] reported a 15 percent mortality rate from invasive mole causing uterine rupture and intraperitoneal hemorrhage. Despite the locally aggressive growth of these tumors, Ewing[4] noted that they usually regressed if death did not result from sepsis or hemorrhage.

Microscopically the tumor is identified by the presence of the villous structure in both primary and metastatic lesions (Fig. 5).[72,73] It is difficult to make a diagnosis from curettage because the lesion is often deep in the myometrium. Many sections of tissue from the uterus, or even a metastatic focus, have to be searched because the villi are often only 2 to 4 mm in diameter.[72] Chorioadenoma destruens comprises about 15 percent of all gestational trophoblastic neoplasia in the United States.

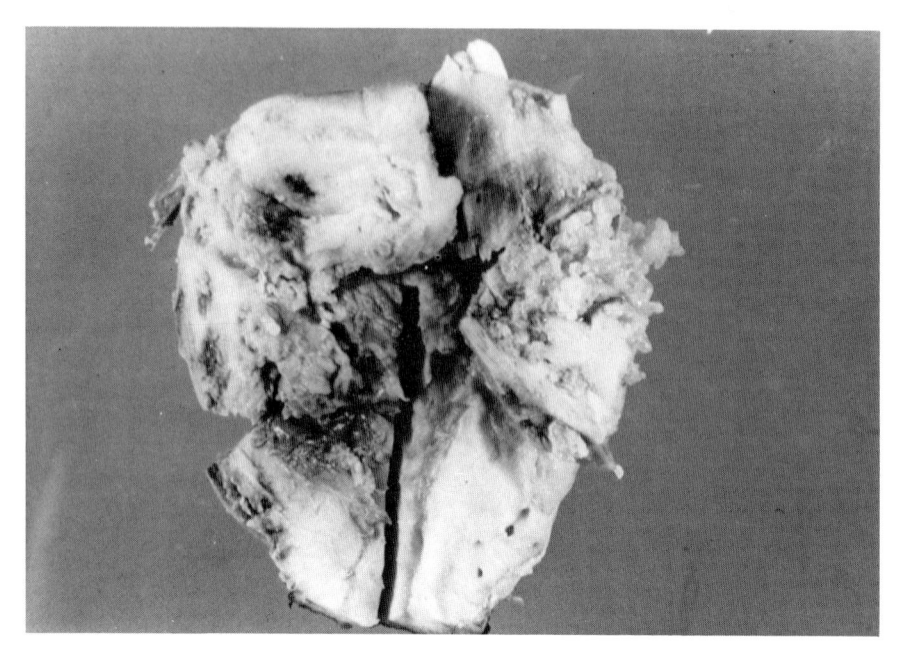

Figure 4. Chorioadenoma destruens. Hysterectomy specimen demonstrating invasion and complete penetration of lateral myometrial wall by typical molar tissue.

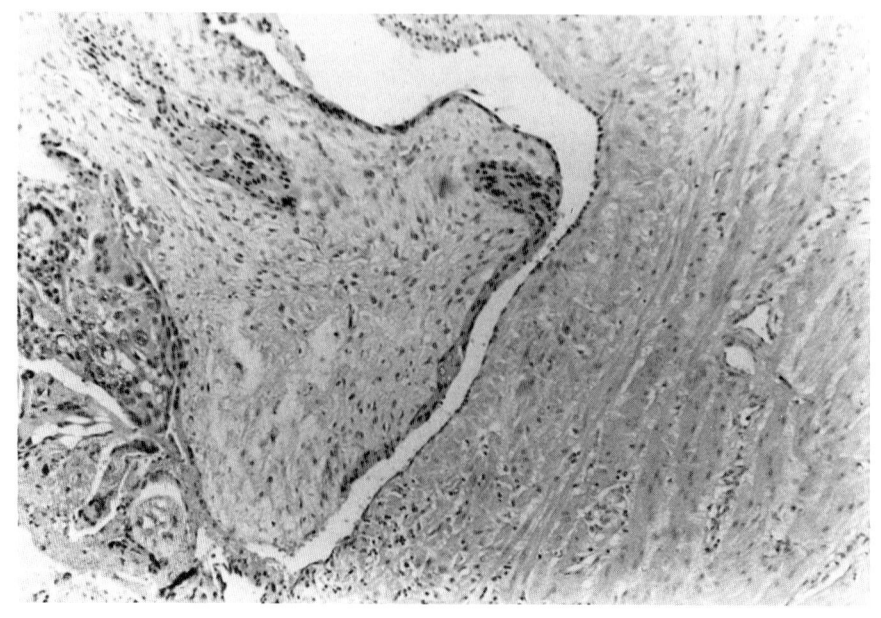

Figure 5. Chorioadenoma destruens. Photomicrograph depicting invading molar tissue deep in the myometrium. Note preservation of villous structures and lack of necrosis. H&E. ×40.

Choriocarcinoma

Gestational choriocarcinoma may follow or develop with any form of pregnancy. Its biologic behavior is distinct from that of nongestational choriocarcinoma which may appear as a germ cell gonadal neoplasm in either sex.[73] Approximately 1 in every 40 molar gestations is followed by choriocarcinoma, while approximately 1 in every 160,000 normal term pregnancies is followed by a choriocarcinoma. An occasional case of choriocarcinoma has no history of previous gestation, but these cases probably represent the existence of an unrecognized previous ectopic pregnancy or spontaneous abortion. The time interval between the antecedent pregnancy and the diagnosis of choriocarcinoma is usually short. However, there are occasional patients with documented asymptomatic periods of 5 to 17 years between the last known pregnancy and the diagnosis of choriocarcinoma.[9,74-77]

Gross Appearance. Choriocarcinoma may be localized anywhere in the uterus. It usually has a red, hemorrhagic necrotic appearance. It may occupy a circumscribed area of the fundus of the uterus or present as a diffuse involvement of the entire myometrium (Fig. 6). The full term placenta may contain a small focus or a diffuse choriocarcinoma. The neoplasm often develops in the uterine wall with the endometrial surface remaining intact. This makes the diagnosis by curettage very unlikely.[78]

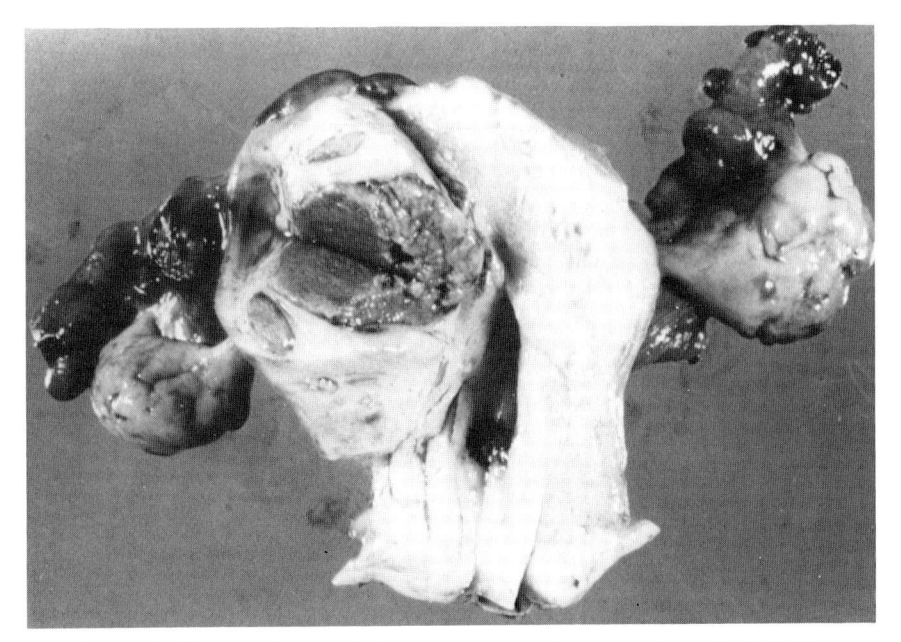

Figure 6. Choriocarcinoma. A discrete hemorrhagic nodule of tumor within the myometrium.

Microscopic Appearance. Choriocarcinoma is extremely vascular and prone to blood-borne metastasis. There is uncontrolled growth of both cytotrophoblast and syncytiotrophoblast in anaplastic sheets and columns invading the uterine musculature (Fig. 7). Hemorrhage and necrosis are invariably present and may make it difficult to distinguish the growth pattern. Chorionic villi are absent in choriocarcinoma.[74]

Natural History of Choriocarcinoma. Choriocarcinoma is more likely to be diagnosed promptly following a hydatidiform mole than following a term delivery, spontaneous abortion, or ectopic pregnancy. Gestational trophoblastic neoplasia diagnosed following a term delivery is almost always choriocarcinoma, whereas GTN following mole, spontaneous abortion, or ectopic pregnancy may be either chorioadenoma destruens or choriocarcinoma. In general, the longer the time interval between evacuation of a mole and the discovery of persistent GTN, the greater is the probability of choriocarcinoma. Up to 6 months after the antecedent pregnancy, chorioadenoma destruens is often present. After 6 months, the lesion is usually choriocarcinoma.[22] Choriocarcinoma has been reported 17 years following a hysterectomy for hydatidiform mole.

Clinical Picture in Choriocarcinoma

The propensity for widespread metastases gives choriocarcinoma a variety of clinical pictures that mimic other medical and surgical conditions. Clinical

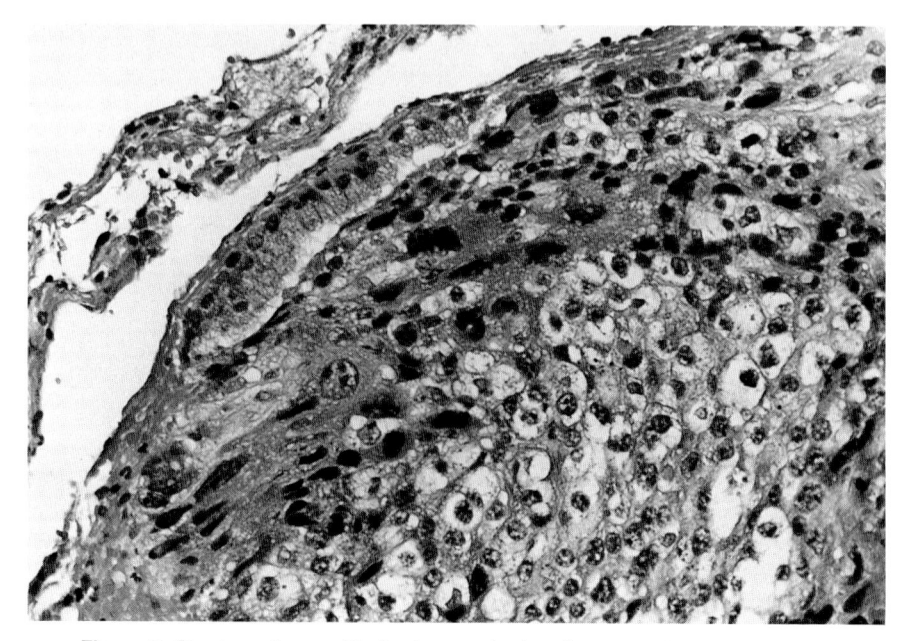

Figure 7. Choriocarcinoma. Photomicrograph of malignant cyto- and syncytiotrophoblast invading myometrium. Note necrosis of muscle in lower left. H&E. ×40.

manifestations usually relate to the location of the metastases. Lung metastases are the most common site of extrauterine spread, followed in order of decreasing frequency by brain, liver, kidneys, small intestine, spleen, and vagina.[49] Bony metastases are rare and even breast metastases have been reported.[79]

A patient with pulmonary metastases may present with progressive dyspnea, cough, hemoptysis, pleuritic pain, or respiratory failure. An x-ray of the chest may show a solitary coin lesion, or multiple scattered lesions, or a diffuse miliary spread. Even in the face of extensive metastases chemotherapy is still highly effective (Figs. 8A, B and C). Several metastases may account for a clinical presentation suggesting epilepsy, stroke, psychosis, or brain tumor in the absence of gynecologic complaints. Fatal, sudden intracranial hemorrhage may occur. The more gradual onset of a dull headache, behavioral changes, confusion, or dizzy spells could present in a patient with multiple microscopic metastases, with surrounding necrosis and edema causing a gradual rise in intracranial pressure. The diagnosis of metastatic choriocarcinoma in the central nervous system should be considered in any woman of reproductive age presenting with neurologic signs and complaints.[80] A chest film will usually detect pulmonary metastasis in a patient with brain metastasis, but sometimes whole lung tomography, or a pulmonary CT scan is necessary.[81]

Diagnostic Methods in Choriocarcinoma

These are similar to those outlined for benign GTN, but when a tissue diagnosis of choriocarcinoma has been made the search for metastases should be more intense. While all malignant GTN should be considered seriously, most of the deaths are in patients with choriocarcinoma. Begent and Bagshawe[82] recently reviewed available diagnostic studies.

1. *Biochemical markers.* Human chorionic gonadotrophin (hCG) remains the principal marker, but placental glycoprotein (SPI) may give additional information in a few cases.[83] A good assay for beta hCG will indicate a value of less than 2 milli international units (mIU) per ml in normal serum. Any excess of beta hCG not accounted for by pregnancy is likely to be due to gestational trophoblastic neoplasia although rarely it may be associated with a malignant teratoma. Immunofluorescent and peroxidase studies suggest that hCG synthesis is more active in syncitial than in cytotrophoblastic tissue. In patients under treatment assays should be done twice weekly. After treatment is completed assays should be performed every 1 to 2 weeks for 3 months. Thereafter, they should be performed every 3 months up to 3 years, and then every 6 months. Although CT scanning is now used routinely to detect brain metastases, when the ratio of hCG in spinal fluid/hCG in serum is greater than 1:60 a metastatic brain lesion should be suspected. Urinary nucleic acid breakdown products appar-

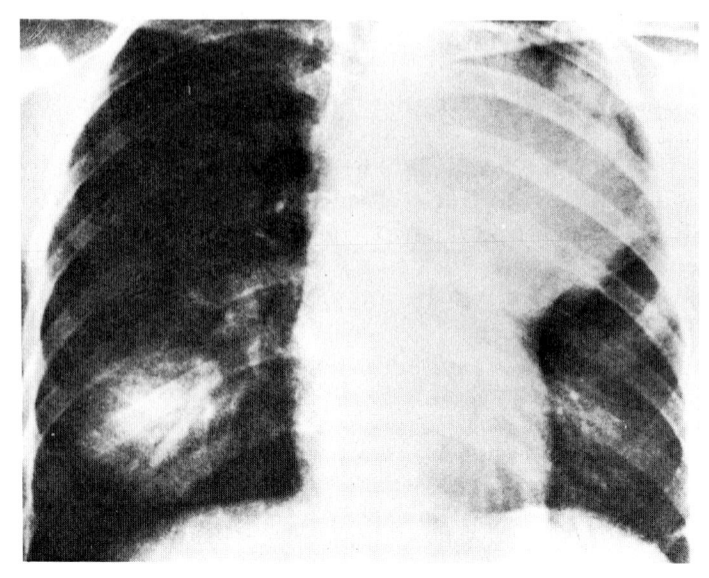

Figure 8A. Initial chest radiograph of patient with metastatic choriocarcinoma.

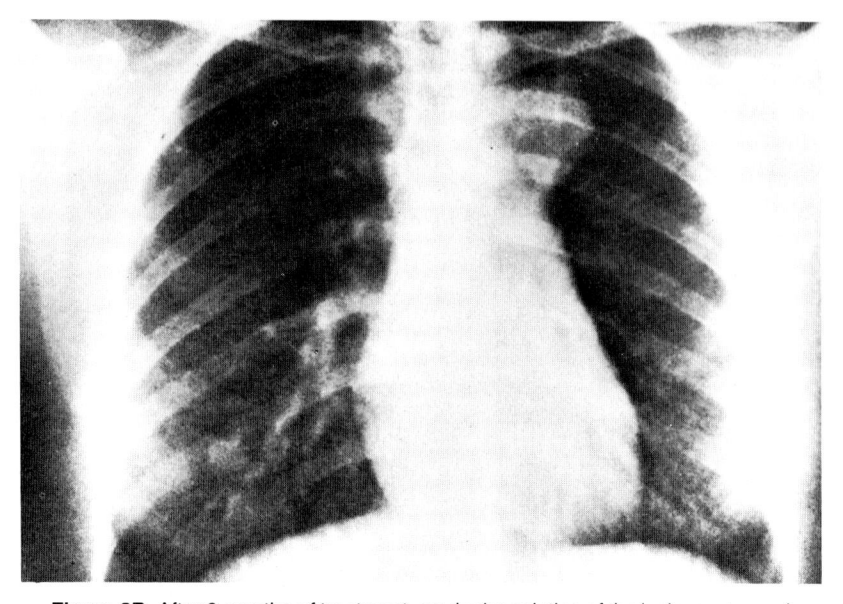

Figure 8B. After 9 months of treatment, gradual resolution of the lesions occurred.

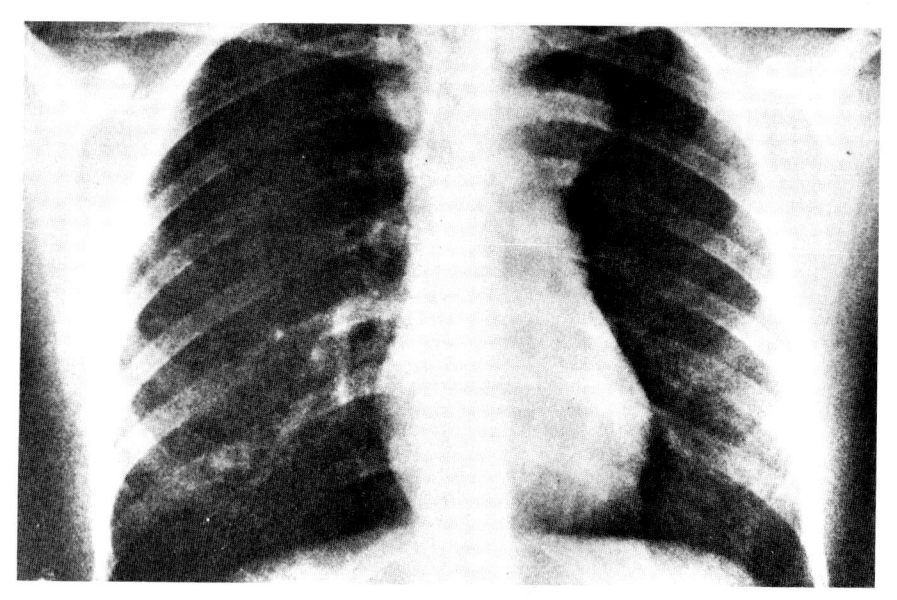

Figure 8C. No change is seen in left hilar or right lower lobe metastases over 4 additional months. Only necrosis and fibrosis were noted in resected left hilar lesion. (*From Libshitz HI, et al: Obstet Gynecol 49:415, 1977, with permission.*)

ently return to normal more rapidly than the hCG levels in the presence of regression.[84] If this finding is borne out by further studies, patients will be saved needless continuation of chemotherapy.

2. *Ultrasonography* can be used to monitor progress in GTN,[85] but it is of most value in differentiating GTN from a normal pregnancy.
3. *Pelvic arteriography* is occasionally useful but now has been almost completely replaced by ultrasonography for making the initial diagnosis.
4. *Chest radiography* is essential in all patients with GTN, and CT scanning is now more useful than whole lung tomography.
5. *Brain scanning* is now done with CT scans because they are superior to isotope scans.
6. *Liver scanning* can be done using colloidal isotopes, CT scanning, or ultrasonography.
7. *Thyroid function* studies, especially T3 and T4, may be worthwhile in patients presenting with features of thyrotoxicosis. This is apparently caused by the similarity between the alpha subunit of hCG and thyroid stimulating hormone (TSH).[86]
8. *Radioimmunolocalization* is achieved by the intravenous injection of radiolabeled antibodies against hCG, so that these antibodies become concentrated in trophoblastic tumors. The tumors can then be detected by external scintigraphy. It is likely that with the use of monoclonal antibodies this technique will prove very valuable in the future.

Staging Studies

Once the diagnosis of choriocarcinoma is established or suspected, hospitalization with full staging and investigation is mandatory. The appropriate studies have been described in the ACOG Technical Bulletin No. 59 (December, 1980).[14] Such staging studies are summarized in Table 5 and should include physical examination, evaluation of the pelvis with ultrasound, intravenous urography, evaluation of the liver with either radionucleotide scanning or CT scan, localization of possible brain metastases with CT scan, with possible use of lumbar puncture (simultaneous serum and CSF hCG levels), and electroencephalogram. Chest x-ray is important as approximately 75 percent of metastases from choriocarcinoma occur in the lungs, and thorough physical examination including careful examination of the vaginal wall, rectovaginal septum, and pelvis is necessary to rule out the second most common site of metastases. A 24-hour urine or serum specimen for hCG should be obtained at the time of initial staging.

Following initial staging work-up, the patient is categorized as to nonmetastatic or metastatic disease with further subcategorization of this latter group into "good" and "poor" prognosis. This categorization will determine the eventual choice of therapy (see Table 3).

TABLE 5. MALIGNANT GTN

I. Staging studies
  A. History and physical examination
  B. Blood studies
    1. CBC, differential, platelet count
    2. APTT, prothrombin time
    3. VDRL
    4. Serum electrolytes, BUN, glucose, creatinine, bilirubin, transaminases, LDH, proteins, uric acid, cholesterol, alkaline phosphatase, Ca, PO$_4$
    5. Blood type and Rh
    6. HLA typing (optional)
    7. Thyroid panel
  C. Urinalysis and urine culture
  D. Papanicolaou smear
  E. Chest x-ray, AP and lateral; chest tomography, if indicated
  F. Pelvic sonogram
  G. Intravenous pyelogram
  H. Liver scan (radionucleotide or CT)
  I. Brain CT scan (or radionucleotide if CT unavailable)
  J. 24-hour urine for hCG or serum hCG level
  K. Electrocardiogram
  L. Indicated medical consultations

II. Optional staging studies
  A. EEG
  B. Selective arteriography
  C. Lumbar puncture and CSF hCG level

(From ACOG Tech Bull No. 59, Dec. 1980, with permission.)[14]

Management of Nonmetastatic GTN. Essentially four treatment options exist for treatment of nonmetastatic GTN (Table 6). It has been shown that early hysterectomy in this group (surgical therapy) will shorten the hospitalization and the amount of chemotherapy needed. Thus, the patient's desire for further fertility should be evaluated at the onset of therapy; and if future childbearing is not desired, then abdominal hysterectomy (usually sparing the adnexa) may be done on the third day of a 5-day course of treatment. Continued chemotherapy remains mandatory until three consecutive hCG titers are negative.

Chemotherapy protocols for *nonmetastatic* GTN include single agent methotrexate therapy 15 to 25 mg daily for 5 days, actinomycin D 10 to 13 µg/kg IV for 5 days, or high-dose intermittent methotrexate with citrovorum rescue. The latter regimen has extremely low toxicity and, in many instances, is now the treatment of choice for nonmetastatic GTN. An interval of 7 days between repetitive chemotherapy courses is utilized provided toxicity is not prohibitive.

During chemotherapy, daily blood counts with measurements of liver and kidney function are essential. Biweekly chest x-rays are likewise important and weekly serum hCGs are used to monitor the response to therapy. In general, no treatment course should be begun if the white blood count is less

TABLE 6. NONMETASTATIC GTN

Treatment Regimen Options

1. Methotrexate 15–25 mg IM. (0.4 mg/kg) daily × 5 days
   Monitor toxicity daily
   Repeat on 7th to 9th nontreatment day if toxicity permits
                 OR
2. Actinomycin D 10–13 µg/kg IV daily × 5 days
   Monitor toxicity daily
   Repeat on 7th to 9th nontreatment day if toxicity permits
                 OR
3. Methotrexate 1 mg/kg IM on days 1, 3, 5, 7 at 7 P.M.
   Folinic acid 0.1 mg/kg IM on days 2, 4, 6, 8 at 7 P.M.
   Monitor toxicity on days of methotrexate
   Repeat on nontreatment day 6 or 7 depending on toxicity
   Folinic acid should be available on unit prior to giving methotrexate dose
4. Treatment limitations
   No treatment regimen to be started or continued if:
      WBC is less than 3000/millimeter^3
      Segs less than 1500/millimeter^3
      Platelets less than 100,000/millimeter^3
      SGPT—significant elevation
      BUN—significant elevation
5. All patients followed with weekly hCG determinations and exams
6. Continue treatment until three consecutive negative weekly hCG titers

(From ACOG Tech Bull No. 59 Dec. 1980, with permission.)[14]

than $3000/mm^3$, polymorphonuclear leukocytes less than $1500/mm^3$, or platelet count less than $100,000/mm^3$, or if a significant elevation of BUN and liver function studies exists.

Treatment is continued with one of the above regimens until three consecutive negative hCG titers have been obtained. The hCG titers are then repeated at 2-week intervals for 3 months, every month for 3 months, every 2 months for 6 months, and then every 6 months for life. Fastidious contraception is required for at least 1 year and oral contraceptives are the method of choice unless there is contraindication to their use.

Patients who have plateauing of hCG titer while on therapy for nonmetastatic GTN can be considered for alternate therapy with either actinomycin D or methotrexate, depending on which was used initially. If, during the course of chemotherapy, there is a significant elevation in hCG titer or the development of new metastases, the patient should probably be begun on multiagent therapy, with the assistance of a gynecologic oncologist. Delayed or secondary hysterectomy should be considered. Continued treatment with single agent therapy in the light of new metastases or marked elevation in titer is hazardous.

Management of Metastatic GTN: "Good" Prognosis. Patients with metastatic GTN are classified as "poor" prognosis or "good" prognosis patients based on the criteria in Table 3. In general, patients with "good" prognosis metastatic disease can be treated with either single agent methotrexate or actinomycin D as initial treatment. The use of adjunctive surgical therapy depends upon the desires of the patient as to future fertility. Even in patients with metastatic disease there is evidence to show that when there is disease in the uterus, hysterectomy may shorten the duration and amount of chemotherapy required to achieve remission. In some centers methotrexate with citrovorum rescue is also used for "good" prognosis metastatic disease but, to date, we have reserved its use for patients without evidence of dissemination. Close follow-up with physical examinations and chest x-rays is essential. Monitoring of hCG titers, and hematologic and hepatic indices are done as for nonmetastatic disease.

In patients with "good" prognosis metastatic disease, the appearance of new metastases or failure of hCG titer to drop is an indication for changing to multiagent chemotherapy. Again, if uterine disease is present, a hysterectomy should be considered.

Management of Metastatic GTN: "Poor" Prognosis. Patients with "poor" prognosis gestational trophoblastic neoplasia require sophisticated medical support, constant intensive monitoring, and potent multiagent chemotherapeutic regimens administered by experienced personnel. Surgery and radiotherapy also play important roles in management.

Multiagent chemotherapy is of primary importance in the treatment of metastatic gestational trophoblastic disease. Triple therapy with methotrexate, actinomycin D, and chlorambucil, as outlined in Table 7, has been the stan-

TABLE 7. MANAGEMENT OF HIGH-RISK GTN

1. Standard triple therapy (MAC)
   Methotrexate 12–15 mg IM ⎫
   Actinomycin D 8–10 μg/kg IV ⎬ daily × 5 days
   Chlorambucil 8–10 mg PO ⎭
   Monitor toxicity daily
   Repeat treatment course as soon as toxicity
     permits after 10 days without treatment

2. Modified Bagshawe regimen (CHAMOCA)
   Day 1: Hydroxyurea 500 mg PO at 0600, 1200, 1800, 2400
          Actinomycin D 0.2 mg IV at 1900
   Day 2: Vincristine 1 mg/m² IV at 0700
          Methotrexate 100 mg/m² IV push at 1900
          Methotrexate 200 mg/m² infusion over 12 hr at 1900
          Actinomycin D 0.2 mg IV at 1900
   Day 3: Actinomycin D 0.2 mg IV at 1900
          Cytoxan 500 mg/m² IV at 1900
          Folinic acid 14 mg IM at 1900
   Day 4: Folinic acid 14 mg IM at 0100
          Folinic acid 14 mg IM at 0700
          Folinic acid 14 mg IM at 1300
          Folinic acid 14 mg IM at 1900
          Actinomycin D 0.5 mg IV at 1900
   Day 5: Folinic acid 14 mg IM at 0100
          Actinomycin D 0.5 mg IV at 1900
   Days 6
   and 7: No treatment
   Day 8: Cytoxan 500 mg/m² IV at 1900
          Adriamycin 30 mg/m² IV at 1900
   Monitor toxicity daily
   Repeat treatment course as soon as toxicity
     permits after 10 days without treatment

(From ACOG Tech Bull No. 59, Dec. 1980, with permission.)[14]

dard in many centers. Despite sometimes life-threatening toxicity, this combination has worked well. Recently, a modification of Bagshawe's multiagent regimen has been used, and this appears to have good success with poor prognosis disease while toxicity is lessened. At the present time, a randomized study comparing these two regimens is under investigation. Both regimens require intensive management as life-threatening complications from chemotherapy are common. Severe leukopenia, thrombocytopenia with resultant sepsis, and bleeding are common complications and bleeding into the chest, brain, and liver may occur. A list of common complications from treatment of GTN is included in Table 8.

If cerebral or hepatic metastases are detected, irradiation therapy (2000 rads—liver; 3000 rads—brain) is begun simultaneously with the start of chemotherapy. Even with intensive chemotherapy and radiation, additional

TABLE 8. COMPLICATIONS OF THERAPY OF GTN

1. Intracavitary bleeding from metastasis (chest, liver, brain, intraperitoneal)	11. Paralysis secondary to spinal metastasis
2. Arteriovenous fistula with high-output cardiac failure	12. Pathologic fractures
3. Pleurodynia	13. Stomatitis and ulcerations
4. Agranulocytosis	14. Severe malnutrition
5. Septic shock	15. Hepatitis and/or nephritis
6. Thrombocytopenia	16. Alopecia
7. Cerebral edema	17. Dermatologic eruptions
8. CVA	18. Photosensitivity
9. Intestinal obstruction	19. Immunosuppression
10. DIC	

(From ACOG Tech Bull No. 59, Dec. 1980, with permission.)[14]

adjunctive surgery may be necessary to control bleeding, extirpate isolated metastases, or relieve obstruction from metastases. Additionally, experimental chemotherapy protocols may be required for patients with resistant disease.

Long-term chemotherapy leads to severe nutritional depletion and immunologic incompetence. The aggressive use of total parenteral nutrition or other forms of hyperalimentation may improve the overall condition of such patients and actually increase the patient's ability to withstand toxic chemotherapy. Improvement in immunologic status may also occur with vigorous nutritional support.

Chemotherapy is continued until three consecutive negative titers are reached, and this is usually followed by several courses of chemotherapy in the hopes of destroying all viable tumor cells. Even with the sensitive beta subunit radioimmunoassay, a subset of 10^4 and 10^5 cells could probably continue to exist despite negative hCG titers. Following the initial negative titers and following the completion of therapy, hCG titers should be obtained every 2 weeks for 3 months, every month for 3 months, every 2 months for 6 months, and every 6 months for life. Only after 1 year of completely negative titers should pregnancy be permitted.

Prognosis

Lurain and associates[87] identified five factors influencing prognosis. These were:

1. Clinicopathologic diagnosis of choriocarcinoma versus invasive mole (71 versus 100 percent, $p < .0005$).
2. Pretreatment human chorionic gonadotropin titer greater than 100,000 IU/liter and time greater than 4 months from pregnancy event to treatment (62 versus 93 percent, $p < .005$).
3. Metastases to sites other than lung and/or vagina (37 versus 92 percent, $p < .0005$).
4. Antecedent term gestation compared with hydatidiform mole, abortion, and ectopic pregnancy (56 versus 79 percent, $p < .02$).

5. Prior unsuccessful chemotherapy compared with no previous treatment (48 versus 83 percent, p < .0005).

Lurain and associates[88] reported that 48 of 399 patients referred to the John I. Brewer Trophoblastic Center of Northwestern University Medical School from 1962 to 1979 for treatment of gestational trophoblastic disease (invasive mole or choriocarcinoma) died. All patients who died had histologically documented metastatic choriocarcinoma. The time from pregnancy event to treatment was 4 months and/or the pretreatment hCG titer was 100,000 IU/L in 64 percent of these patients. Seventy-one percent of fatal cases developed in association with term pregnancies, abortions, or ectopic pregnancies rather than hydatidiform moles. Fifty percent of patients who died had metastases to the liver, brain, and/or peritoneal cavity when they first presented for treatment. The most common causes of death were hemorrhage from one or more metastatic sites (42 percent) and pulmonary insufficiency (31 percent). Factors primarily responsible for the treatment failures in these patients were the presence of extensive disease at the time of initial treatment, inadequate initial treatment, and failure of presently used chemotherapy protocols in advanced disease. Secondary chemotherapy, radiation therapy to sites other than the brain, and adjuvant surgical procedures failed to improve survival in these high-risk patients. In an effort to individualize the management of GTN, Bagshawe[9] introduced a prognostic scoring system based on factors known to affect tumor drug resistance (Table 9).

On the basis of the magnitude of the various factors a group could be defined with 100 percent survival (low score) and at the other extreme a group with no survivors (high score).

Recently, Begent and Bagshawe[89] reported on 72 patients in a high-risk group of patients treated at Charing Cross Hospital (London, England) since 1973. They found metastatic disease outside the pelvis was present at the start of treatment in 64 (89 percent). The lungs were the most common site (79 percent), followed by the brain (15 percent) and liver (8 percent). They point out that although it is tempting to deal with such presentations by local surgery or radiotherapy, this is rarely wise, because such action usually prohibits effective chemotherapy for up to 3 weeks. Also, large masses of choriocarcinoma are usually enmeshed in a network of large and delicate vessels so that surgery may be hazardous prior to the completion of chemotherapy. However, neither is chemotherapy without its problems and a rapid tumor response may be associated with increasing edema around the tumor or hemorrhage into it. Thus, discrete pulmonary metastases may become diffuse as a result of chemotherapy, with the patient developing respiratory failure. In these circumstances care must be taken to see that fluid overloading does not occur and diuretics may produce temporary improvement. In such conditions infection readily supervenes and must be treated vigorously. Despite their extensive experience in the management of GTN, Begent and Bagshawe[82] found that between 5 and 10 percent of "high-risk" patients died as a result of the initial extent of the disease.

TABLE 9. BAGSHAWE'S PROGNOSTIC SCORING SYSTEM

Risk Factors	Prognostic Score[a]			
	0	10	20	40
Age	<39	>39		
Parity	1 or 2	3 or 4		
Antecedent pregnancy (AP)	Mole	Abortion	Term	
Interval (AP-chemotherapy) in months	<4	4–6	7–12	>12
HCG (plasma IU/L or urine IU/day)	<10^3	10^3–10^4	10^4–10^5	>10^5
ABO (mother × father)	A × A × B × AB	0 × 0 A × 0	B × AB ×	
No. of metastases	Nil	1–4	5–8	>8
Site of metastases	Not detected Lungs Vagina	Spleen Kidney	GI tract Liver	Brain
Largest tumor mass	<3 cm	3–5 cm	>5 cm	
Lymphocytic infiltration	Marked	Moderate Unknown	Slight	
Immune status	Reactive	Unknown	Unreactive	
Previous chemotherapy	Nil	Unknown	Single drug	Two drugs or more

[a]Scored for individual risk factors are added and risk group determined by the total score as follows: low risk 50 or less; medium risk 50–100; and high risk >100.
(From Begent RHJ, Bagshawe KD: Gynecologic Oncology, Hingham, Mass., Martinus Nijhoff Publishers, 1983, with permission.)[82]

RECENT ADVANCES IN THE MANAGEMENT OF HIGH-RISK GTN

Drug resistance leads to death in approximately 10 percent of patients with "high-risk" choriocarcinoma. Attempts to improve the results are based on the use of new drugs, better use of surgery, and special attention to the treatment of metastases in the central nervous system.

New Drug Regimens

The MECA Regimen. This is presently being considered by Begent and Bagshawe[82] as the initial treatment for patients in the "high-risk" group. They feel it is less toxic than CHAMOCA and has good antitumor effect. However, it is too early to know whether survival of patients treated in this way will be as good as that achieved when CHAMOCA is given as the initial treatment (Table 10).

Cis-Platinum. This agent has been studied both alone and in combination with vincristine and methotrexate.[90] The combination was found to be more

TABLE 10. BAGSHAWE'S CHAMOCA REGIMEN

Day 1		Hydroxyurea 1 g q.d.s. for 24 hours
Day 2	10.00 A.M.	Vincristine 1.0 mg/m² stat IV
	3.00 P.M.	Methotrexate 100 mg/m² stat IV
		Methotrexate 200 mg/m² 12-hour infusion IV
Day 3	3.00 P.M.	Folinic acid 15 mg IM or PO
Day 4	8.00 A.M.	Folinic acid 15 mg IM or PO
	10.00 A.M.	Cyclophosphamide 600 mg/m² IV
		Actinomycin-D 0.5 mg IV
	8.00 P.M.	Folinic acid 15 mg IM or PO
Day 5	8.00 A.M.	Folinic acid 15 mg IM or PO
	10.00 A.M.	Actinomycin-D 0.5 mg IV
Day 6	10.00 A.M.	Actinomycin-D 0.5 mg IV
Day 7		No treatment
Day 8		No treatment
Day 9		Adriamycin 30 mg/m² IV[a]
		Cyclophosphamide 400 mg/m² IV[a]

[a]Check WBC and platelets before giving.
(From Begent RHJ, Bagshawe KD: Gynecologic Oncology, Hingham, Mass., Martinus Nijhoff Publishers, 1983, with permission.)[82]

effective. Vincristine was given in a dose of 1 mg/m² at 10.00 A.M. on day 1 and methotrexate 100 mg/m² IV stat at 3.00 P.M. on the same day, followed by methotrexate 200 mg/m² over the next 12 hours by IV infusion. Folinic acid rescue was started in the dose of 15 mg IM 24 hours after the start of the methotrexate and continued 12 hourly for a further three doses. *Cis*-platinum was given in the dose of 120 mg/m² on the third day with intense hydration. Based on the work of Hayes and associates[91] mannitol was given in a dose of 10 grams hourly for each of 6 hours. One liter of IV fluids (alternating normal saline with 5 percent dextrose, each containing 1 gram of KCl) was given hourly for 3 hours before *cis*-platinum administered by intravenous infusion. Intravenous fluids were continued at a rate of 1 liter hourly for a further 3 hours. Hydration was continued until all vomiting had stopped. When the drugs were used in this way two courses could usually be given without significant nephrotoxicity. Ototoxicity is usually measurable by audiogram after one course, and four courses tend to produce measurable deterioration in glomerular filtration and high frequency hearing loss. Significant hypomagnesemia commonly occurs after repeated courses due to renal tubular losses. Unless anticipated this may be sufficiently severe to produce tetany. Platinum may also be given in a dose of 20 mg/m² daily, for 3 to 5 days in succession. This may also be combined with vincristine and methotrexate. Schlaerth and associates[92] have reported sustained remission of choriocarcinoma with *cis*-platinum, vinblastine, and bleomycin after MAC chemotherapy failed. Rustin and associates[93] found no increase in secondary tumors after cytotoxic chemotherapy for gestational trophoblastic disease.

Surgery for Drug-Resistant Disease

If tumor appears to be restricted to resectable sites surgery should be considered. In the absence of known active tumor at other sites, hysterectomy should be performed and if hCG is not normal within 2 weeks, it has to be assumed that there is tumor elsewhere. The value of hysterectomy in selected patients is well established.

Thoracotomy may be successful in removing solitary or even multiple lesions. Solitary lesions within the abdomen can sometimes be excised successfully though it is wise to perform arteriography beforehand to determine the extent of the vascular supply. Begent and Bagshawe[82] give methotrexate 50 mg IV at the time of operation to reduce metastases caused by manipulation of the tumor. The dose is reduced and folinic acid rescue given if renal function is impaired. Methotrexate is less likely to cause vomiting than some other cytotoxic agents but other drugs may be appropriate. Chemotherapy is restarted as soon as possible after surgery but rarely is this advisable before 10 to 14 days have passed. Two weeks rest is usually necessary between the preceding chemotherapy and surgery. Thus, about 4 weeks pass during which little or no systemic chemotherapy is given to these high-risk patients. Also, as pointed out by Begent and Bagshawe,[82] if all the tumor is not removed the patient may have a larger tumor burden by the time she receives her next course of chemotherapy than she had before surgery. However, in drug-resistant disease the effects of surgery may be dramatic and undoubtedly contribute to cure in selected patients. Hammond and associates[94] advocate operation at the start of treatment, usually hysterectomy, and we agree with their general approach.

Radiotherapy for Drug-Resistant Disease

Radiotherapy is useful for preventing hemorrhage from both brain and liver metastases in patients having concomitant chemotherapy.[95] Radiotherapy is also effective in treating localized choriocarcinoma. In this respect, however, it has less to offer than surgery while compromising the results of chemotherapy to a similar degree because of delay.

Central Nervous System (CNS) Metastases (Bagshawe's Method)

CNS metastases of choriocarcinoma were associated with pulmonary deposits in 65 of 69 patients treated at Charing Cross Hospital (London, England).[82] Some were present on referral, but others developed during chemotherapy. For this reason, all patients with lung deposits or high-risk choriocarcinoma are given prophylactic intrathecal methotrexate 12.5 mg with each course of chemotherapy which does not contain a moderately high dose (0.3 g/m^2 or more) of systemic methotrexate. For this purpose, intrathecal or high-dose systemic methotrexate is given no less frequently than every 2 weeks. When these measures have been employed by Bagshawe and associates no patient has developed CNS metastases, unless disease elsewhere had become drug-resistant and presumably reseeded the brain. By contrast, brain metastases were the only site of progressive disease in 19 patients who did not receive CNS prophylaxis. Thus, in these patients the disease outside the CNS was responding to systemic chemotherapy while that in the brain was progressing, presumably due to inadequate penetration of cytotoxic drugs into the central nervous system.

When central nervous system metastases are evident at the start of treatment, the poor access of drugs into the CSF is overcome by the use of high-dose methotrexate together with intrathecal methotrexate in standard doses (12.5 mg). An intravenous infusion of 3 g/m^2 over 24 hours gives CSF methotrexate concentrations of 10^{-6} molar at the end of the infusion and the data of Tattersall[96] indicate that 1 g/m^2 also gives therapeutic concentrations. Although lower doses sometimes produce responses, it is Bagshawe's policy to give methotrexate 1 g/m^2 as a 24-hour infusion with folinic acid (Leucovorin) 30 mg, 12-hourly for 3 days, starting 32 hours after the start of the infusion. With this regimen it is essential to maintain a urinary output of 2.5 liters per day. The dose of intravenous methotrexate and folinic acid in the CHAMOCA and MECA regimens may be increased to these levels. Provided that there is no evidence of raised intracranial pressure, intrathecal methotrexate is given approximately once every 2 weeks, either between courses of systemic chemotherapy or concurrent with those regimens which do not contain intravenous methotrexate.

The time of greatest risk to patients presenting with CNS metastases is during the first month of treatment. Eight of 33 patients in Bagshawe's series died during this time.[82] These patients all had severe neurologic damage when first seen. Cerebral edema can sometimes be improved with dexamethasone administration. High-dose methotrexate at the onset may exacerbate cerebral edema or cause cerebral hemorrhage as the tumor becomes necrotic. On the other hand, using a lower dose may predispose to drug resistance. Apart from the eight patients dying in the first month, another nine died of drug-resistant disease during the ensuing 43 months. Sixteen patients in this series had been off treatment for a mean interval of 111 months. Since 1974 when treatment was based on the principles outlined above, only one of eight patients has died of drug resistance, but mortality during the first month of treatment has remained at 25 percent.

For patients developing CNS metastases while on chemotherapy the prognosis is grave. The disease is usually drug resistant from the outset and only 3 of 36 patients in Bagshawe's series have survived, although 2 are still on treatment. The remaining patient is worthy of note in that a solitary metastasis was localized by CT scan and successfully resected.

IMMUNOTHERAPY

The results with immunotherapy have been disappointing to date. However, the demonstration by radioimmunolocalization that antibody to hCG can be concentrated in choriocarcinomatous tissue has stimulated further interest in this type of treatment.[97] A recent report by Berkowitz and associates[98] showed that circulating immune complexes remained elevated during gonadotrophin remission from 6 to 16 weeks and then declined to initial values. Further investigation should be undertaken to evaluate possible interactions between circulating immune complex and host immune defenses.

REFERENCES

1. Schmorl G: Demonst ein syncytialen scheidentumors. Cent f Gynak 21:1217, 1897
2. Gottschalk S: Das sarcom der chorionzotten. Arch Gynak 46:1, 1894
3. Marchand F: Uberdie sogenannten "decidualen" geschwulste in anschluss an normale geburt, abort, blasenmole, and extrasuterin monatsschr. Gerburtshilfe Gynakol 1:419, 1895
4. Ewing J: Chorioma, a clinical and pathological study. Surg Gynecol Obstet 10:366, 1910
5. Ross GT, Hammond CB, Hertz R, et al: Chemotherapy of metastatic and nonmetastatic gestational trophoblastic neoplasms. Tex Rep Biol Med 24:326, 1966
6. Tomoda Y, Kaseki S, Goto S, et al: Rh-D factor in trophoblastic tumors: A possible cause of the high incidence in Asia. Am J Obstet Gynecol 139:742, 1981
7. Wei P, Ouyang P: Trophoblastic disease in Taiwan. Am J Obstet Gynecol 85:844, 1961
8. Hammond CB, Parker RT: Diagnosis and treatment of trophoblastic disease. A report from the Southeastern Regional Center. Obstet Gynecol 35:132, 1970
9. Bagshawe KD: Risk and prognostic factors in trophoblastic neoplasia. Cancer 38:1373, 1976
10. Stone M, Bagshawe KD: An analysis of the influences of maternal age, gestational age, contraceptive method, and the mode of primary treatment of patients with hydatidiform moles on the incidence of subsequent chemotherapy. Br J Gynaecol 86:782, 1979
11. Fasoli M, Ratti E, Franceschi S, et al: Management of trophoblastic disease: Results of a cooperative study. Obstet Gynecol 60:205, 1982
12. Acosta-Sison H: Statistical study of chorionephithelioma in the Philippine General Hospital. Am J Obstet Gynecol 58:125, 1949
13. Marquez-Monter H, de la Vega G, Robles M, Bolio-Cicero A: Epidemiology and pathology of hydatidiform mole in the General Hospital of Mexico. Am J Obstet Gynecol 85:856, 1963
14. American College of Obstetricians and Gynecologists Technical Bulletin No. 59, December 1980
15. Cohen BA, Burkman RT, Rosenshein NB, et al: Gestational trophoblastic disease within an elective abortion population. Am J Obstet Gynecol 135:452, 1979
16. Surwit EA, Hammond CB: Gestational trophoblastic neoplasia. In Pitkin RM, Zlatnik FJ (eds): 1980 Yearbook of Obstetrics and Gynecology. Chicago: Year Book, 1980, p 275
17. Lurain JR, Brewer JI, Torok EE, Halpern B: Natural history of hydatidiform mole after primary evacuation. Am J Obstet Gynecol 145:591, 1983
18. Ross GT, Goldstein DP, Hertz R, et al: Sequential use of methotrexate and

actinomycin D in treatment of metastatic choriocarcinoma and related trophoblastic disease in women. Am J Obstet Gynecol 92:223, 1965
19. Curry SL, Hammond CB, Tyrey L, et al: Hydatidiform mole: Diagnosis, management and long-term followup of 347 patients. Obstet Gynecol 45:1, 1975
20. Odell WD, Hertz R, Lipsett MB, et al: Endocrine aspects of trophoblastic neoplasms. Clin Obstet Gynecol 10:290, 1967
21. Vaitukaitis JL, Braunstein GD, Ross GT: A radioimmunoassay which specifically measures human chorionic gonadotropin in the presence of human luteinizing hormone. Am J Obstet Gynecol 133:751, 1972
22. Bagshawe KD: Trophoblastic disease. In Caplan RM, Sweeney WJ (eds): Advances in Obstetrics and Gynecology. Baltimore: Williams & Wilkins, 1978, p 225
23. Bakri Y, Lee JH Jr, Jahshan AE, Lewis GC Jr: Uterine choriocarcinoma with negative specific serum radioimmunoassay for human chorionic gonadotropins. Gynec Oncol 14:112, 1982
24. Hammond CB, Borchert L, Tyrey L, et al: Treatment of metastatic trophoblastic disease: Good and poor prognosis. Am J Obstet Gynecol 115:451, 1973
25. Hertig AT, Edmonds HW: Genesis of hydatidiform mole. Arch Pathol 30:260, 1940
26. Park WW: Choriocarcinoma. A study of its pathology. Philadelphia: FA Davis, 1971
27. Stone M, Bagshawe KD: Hydatidiform mole: Two entities. Lancet 1:535, 1976
28. Vassilakos P, Riotton G, Kajii T: Hydatidiform mole: Two entities. Am J Obstet Gynecol 127:167, 1977
29. Kajii T, Ohama K: Androgenetic origin of hydatidiform mole. Nature 268:633, 1977
30. Szulman AE, Surti U: The syndromes of hydatidiform mole. I. Cytogenetic and morphologic correlations. Am J Obstet Gynecol 131:665, 1978
31. Lavecchia C, Franceschi S, Fasoli M, Mangioni C: Gestational trophoblastic neoplasms in homozygous twins. Obstet Gynecol 60:250, 1982
32. Surti U, Szulman AE, O'Brien S: Dispermic origin and clinical outcome of three complete hydatidiform moles with $46 \times \times$ karyotype. Am J Obstet Gynecol 144:84, 1982
33. Szulman AE, Ma KH, Wong LC, Hsu C: Residual trophoblastic disease in association with partial hydatidiform mole. Obstet Gynecol 57:392, 1981
34. Hertig AT, Sheldon WH: Hydatidiform mole: A pathologico-clinical correlation of 200 cases. Am J Obstet Gynecol 53:1, 1947
35. Hertig AT, Mansell H: Tumors of the female sex organs. Part I. Hydatidiform mole and choriocarcinoma. Atlas of Tumor Pathology, Armed Forces Institute of Pathology, Washington DC, sect. 9, fasc. 33, 1956
36. Elston CW, Bagshawe KD: The value of histological grading in the management of hydatidiform mole. J Obstet Gynaecol Br Commonw 79:717, 1972
37. Beischer NA: Hydatidiform mole with coexistent foetus. Aust NZ J Obstet Gynaecol 6:127, 1966
38. Bowles HE: Extensive hydatidiform mole formation with a living child. Am J Obstet Gynecol 46:154, 1943
39. Jones WB, Laursen NH: Hydatidiform mole with coexistent fetus. Am J Obstet Gynecol 122:267, 1975
40. Ruffolo EH: Hydatidiform mole and a seven-month fetus. Obstet Gynecol 8:296, 1956

41. Suzuki M, Matsunobu A, Wakita K, et al: Hydatidiform mole with a surviving coexisting fetus. Obstet Gynecol 56:384, 1980
42. Hershman, JM: Hyperthyroidism induced by trophoblastic thyrotropin. Mayo Clin Proc 47:913, 1972
43. Hershman JM, Higgins P: When mole causes thyroid dysfunction. Contemp OB/GYN 12:79, 1978
44. Twiggs LB, Morrow CP, Schlaerth JB: Acute pulmonary complications of molar pregnancy. Am J Obstet Gynecol 135:189, 1979
45. Morrow CP, Kletzky OA, DiSaia PJ, et al: Clinical and laboratory correlates of molar pregnancy and trophoblastic disease. Am J Obstet Gynecol 128:424, 1977
46. Kiyoshi T, Shigeo Y, Ryousuke N: Increased risk of malignant transformation of hydatidiform moles in older gravidas: A cytogenetic study. Obstet Gynecol 58:351, 1981
47. Kohorn EI: Theca lutein ovarian cyst may be pathognomonic for trophoblastic neoplasia. Obstet Gynecol 62:805, 1983
48. Stone M, Dent J, Kardana A, Bagshawe KD: Relationship of oral contraceptives to development of tumor requiring treatment after hydatidiform mole. Br J Obstet Gynaecol 83:913, 1976
49. Goldstein DP, Berkowitz RS: The diagnosis and management of molar pregnancy. In Gestional Trophoblastic Neoplasms. Philadelphia: Saunders, 1982, p 143
50. Hammond CB, Surwit EA: Achieving a high cure rate for GTN. Contemp OB/GYN 17:163, 1981
51. Eddy GL, Schlaerth JB, Nalick RH, et al: Postmolar trophoblastic disease in women using hormonal contraception with and without estrogen. Obstet Gynecol 62:736, 1983
52. Delfs E: Quantitative chorionic gonadotropin: Prognostic value in hydatidiform mole and chorioepithelioma. Obstet Gynecol 9:1, 1957
53. Novak E, Seah CS: Choriocarcinoma of the uterus. Am J Obstet Gynecol 67:933, 1954
54. Park WW, Lees JC: Choriocarcinoma. A general review with an analysis of 516 cases. Arch Pathol 49:73, 205, 1950
55. Federschneider JM, Goldstein DP, Berkowitz RS, et al: Natural history of recurrent molar pregnancy. Obstet Gynecol 55:457, 1980
56. MacGregor C, Ontiveros E, Vargas E, Valenzuela S: Hydatidiform mole—Analysis of 145 patients. Obstet Gynecol 33:343, 1969
57. Matalon M, Modan B: Epidemiologic aspects of hydatidiform mole in Israel. Am J Obstet Gynecol 112:107, 1972
58. Yen S, MacMahon B: Epidemiologic features of trophoblastic disease. Am J Obstet Gynecol 101:126, 1968
59. Pastorfide GB, Goldstein DP: Pregnancy following hydatidiform mole. Obstet Gynecol 42:67, 1973
60. Walden PAM, Bagshawe KD: Reproductive performance of women successfully treated for gestational trophoblastic tumors. Am J Obstet Gynecol 125:1108, 1976
61. Lewis JL Jr: Chemotherapy of gestational choriocarcinoma. Cancer 30:1517. 1972
62. VanThiel D, Grodin JM, Ross GT, Lipsett MB: Partial placenta accreta in pregnancies following chemotherapy for gestational trophoblastic neoplasms. Am J Obstet Gynecol 122:54, 1972
63. Lurain JR, Sand PK, Carson SA, Brewer JI: Pregnancy outcome subsequent to consecutive hydatidiform moles. Am J Obstet Gynecol 142:1060, 1982

64. Sand PK, Lurain JR, Brewer JI: Repeat gestational trophoblastic disease. Obstet Gynecol 63:140, 1984
65. Goldstein DP: Five years' experience with the prevention of trophoblastic tumors by the prophylactic use of chemotherapy in patients with molar pregnancy. Clin Obstet Gynecol 13:945, 1971
66. Franke HR, Risse EKJ, Kenemans P, et al: Plasma human chorionic gonadotropin disappearance in hydatidiform mole: A central registry report from the Netherlands. Obstet Gynecol 62:467, 1983
67. Hertig AT, Gore HM: Tumors of the female sex organs. Part 2. Tumors of the vulva, vagina, and uterus, sect. 9, fasc. 33 of Atlas of Tumor Pathology, Armed Forces Institute of Pathology, Washington, DC 1960
68. Berkowitz RS, Goldstein DP, Bernstein MR: Choriocarcinoma following term gestation. Gynec Oncol 17:52, 1984
69. Brewer JI, Mazur MT: Gestational choriocarcinoma: Its origin in the placenta during seemingly normal pregnancy. Am J Surg Pathol 5:267, 1981
70. Wilson RB, Hunter JS, Dockerty MB: Chorioadenoma destruens. Am J Obstet Gynecol 81:546, 1961
71. Green RR: Chorioadenoma destruens. Ann NY Acad Sci 80:143, 1959
72. Wilson RB, Dockerty MB: Management of trophoblastic disease. In Marcus SL, Marcus CC (eds): Advances in Obstetrics and Gynecology, vol. 1. Baltimore: Williams & Wilkins, 1967, p 292
73. McDonald TW, Ruffolo EH: Modern management of gestational trophoblastic disease. Obstet Gynecol Survey 38:67, 1983
74. Bigelow B: Gestational trophoblastic disease. In Blaustein A (ed): Pathology of the Female Genital Tract. New York: Springer-Verlag, 1977, p 698
75. DiSaia PJ, Morrow CP, Townsend DE: Gestational trophoblastic disease. In Synopsis of Gynecologic Oncology. New York: John Wiley, 1975, p 230
76. Dockerty MB, Craig WM: Chorionephithelioma. An unusual case in which cerebral metastasis occurred four years after hysterectomy. Am J Obstet Gynecol 44:497, 1942
77. Wilde WL, Armstrong S, Byrne JJ: Metastatic choriocarcinoma masquerading as acute cholecystitis six years after hysterectomy. Am J Surg 113:414, 1967
78. Novak ER, Woodruff JD: Hydatidiform mole and choriocarcinoma. In Novak's Gynecologic and Obstetric Pathology, 7th ed. Philadelphia: Saunders, 1974, p 599
79. Tsukamoto N, Kashimura Y, Masatoshi S, et al: Choriocarcinoma occurring within the normal placenta with breast metastasis. Gynec Oncol 11:348, 1981
80. Sengupta BS, Chatterjee D, Persaud V, Wynter HH: Primary neurological manifestations of choriocarcinoma. International Surg 61:88, 1976
81. Smith EB, Weed JC, Tyrey L, et al: Treatment of nonmetastatic gestational trophoblastic disease: Results of methotrexate alone versus methotrexate-folinic acid. Am J Obstet Gynecol 144:88, 1982
82. Begent RHJ, Bagshawe KD: Treatment of advanced trophoblastic disease. In Griffiths CT, Fuller AF (eds): Gynecologic Oncology. Boston: Martinus Nijhoff, 1983
83. Searle F, Leake BA, Bagshawe KD, Dent J: Serum-SPI-pregnancy specific glycoprotein in choriocarcinoma and other neoplastic disease. Lancet 1:579, 1978
84. Borek E, Sharma OK, Brewer JI: Urinary nucleic acid breakdown products as markers for trophoblastic diseases. Am J Obstet Gynecol 146:906, 1983
85. Berkowitz RS, Birnholz J, Goldstein DP, Bernstein MR: Pelvic ultrasonography

and the management of gestational trophoblastic disease. Gynec Oncol 15:403, 1983
86. Nisula BC, Taliadouros GS: Thyroid function in gestational trophoblastic neoplasia: Evidence that the thyrotropic activity of chorionic gonadotropin mediates the thyrotoxicosis of choriocarcinoma. Am J Obstet Gynecol 138:77, 1980
87. Lurain JR, Brewer JI, Torok EE, Halpern B: Gestational trophoblastic disease: Treatment results at the Brewer Trophoblastic Disease Center. Obstet Gynecol 60:354, 1982
88. Lurain JR, Brewer JI, Mazur MT, Torok EE: Fatal gestational trophoblastic disease: An analysis of treatment failures. Am J Obstet Gynecol 144:391, 1982
89. Begent RHJ, Bagshawe KD: The management of high risk choriocarcinoma. Sem Oncol 9:198, 1982
90. Newlands ES, Bagshawe KD: Activity of high dose *cis*-platinum (NCI 119875) in combination with vincristine and methotrexate in drug-resistant choriocarcinoma. A report of 17 cases. Br J Cancer 40:943, 1979
91. Hayes DM, Cvitkovic E, Golbey RB, et al: High dose *cis*-platinum diammine dichloride. Amelioration of renal toxicity by mannitol diuresis. Cancer 39:1372, 1977
92. Schlaerth JB, Morrow PC, DePetrillo AD: Sustained remission of choriocarcinoma with *cis*-platinum, vinblastine and bleomycin after failure of conventional drug therapy. Am J Obstet Gynecol 136:983, 1980
93. Rustin GJS, Rustin F, Dent J, et al: No increase in second tumors after cytotoxic chemotherapy for gestational trophoblastic tumors. N Engl J Med 308:473, 1983
94. Hammond, CB, Weed JC, Curry SL: The role of operation in the current therapy of gestational trophoblastic disease. Am J Obstet Gynecol 136:844, 1980
95. Lacey CG, Barnard D, Degefu S, et al: Irradiation of liver metastases due to gestational choriocarcinoma. Obstet Gynecol 61:71S, 1983
96. Tattersall MHN, Parker LM, Pittman SW, Frei E: Clinical pharmacology of high dose methotrexate. Cancer Chemother Rep 6:25, 1975
97. Begent RHJ, Searle F, Stanway G, et al: Radioimmunolocalization of tumours by external scintigraphy after administration of ^{131}I antibody to human chorionic gonadotrophin. J Roy Soc Med 23:624, 1980
98. Berkowitz RS, Lahey SJ, Rodrick ML, et al: Circulating immune complex levels in patients with molar pregnancy. Obstet Gynecol 61:165, 1983

Index

Letters after page numbers represent figures (f) and tables (t).

Adenocarcinomas
  cervical intraepithelial neoplasia (CIN), primary, 110
  incidence of, 110
  invasive, 86, 89f, 90f
  prognosis, 110
  treatment, 110
  endometrial carcinomas
    clear cell, 155, 158f
    secretory, 155
  vagina, cancers of
    clear cell from, 50
Age as factor. *See specific cancer*

Bartholin's gland. *See Vulva, cancers of*

Carcinomas. *See specific cancer*
Cervical cancers
  Cervical intraepithelial neoplasia (CIN)
    adenocarcinomas. *See Adenocarcinomas*
    age, neoplastic lesions and, 66t
    carcinoma in situ, 63–66
      invasive cancer developing, 63–66
    colposcopy, 69
    concept of, 61–63
    condoms as treatment, 77
    cone biopsy as treatment, 72–74
      accuracy of prediction of residual disease in hysterectomy specimen based on histological examination of cone markings, 73f
    childbearing, effect on, 73

    incidence of recurrent carcinoma in situ and of invasive carcinoma of the cervix following, 72t
    need for conization, 70
  cryosurgery, use of, 74–75
    success rate, 75
  cytologic screening, 68–69
    Papanicolaou smear and, 68
  diagnosis, 68–70
    colposcopically directed biopsies reducing need for diagnostic cone biopsies, 70
    histopathologic diagnosis, correlation of on colposcopically directed punch biopsy and cold knife conization, 70t
  dysplasia
    mild; transit time to carcinoma in situ, 62f, 65
    moderate; transit time to carcinoma in situ, 63f
    severe; transit time to carcinoma in situ, 64f, 65
  early detection techniques, 59–61, 61f
  electrocautery as treatment, 75–76
  epidemiology, 66–67
  etiology, 67–68
  folic acid as treatment, 77
  follow-up after treatment, 112–113
    Papanicolaou smear and, 113
    tracking, 111–113
  freezing techniques, use in treatment, 74–75
  genital herpes, presence of, 67
  hysterectomy as treatment, 71, 72f

Endometrial carcinomas (cont.)
  lymph node involvement, 158, 163
    exenteration not indicated by, 170
      Stage I carcinoma, relationship between tumor stage and incidence of lymph node involvement, 165t
  menstrual abnormalities and, 147
  myometrial invasion
    5-year survival rates, varying combinations of tumor differentiation and, 164f, 165t
    lymph node involvement; Stage I carcinoma and, relationship, 165t
    prognostic significance, 157
    tumor grade and, relationship, 164t
  nulliparity, association with, 138
  obesity as factor, 133
  ovarian dysgenesis and (Turner's Syndrome), 135
  papillary, 155, 158f, 159fs
  parity as factor, 138
  peritoneal cytology, 163, 164, 166
  polycystic ovarian disease and, 134–135
  precursors of, 139
  presentation, mode of, 145, 147–148
  pretreatment work-ups, 164–167
  prognosis, significant factors
    myometrial invasion, 157, 164t, 165f, 165t
    tumor differentiation, 157, 160f, 161fs, 162fs, 163f
    tumor types, 156
  racial factors, survival and, 130–131
  radiation therapy and. See Radiation therapy, use of
  recurrence, 168, 170
  relative risk of developing, 136t, 137t
  secretory adenocarcinoma, 155
  Stage I patients, death rate, North American series, 131t
  Staging; FIGO system and. See FIGO staging
  surgery as treatment
    Stages I and II, 167–168
    Stage III, 169
    Stage IV, 169–170
  survival by stage. See FIGO staging in
  survival rates, 129–130, 130t
  symptomatic patients, evaluation, 148–149
    investigation of symptoms, 145–149
    office biopsy, 148–149
  treatment, 167–170
  tumor differentiation, prognostic significance, 157, 160fs, 161fs, 162fs, 163f
  tumor subtypes, 153–154
    frequency of, recent studies, 154t
  tumor types
    prognostic significance, 156
    survival rates and, 156
  unopposed estrogen action and, 134–138
    functioning ovarian tumors and, 134
    ovarian dysgenesis (Turner's Syndrome), 135
    polycystic ovarian disease and, 134–135
    sequential oral contraceptives, effect, 135
Electrocautery as treatment for cervical cancers, 75–76
Exenteration as treatment in endometrial carcinomas, 170

Fallopian tube, cancers of
  choriocarcinomas. See Choriocarcinomas
  ectopic pregnancies, 211
  extrauterine pregnancies, 211
  immature malignant teratomas, 211fs
  malignant teratomas, 211
  metastatic cancer. See Metastatic cancers
  primary carcinomas, 205–209
    age as factor, 205
    CT scanning, diagnostic use, 209
    chemotherapy, use of, 208–209
    clinical picture, 206–207
    clinical staging; FIGO classification for ovarian cancer, unofficial use of, 208
    diagnosis, conditions affecting accuracy, 207
    epidemiology, 205
    histology, 206
    identification, criteria for, 206
    incidence of, 205
    lymph node involvement and, 206
    management, 208–209
      ovarian cancers, similarities to, effect, 208
    Papanicolaou smear showings, 207
    papillary adenocarcinoma, 207f
    pathology, 206
    prognosis, 209
    routes of spread, 206
    symptoms, 207
    treatment, 208
  sarcomas, 211
    Müllerian tumors, 211

FIGO classification
  fallopian tube, cancers of
    ovarian cancer, clinical staging; unofficial use of, 208
  vagina, cancers of
    clinical classification, FIGO adoption, 41, 42t
  vulva, cancers of
    invasive squamous cell carcinoma, 18–19
FIGO staging
  cervical intraepithelial neoplasia (CIN) invasive cervical cancers
    clinical staging and pretreatment; investigations, 92–94
    FIGO adopted system, 92
  endometrial cancer
    prognostic significance, 153, 153t
    survival by, 153t

Geographical factors in incidence of cancers. *See specific cancer*
Gestational trophoblastic neoplasia (GTN)
  benign, 309–319
    associated medical problems, management, 315
    bleeding as symptom, 313
    chemotherapy, prophylactic, 319
    clinical picture, 313–314, 315t
    contraception, adequacy of, follow-up management and, 317–318
    diagnostic steps, 314
    follow-up management and, 317–319
    grading, effect, 313
    hydatidiform mole. *See* Primary hydatidiform mole
    hysterectomy, 316
    hysterotomy, 316
    large uterus, evacuation of, 316
    living children born from these pregnancies, 314
    management, 315–319
    ovarian enlargement, 317
    procedure as to, 316–317
    prognostic indicators, 311, 313
    serial hCG determination, 318–319
    small uterus, evacuation, 315–316
    spontaneous abortion and, 313
    treatment, 315–319
    trophoblast, range from benign to malignant based on, 311
    ultrasonography, diagnosed by, 314
    variants, 310

chorionic tissue as tumor source, 305
    histopathological features predicting malignancy, 305
    neoplasms arising from, 305
  classification, 309, 309t
    ACOG classification, 309
  human gonadotropin assay, 307
    chemotherapy for, 308
    hCG determination, techniques, 308t
    measurement of, 308
    molar pregnancies, incidence, 306f
    pregnancy tests, usefulness, 308
    prevalence of, 307
  incidence of, 305–306
  malignant, 319–332, 326t
    chemotherapy and surgery for drug resistant diseases, 334
    choriocarcinoma. *See* Choriocarcinomas
  natural history of, 306–307, 307t
  primary hydatidiform mole, 309–319, 311f, 312fs, 313f
    characteristics of, 309
    complete moles, 310
      partial mole, usefulness of distinguishing from, 310
    frequency of, 305–306
    histologic grading linked to prognosis, 311, 313
    partial moles, 310
      complete moles, usefulness of distinguishing from, 310
    pathology, 311, 311f
    prognosis, histologic grading linked to, 311, 313
  therapy, 328, 330
    complications, 330t
  variants, 310
    distinguishing between partial and complete moles, usefulness, 310
Granulosa cell tumors. *See* Ovarian; nonepithelial cancers; primary

Hydatidiform moles. *See* Gestational trophoblastic neoplasia; primary hydatidiform mole
Hysterectomy as treatment, 71, 72f, 316
  radical hysterectomy, 103, 104f, 105f
    associated procedures, 104
    role of, 105
    survival rates, 104, 106, 106t
      operative mortality for, 107t

Hysterectomy as treatment (*cont.*)
    patients with Stage IB and Stage IIA cervical carcinoma treated by pelvic lymphadenectomy and, 105, 106t
    time for, 105–106

Immature malignant teratomas, 210f, 211
Incidence of varying cancers. *See specific cancer*
Interferon, treatment of cervical cancers, 77
Invasive carcinomas. *See specific cancer*

Laparoscopy, 256–257
Laparotomy, 227, 257
Laser therapy as treatment, 76, 76t
Lymph node involvement. *See specific cancer*

Melanomas. *See* Vulva, cancers of
Metastatic cancers of
  fallopian tube, 209–211
    adenomatoid tumor, 209f
    benign mesothelioma as, 211
    incidence of, 209
    lymphocytes, presence of, 209f, 211f
    prognosis, 209
  See also. Choriocarcinomas; malignant gestational trophoblastic neoplasia (GTN); metastases
Microinvasive carcinomas
  invasive cervical cancers, 78–83
    borderline tumors, 82
    cone biopsy, need for, 81
    diagnosing, 78–81
    early identification, 78
    early stromal invasion, 82f
    lymph node involvement, 78
      incidence of pelvic lymph node involvement in relationship to depth of stromal invasion, 79t
    pattern of invasion, 80
    treatment, 81–82
    what constitutes, 78–79
  vulva, 9, 10f
    age factors, 1, 5
    lymphatic and vascular permeation, significance, 11–12
    7th International Congress International Society for the Study of Vulvar Diseases, recommendations as to terminology, 13
    stromal invasion, effect of depth, 11
    treatment, 9–10, 12–13
Müllerian tumors, 193fs, 194fs, 211, 219–220

Noninvasive cancers. *See specific cancer*
Nulliparity as a factor in gynecologic cancers, 138, 179, 217

Ovarian cancers
  differentiating invasive from noninvasive masses, 225
  epithelial carcinomas, 213–263
    adjunctive therapy to surgery, 249–258
    age as factor, 215, 224
      age standardized death rates, 215t
      malignancy rates at different ages, 258f
      young woman with ovarian cancer, 258–262
    bilateral serous cystadenocarcinomas with extracystic excrescences, 245f
    borderline, 228
    chemotherapy and, 251–254
      complications of, 253
      immunotherapy and, 254
      repetition of use, 253
      second look surgery and, 255–256
    classification; World Health Organization, 227t
    criteria, 228
    clear cell carcinoma, 233f
    clinical picture, 221–227
    clinical staging based on findings at surgery, 240t
    CT scanning, diagnostic use, 225–226
    conditions creating, 213
    contraceptive methods, effect, 218
    contralateral ovary with tumor on ovarian surface, 244f
    current knowledge and techniques, 214–215
    diagnosis
      extent of disease, 221, 221t, 222fs
      in early stage, 221, 221t, 221f
    endogenous hormone levels, 218–219
    endometrioid adenoacanthoma of the ovary, 235f
      sample from, 235f
    endometrial carcinoma, 232f
    endometriosis and, 219
    epidemiology, 215–221
    extensive disease, surgery for, 243–247

INDEX 347

extent of tumor, double contrast enemas ascertaining, 226
5-year survival rates, 260
 Stage I cancers, gross characteristics at surgery, 259t
 various Stage I malignancies, relative rates, 261t
foreign matter particles and, 218
frozen section reports, use in staging and, 218
geographical factors, 215–216
high risk factors, common, 220–221
histologic classification; World Health Organization, 227t
 criteria, 228
histologic grading, 237
 mucinous tumors and, 238
 prognosis related to, 238
histologic tumor types, 232–236
 common types of primary ovarian malignancies, relative frequency, 234t
hormonal factors, 217–219
host response to the tumor, 238
 immunocompetence in patients with ovarian cancers, reduction in, 238
immunotherapy and, 254
 chemotherapy, as aid to, 254
inadequate ovarian function, 220–221
"incessant ovulations", 217–218
incidence of, 213, 217
 environmental factors and, 217
 retrospective studies, 216–217
intraperitoneal radiocolloids as adjunctive therapy, 249–250
"in vitro" tumor sensitivity studies, 254–255
liver metastases from ovarian carcinoma, 242f
management, considerations, 231
median survival time, 223, 223t
metastatic adenocarcinoma to the ovary from primary breast tumor, 236f
mucinous cytadenocarcinomas with multiocular cut surface, 245f
mucinous tumors, time seen, 233
Müllerian tissue, differentiation, effect, 219–220
nonepithelial, proportions, 234
noninvasive tests for, 225–226
nulliparity, 217
ovarian enlargement, age as factor, 224–225
ovulation as factor, 217–218

papillary mucinous carcinoma of low malignant potential, 230f
papillary serous tumor of low malignant potential, 229f
pathologist's role, 236–237
pathology, 227–240
peritoneal irritants, effect, 218
pluripotential "secondary Müllerian system", 219–220
pregnancy, possible effects, 217–219
pregnant patients, 217–219, 262
preoperative assessments, 226
primary malignancies, frequency, 234t
primary tumor producing ovarian metastases, common sites, 236
racial factors and, 215–216
radical surgery and, 243–247
radiotherapy as adjunctive therapy, 250–251
range of tumors, 213
reproductive years, ovarian enlargement in, 224–225
retrospective studies, 216–217
screening for, 223–224
"secondary Müllerian system", 219–220
serous cystadenoma, 228f
sexual activity, effect, 217
sigmoid colon, external compression of, barium enema in patient with ovarian carcinoma, 246f
small cell ovarian carcinomas, 234f
specimens thought to be benign, malignancies found, 248–249
 frozen sections, use, 248–249
staging, critical importance of, 233
 clinical staging based on findings at surgery, 240t
 frozen sections, use, 236–237
 pathologist's role, 236
 surgery, role of, 240–249
stromal invasion, 228
surgery, role of, 240–258
 adjunctive therapy, as, 249–255
 extent of, factors, 243–247
 radical, 243–247
 second look surgery, 255–258, 257f
 staging, restaging and major mode of treatment, surgery as, 240–249
survival rates, 214, 221, 258
symptomatology of early disease, 221
"tumors of low malignant potential", 228, 229f
 stage and prognosis, 238, 239t

348   INDEX

Ovarian cancers (*cont.*)
    tumors to be considered as, proportions of; 990 epithelial malignancies of the ovary, 239t
    typical intracystic papillations of serous cystadenocarcinoma, 244f
    well-differentiated mucinous adenocarcinoma, 231f
    well-differentiated papillary serous cystadenocarcinoma, metastatic to the omentum, 237f
    young woman with, 258–262
        malignancy rates at different ages, 258f
  etiology, 215–221
  5-year survival rates, 214t, 221
  mucinous tumors, multilocular, 238
  nonepithelial ovarian cancers, primary
    age factors, 271–272f
    androblastomas (Sertoli-Leydig), 285–288
      tumors of intermediate and poor differentiation, 285–287
      survival rate, 287–288
    children, in, 271–272, 272t
    classification, 271–274
      FIGO, 273t
      frequency of diagnosis of forms within major subgroups, 274t
    combination chemotherapy, 271–272
    dysgerminomas, 287–291, 289f
      clinical features, 288
      pathology, 288
      pattern of spread, 289, 290
      prognosis, 289–290
      staging, 290
      treatment, 290–291
    embryonal carcinoma, 295
    endodermal sinus tumor, 291–294, 293f
      pathology, 292–293
      pregnancy during, 293
      prognosis, 293
      treatment, 293–295
    girls under 15, incidence in, 271–272, 272f
    granulosa cell tumors, 272–281
      associated abnormalities, 277–278
      bleeding as sign, 275
      cell patterns, 275, 277, 276f, 277f
      coexistent endometrial hyperplasia of carcinomas, incidence, 277, 287f
      histology, 275–277
      pregnancy, effect, 275–280
      prognosis, 278–279
      staging, 278, 279t
      treatment, 279–281
    Hilus cell tumor (Leydig cell tumor), 285
    immature teratomas, 296–300
      pathology, 297–298
      survival, 298
      treatment, 298–299
    incidence, 271–272, 274
      by age, 272f
    malignant germ cell tumors 287–300
    mixed germ cell tumors, 299–300
    ovarian choriocarcinomas. *See* Choriocarcinomas
    polyembryomas, 295
    thecomas, 281–283
      management, 282–283
      pathology, 281, 281f
    tubular adenoma with Leydig cells, 283–285
      pathology, 284
      symptoms, 284
      tubular androblastoma (Sertoli cell tumor), 283–284
      well-differentiated, 283–285
  nonovarian masses, differentiating from ovarian masses, 225
  oophorectomy, prophylactic desirability, 262–263

Papanicolaou smear, use of, 45, 68, 207
Pregnancy as a factor in gynecologic cancers, 32, 110–112, 111f, 217–219, 262

Racial factors. *See specific cancer*
Radiation therapy, use of, 97–108, 102t, 103f, 166–167
  endometrial cancer; treatment of
    Stages I and II, 169
    Stage III, 169
    Stage IV, 169, 170

Sarcomas
  fallopian tube, cancers of, 211
  Müllerian tumors, 211
  invasive cervical cancer, 86–88
  vulva, cancers of, 36
  uterus. *See also. Uterus, sarcomas of*
Second look surgery, 255–258, 257f
Sexual aspects of conditions. *See specific cancers*
Squamous cell carcinomas

invasive cervical cancer, 85–86, 88f, 90f
  incidence of, 85
  prognosis, 85
  supplementary parametrial irradiation, management by, 98
  surgical staging, 94–96
    para-aortic node involvement in the various stages of cervical carcinoma, incidence of, 96t
  tests as adjuncts to pretreatment evaluation, 93–94
  treatment, surgical, 102–107
  tumor grading and, 86
  ulcerative lesions, 84, 86f
  whole pelvis radiotherapy, 98
vagina, cancers of, 41–42
vulva, cancers of; invasive, 14–28
  classification, FIGO, 18–19
  clinical course, 19, 20f
  5-year survival, 25, 26t
  "high-risk patient", 14
  histopathology, 15, 15t, 16, 16t
  incidence, 14
  management, 21–24
  morbidity and postoperative mortality, 24, 24t, 25f
  radical vulvectomy, survival following, 25, 26t
    positive pelvic nodes, 26t
  recurrence, 27
  spread, 16–19, 20f
    nodal metastases, 18, 18t
  symptoms, 14, 15
  treatment, 19–24, 22t
  vulvar dystrophy associated, 14
  well-differentiated keratinizing carcinoma, 17f
Staging. *See specific cancer*
Surgery. *See specific cancer*
Survival rates for. *See specific cancer*

Therapies used. *See specific cancer*
Tumors, types. *See specific cancer*

Uterus, sarcomas of
  age factors, 179
  classification, 180–181, 181t
    Gynecologic Oncology Group (GOG) endorsement, 181
  composition of, 180–181
  diagnosis, accuracy, 180

endometrial stromal sarcomas, 186–188, 187f, 188f
  histopathology, 186
  management, 186–187
  survival rates, 186, 188
endometrial stomatosis (endolymphatic stromal myosis), 189–191, 189f, 190f
  therapy, 191
heterologous tumors, 180
histopathologic types, treatment, 179–180
homologous tumors, 180–191, 184f, 187f, 188f, 189f, 190f
incidence of, 179
lethal nature of, 179
leiomyosarcoma, 181–186, 184f
  clinical picture, 182–183
  management, 185–186
  prognosis, 183–184
  symptoms, 182
  therapy, 185
malignant lymphoma, 200–201, 199fs, 200f
mixed mesodermal tumors, 191–200
  histopathology, 192–195
  incidence, 192
  prognosis, 199
  recurrence, 200
  survival
    different therapies, effect, 197t
    extrauterine disease and, 198, 198t
morbidity, 179
Müllerian tumors, 193fs, 194f
nulliparous women, incidence in, 179
prognosis and classification, 180
pure sarcomas, 181–191
  homologous, 181–191, 184f, 187f, 188f, 189f, 190f
sarcoma botryoides, 200
staging, formal, lack of, 179
unclassified sarcomas, 201

Vagina, cancers of
  adenosis, progression to clear cell, 50–51
  children, in
    endodermal sinus tumor, 55
    malignant melanoma, 55–56
    metastatic cancer of the vagina, 56
    rhabdomyosarcoma (Sarcoma botryoides), 53f, 54
  clear cell adenocarcinoma. *See* Clear cell adenocarcinomas
  clinical classification, 41. *See also* FIGO classification

Vagina, cancers of (cont.)
  DES syndrome, 49
  intraepithelial carcinoma (VAIN), 42–44
    mild dysplasia (VAIN 1), 43–43
    moderate dysplasia (VAIN 2), 43
    severe dysplasia and carcinoma in situ
      (VAIN 3), 43
  invasive carcinoma, 44–49
    clinical staging, 47, 47t
    histopathology, 46, 46f
    lymphatic spread, 46
    management, 47
    Papanicolaou smear and, 45
    prognosis, 48
    routes of spread, 45–46
    symptoms, 45
    treatment, 47–48
  mild dysplasia (VAIN 1), 43–44
  moderate dysplasia (VAIN 2), 43
  primary, 41–42
  severe dysplasia and cancer in situ (VAIN
    3), 43
  squamous cell carcinoma, 41–42
Vulva, cancers of
  adenocarcinomas, 30
  Bartholin's gland, 30, 31f, 32f
  basal cell carcinoma, 30, 31f, 32f
    microscopic picture, 31f
  dystrophies of, 2–4, 2t, 3f
    atrophic, 3f
    management, 4
    treatment, 4
  incidence of, 1
  invasive squamous cell carcinoma.
    See Squamous cell carcinomas
    Vulva; cancers of; invasive
  melanomas, 32–36
    diagnosis, 31–32
    incidence of, 31
    massive malignant melanoma, 34f
    pregnancy and, 32
    prognosis, 32–33, 35
    racial factors, 32
    staging, 33–34
    survival rates, 35
    symptoms, 32
    treatment, 34–35
  microinvasive carcinomas. See Microinva-
    sive carcinomas
  Paget's disease, 8–9, 8f
    symptoms, 2
  sarcomas, 36
  symptoms, generally, 2
  treatment, generally, 2
  types, 2
  verrucous carcinoma of the vulva, 28–30
    benign condyloma acuminatum and, 29
    incidence of, 29
      symptoms, 28–30
      treatment, 29–30
  vulvar intraepithelial neoplasia, (VIN), 4–8
    age of patients, effect, 5
    incidence, 4–5
    management, 5–8
    sexual aspects of, 5
    squamous cell carcinoma in situ, 5, 6f